Barron's
How to Prepare for the National Council Licensure Examination for Practical Nurses
NCLEX-PN

Second Edition

By
Vashti R. Curlin, M.D.
Hattie L. Allen, R.N., M.A., M.S.

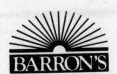

Barron's Educational Series, Inc.

Acknowledgments

The authors acknowledge and express appreciation to Ms. Lee Xippilitos, R.N., M.S. (Clinical Assistant Professor, State University of New York at Stony Brook, School of Nursing), who carefully reviewed the manuscript.

In addition, the authors acknowledge the guidance and assistance of the following people: Mrs. Gabrielle I. Edwards, M.A. (Assistant Principal Emerita, Science Supervision, Franklin D. Roosevelt High School, Brooklyn, New York); Mrs. Bernice Rosner, R.N., M.S. (Executive Director, Visiting Nurse Association, Brooklyn, New York; formerly Professor of Nursing, Cornell University School of Nursing); Dr. Dorothy L. Trice, R.N., M.D., M.P.H. (formerly Deputy Commissioner of Health, New York City Department of Health); Miss Joan V. Hayden, R.N., B.A.; and Mrs. Julia R. Hayden, L.P.N.

All inquiries should be addressed to:
Barron's Educational Series, Inc.
250 Wireless Boulevard
Hauppauge, New York 11788

Library of Congress Catalog Card No. 90-427

International Standard Book No. 0-8120-4385-5

Library of Congress Cataloging-in-Publication Data

Curlin, Vashti R.
  Barron's how to prepare for the national council licensure examination for practical nurses, NCLEX-PN / by Vashti R. Curlin, Hattie L. Allen—2nd ed.
    p. cm.
  Rev. ed. of: Barron's how to prepare for the practical nurse licensing examination / by Hattie L. Allen, Vashti R. Curlin. c1979.
  Includes bibliographical references.
  ISBN 0-8120-4385-5
  1. Practical nursing—Outlines, syllabi, etc. 2. Practical nursing—Examinations, questions, etc. I. Curlin, Vashti R. II. Allen, Hattie L. How to prepare for the national council licensure examination for practical nurses, NCLEX-PN. III. Title. IV. Title: How to prepare for the national council licensure examination for practical nurses, NCLEX-PN.
  [DNLM: 1. Nursing, Practical—examination questions. 2. Nursing, Practical—outlines. WY 18 A426b]
  RT62.A44 1990
  610.73′ 076—dc20
  DNLM/DLC   90-427
  for Library of Congress   CIP

PRINTED IN THE UNITED STATES OF AMERICA

2   100   987654

Contents

CONTENTS

Introduction

When you have completed a state-approved program of studies in practical nursing, you are ready for the next step—taking the NCLEX-PN.

WHAT YOU SHOULD KNOW ABOUT THE NATIONAL COUNCIL LICENSURE EXAMINATION FOR PRACTICAL NURSES (NCLEX-PN)

The NCLEX-PN, administered by the board of nursing in each of the 50 states, the District of Columbia, Guam, the U.S. Virgin Islands, American Samoa, and the Commonwealth of Northern Marianas, is the examination that you must pass in order to be licensed as a practical nurse. The examination reflects the knowledge, skills, and abilities that a practical nurse needs to perform satisfactorily at the entry level, that is, the level expected of a newly licensed practical nurse who has been employed no longer than 6 months.

Application

In most cases, to take the examination you must obtain an application form from the board of nursing in the state where you wish to practice (see the list on pp. 8–12), fill it out completely and correctly, and return it with a certified check or money order for the correct amount. The following information will be required on the form:

1. Name
2. Address
3. Birth date
4. Social Security number
5. Code number for your nursing education program (school name and city)
6. Testing location code
7. Jurisdiction where you wish to be licensed
8. Previous examination history if you have taken the NCLEX-PN before
9. Foreign education or training if applicable
10. Examination type (Practical Nursing) and administration date for which you are applying

The application process may be somewhat different in Florida, Illinois, Nevada, New York, and Wisconsin. The state boards of nursing there can inform you of any special requirements or procedures.

After your application has been processed and judged to be satisfactory, the state board will send you an admissions document specifying the date, time, and place of the examination you will take and authorizing you to enter the test site.

Administration

The NCLEX-PN is given at various locations on a single day in April and in October. You will take half the test at a 2-hour session in the morning; the other half, during 2 hours in the afternoon.

To be admitted, you must present your admissions document. At the test site you will be informed of specific procedures—for example, where notes or calculations can be made, when restroom breaks can be taken, how emergencies are to be handled—that are designed to maintain the integrity of the examination.

The Test Plan

The NCLEX-PN is based on a test plan, developed by the National Council of State Boards of Nursing, that includes two major components:

• Phases of the Nursing Process
• Client Needs

The examination tests the knowledge, skills, and abilities required to apply the four phases of the nursing process described below to meet the needs of clients having commonly occurring health problems characterized by predictable outcomes.

Phases of the Nursing Process
1. *Collecting data.* The practical nurse contributes to the development of a data base by observing the client's needs; collecting information from the client, the health team, and other sources; determining the need for more information; and communicating her/his findings. The nurse then participates in formulating a nursing diagnosis.
2. *Planning.* The practical nurse contributes to the development of a nursing care plan, assists in formulating goals and in identifying client needs and nursing measures to meet the goals, communicates with the client and others in planning the nursing care, and communicates client needs that may require changing the care plan.
3. *Implementing.* The practical nurse carries out basic therapeutic and preventive nursing measures as prescribed, provides a safe and effective environment, helps the client and others to understand the care plan, and records and reports client information.
4. *Evaluating.* The practical nurse participates in evaluating the effectiveness of the nursing care and the client's response to it, helps to implement appropriate changes, evaluates the extent to which specific goals of the care plan are achieved, and records and describes the client's response to care.

The percentages of questions on the NCLEX-PN that are based on the various phases are as follows:

Collecting data: 25–35%   Implementing: 25–35%
Planning: 15–25%   Evaluating: 15–25%

Because the entry-level nurse acts more independently when collecting data and implementing, these phases are given more weight in the examination.

Client Needs
1. *Safe, effective care environment.* The practical nurse must be able to provide nursing care in the following categories:

Coordinated care   Environmental safety
Standards of care   Preparation for treatments and procedures
Goal-oriented care   Safe and effective treatments and procedures

Three examples of the basic knowledge, skills, and abilities included here are (1) client preparation for prescribed treatments and procedures, (2) infection control, and (3) evaluation and general knowledge of community agencies.

2. *Physiological integrity.* The practical nurse must be able to provide nursing care to help meet the following client needs:

Physiological adaptation   Comfort
Reduction of risk potential   Provision of basic care
Mobility

Three examples of the areas of basic knowledge, skills, and abilities included here are (1) knowledge of therapeutic and life-saving procedures, (2) principles of administering medications, and (3) comfort measures.

3. *Psychosocial integrity.* The practical nurse must be able to provide nursing care to help meet the following client needs:

Psychosocial adaptation   Coping/adaptation

Three examples of the areas of basic knowledge, skills, and abilities included here are (1) obvious signs of emotional and mental health problems, (2) chemical dependency, and (3) therapeutic communication.

4. *Health promotion/maintenance.* The practical nurse must be able to provide nursing care to help meet the following client needs:

Continued growth and development   Integrity of support system
Self-care   Prevention and early treatment of disease

Three examples of the areas of basic knowledge, skills, and abilities included here are (1) family interactions, (2) reproduction and human sexuality, and (3) growth and development, including death and dying.

The percentages of questions on the NCLEX-PN related to the various areas of client needs are as follows:

Safe, effective care environment: 24–30%   Psychosocial integrity: 7–13%
Physiological integrity: 42–48%   Health promotion/maintenance: 15–21%

The Test Format

The examination is presented in two booklets, each containing 120–125 multiple-choice questions. Each question is followed by four answer choices, only one of which is correct. In most cases, a nursing situation is described, and the questions that follow are based on it. There may also be some unrelated, individual questions.

A small number of "tryout" questions, not identified as such in the test booklet, are included in each examination but are not counted in determining the score. These questions are being evaluated for use in future examinations.

Scoring the Examination

For each examination a passing standard that represents the lowest level of performance required to function satisfactorily as an entry-level practical nurse is established by a panel of expert nurse judges.

The examination booklets are scored electronically. One point is given for each correct answer; there is no penalty for omitted or incorrect answers. The candidate's score is the total number of correct answers (responses to tryout questions not included). The score is compared to the established point of minimum competency for the examination, and a PASS or FAIL designation is given. To ensure accuracy, booklets at or near the passing point are handscored.

Reporting the Results

The test result (PASS or FAIL) for each candidate is sent to her/his state board of nursing. Only these boards can release the results.

Each candidate who fails is provided with a diagnostic profile that indicates areas of strength and weakness and serves as a guide for further study before retaking the examination. Candidates who fail may request to have their test booklets handscored.

HOW YOU SHOULD PREPARE FOR THE NCLEX-PN

In a very real sense you have been preparing for the NCLEX-PN for many years. From high school courses in biology, chemistry, algebra, and other subjects you have acquired basic scientific knowledge and mathematical skills. From your nursing school program you have received the specialized education required to perform safely and effectively as a practical nurse. From classroom quizzes, midterm and final examinations, and longer and more formal tests such as the ACT or SAT you have gained experience in test taking. Over the years your contacts and relationships with other people, both inside and outside the classroom, have strengthened your understanding of the physical, mental, and emotional needs of human beings and the ways in which they react to a variety of situations. As you can see, you already have a solid foundation of knowledge, skills, and abilities on which to build your program of formal preparation for the NCLEX-PN.

The Purpose and Organization of This Book

The purpose of this book is, quite simply, to help you prepare for the licensure examination in your profession. The book is not intended to replace your standard textbooks in practical nursing. Rather, its aim is to reinforce and perhaps clarify basic concepts you have already studied.

INTRODUCTION

The book begins with a diagnostic test, followed by an answer key, rationales for the correct answers, and a chart that indicates the chapter on which each question is based. Each of the chapters that follow deals with one area of concentration, such as the adult patient, and is divided into parts called units.

At the beginning of each unit is a list of words, with definitions, whose meanings must be understood in order to comprehend the subject matter covered. Throughout the chapters are data summaries of important information that have been tabulated because they are easier to understand and retain in this form.

A mastery test, again with answer key, rationales, and chart, follows the last chapter.

The Effective Use of This Book

First, take the diagnostic test on pages 13–53, which is similar in difficulty and in number and type of questions to the actual test. Allow yourself two uninterrupted 2-hour sessions in a quiet place, and do not refer to notes, textbooks, or other aids.

When you have finished, check your answers against the answer key and read the rationales carefully, even for questions that you answered correctly. It is sometimes possible to select the right answer for the wrong reason. Then plan your review, allowing more time for subject matter on which you did poorly.

Over a period of several weeks, methodically review the material in this book. Where necessary, particularly in your weak areas, refer also to your textbooks and class notes. Try never to leave a topic until you have mastered the basic principles.

When you have finished your review, take the mastery test. Again, score the examination, study the rationales, and determine the subject areas, if any, in which you are still weak and on which you should focus additional review. Don't hesitate to obtain help from other sources—different textbooks, nursing periodicals, classmates, instructors—on topics where clarification or reinforcement is obviously needed.

A Five-Step Study Plan

1. *Allow plenty of time for review.* To determine how much is "plenty," consider the following factors: your grades in classes and clinical work and on school tests; the length of time, if this is considerable, since you completed your nursing education; your performance on the diagnostic test in this book; and your own study skills and work pace. A minimum time for review is 4–8 weeks; if you have been out of school for some time, if you received your nursing education and training in a foreign country, or if you have serious weaknesses in several areas of knowledge, you may need several months. The important thing is to allow enough time so that you can work at a steady, reasonable pace without frantic cramming as examination time nears.
2. *Study at the same fixed time each day.* Select a time period of 1½ to 2 hours for study, preferably early enough in the day so that you will not be tired, and adhere to this schedule as far as possible. Choose a quiet place, without loud music. Explain your study schedule to family and friends, and ask them not to interrupt you with personal visits or telephone calls. Short breaks are helpful to avoid fatigue or tension, but resist the temptation to take the dog for a 2-mile walk. When you are studying, keep your mind firmly on the subject matter, and refuse to be distracted by the blue jay outside your window or the smell of gingerbread from the kitchen.
3. *Study in a systematic way.* Each day, decide what material you want to cover. First *skim* the material quickly, noting only the main ideas. Then go back and begin a thorough *review*. Concentrate on basic principles of nursing that are applicable to a variety of situations. Keep in mind that the NCLEX-PN is intended to test your ability to use subject-area knowledge to make valid nursing judgments. Take the time to look up any terms whose meanings you have forgotten. When you reach a logical stopping place, perhaps at the end of a particular unit in this book, *summarize* on paper the important points in the material you have just reviewed. Then compare your summary with the source material you are using, and note any pertinent facts you omitted.

INTRODUCTION

4. *Think about group study*. Some people study better alone; others, in a group. A study group offers several advantages: companionship, which may mean less tension; a variety of viewpoints and strengths; and the opportunity to summarize out loud rather than in writing, to ask and to answer oral questions, and to clarify ambiguous points. To be successful, however, all members in the study group must be sufficiently self-disciplined to refuse distractions and to concentrate on the job at hand—reviewing for the NCLEX-PN.

5. *Finally, look over old quizzes and tests, including the ones in this book*. Make a list of topics that you have found difficult in the past, and review this material again. Remember: these are your weak areas, and this is your last chance to master them.

HOW YOU CAN MAXIMIZE YOUR SCORE ON THE NCLEX-PN

The following suggestions will help you to do your best on the licensure examination:

1. *Get enough sleep the night before*. Don't cram the evening before the test; instead go to an early movie, visit with friends, or spend the time in some other pleasant, non-tension-creating way. Take a few minutes to collect everything you will need for the examination (see item 3 below). Go to bed at a reasonable time (you're the best judge of when that should be), and set your alarm so that you will not have to rush around in a frenzy the next morning.

2. *Eat an adequate, nutritious breakfast*. Avoid either extreme: no breakfast or so much food that you may become sleepy or have indigestion. Eat some solid food—cereal, toast, a muffin (skip the chocolate-covered doughnuts)—and limit the amount of coffee; too much may increase nervousness and tension.

3. *Check that you have all the items you will need*. You should have a supply of sharpened #2 pencils, one or more erasers, a watch, and your admissions document, without which you will not be allowed to take the test. Unless you know that eating facilities are nearby, you will also need to take your lunch.

4. *Allow plenty of travel time*. Keep in mind that emergencies have a way of happening at the worst possible times. Leave home early enough so that a canceled train, a late bus, extraheavy traffic, or a crowded parking field will not cause you to arrive at the last minute in a huffing, puffing panic or even to be late.

5. *Approach the examination with confidence*. Think of the three important factors in your favor: you have completed a state-approved program in nursing, you have reviewed systematically and thoroughly, and you have had plenty of experience in test taking. Add the fact that the NCLEX-PN is a fair examination that is not designed to humiliate or to trick you, and things should look pretty good.

6. *Pay careful attention to instructions*. These will be printed in the NCLEX booklet, and you should read them carefully. Probably the proctor will also read the instructions aloud, asking you to follow along as he/she does so. Even though you have already read them, you should listen attentively to the oral reading. No one has ever failed a test by understanding the instructions *too* well.

7. *Keep the time limits clearly in mind, and pace yourself accordingly*. You will be required to answer 120–125 questions in 2 hours. This allows you about 1 minute for each question, which is time enough to read the question carefully, consider the four choices, and choose the one correct answer. You will need to check your pace periodically, perhaps every 10 minutes, to ensure that you are answering one question every minute. Too slow a pace means that you will not have time to finish; too fast a pace, that you may be making careless errors.

8. *Don't spend a lot of time on any one question*. Each correct answer, whether to an easy or a difficult question, will add 1 point to your score. It makes sense, therefore, to answer first all the questions to which you know the answers and then to go back to the others. The second time around, you should reread each of these harder questions, select what you consider the most logical choice, indicate your answer, dismiss that question from your mind, and go on to the next one.

9. *Read each question carefully*. If the question relates to a nursing situation, note any of the following details that are given: age and sex of the patient; medical history; symptoms or injuries;

diagnostic procedures performed; medication(s) prescribed and/or administered, including dosages; other therapeutic or comfort measures. Try to visualize the patient and to keep the details about him/her in mind as you answer the series of questions based on the situation described. As you read each question, pay special attention to limiting and negative words such as *always*, *never*, *first*, *initially*, *most*, *least*, *unnecessary*, *not*, and *except*.

10. *Note and promptly eliminate obviously incorrect answers*. Even if you don't know the right answer, you may spot one or two choices that can't be right because they are untrue, irrelevant, ridiculous, too general, or too specific. Cross such choices out immediately so that you can concentrate on the remaining possibilities.

11. *Use all the information you are given*. When a series of questions is based on a nursing situation, sometimes the correct answer can be found, or your choice validated, from information in a subsequent question. Suppose, for example, that you are given a set of symptoms and asked to diagnose the condition as (A) senile dementia, (B) endogenous depression, (C) Parkinson's disease, or (D) manic-depressive disorder. If you learn from a later question that levodopa has been prescribed for the patient, you can be reasonably sure that the correct choice is (C).

12. *Apply your knowledge of nursing principles*. Keep in mind that general principles, such as those governing patients' rights and the control of infection, can be applied to a variety of situations. Although the details change, the basic principles do not, and application of them may lead you to the correct answer in many cases.

13. *Don't waste time looking for trick questions or answer patterns*. Each question means exactly what it says, and only one of the answer choices is correct for the situation described. Bear in mind that a choice may be correct in itself but irrelevant to the question. Also, there is no pattern to the answers. The first answer choice may be the correct answer in several consecutive questions.

14. *Don't keep changing your answers*. As a rule, your first choice, whether based on knowledge, experience, intuition, or a "hunch," is more likely to be correct. Therefore don't change any answer without a sound reason, such as discovering that you misread the question.

15. *Indicate your answers properly*. Using a #2 pencil, fill in completely the circle next to the answer you choose as correct. Answers are recorded directly in the test booklet; there is no separate answer sheet for this examination. Accidental pencil marks or responses that you wish to change (but note item 14!) must be erased completely.

16. *Answer every question*. There is no penalty for guessing. If you can eliminate any choices, fine: choose one from those that remain. If they all look equally good, choose one at random. An omitted answer adds nothing to your score; a wrong answer costs you nothing. By random guessing, you may pick one or two correct answers, each worth 1 point.

SPECIAL TIPS FOR FOREIGN-EDUCATED NURSES

Many foreign-educated nurses like you are presently practicing their profession in the United States, and the number will undoubtedly increase in the years to come. Because of your special training and experience, you can make a valuable contribution to the quality and diversity of health care in this country. On the other hand, differences in culture, in the health problems commonly encountered, and in normative behavior may complicate your task in preparing for and passing the NCLEX-PN. The following suggestions are intended to help you achieve this goal.

1. *Understand the concept of practical nursing*. The United States, unlike many other countries, recognizes two forms of nursing, which are practiced by the registered nurse and the licensed practical nurse, respectively. In general, the practical nurse is not called upon to exercise the same degree of judgment as is the registered nurse. Moreover, in many states the practical nurse is subject to supervision by registered nurses and other medical professionals. It is possible that you functioned as a practical nurse in another country but worked under a different title.

2. *Bear in mind that the purpose of the licensure examination is to protect the public*. No matter how excellent your education or how extensive your experience, you must demonstrate your ability to function satisfactorily as a practical nurse in the United States before being allowed to practice. The hard truth is that any special problems you may encounter because of your foreign background cannot be allowed to jeopardize the patient's right to receive safe, effective nursing care.

INTRODUCTION

3. *Study the test plan for the NCLEX-PN.* It is essential that you become familiar with the four phases of the nursing process and the practical nurse's role in meeting client needs. The nursing process describes the contributions to patient care expected of the practical nurse in the United States; these may be somewhat different from those to which you are accustomed. Also, cultural differences may be evident in the understanding of client needs.

4. *Make a special effort to master medical terminology in the English language.* Relatively simple vocabulary is used on the NCLEX-PN, and the reading difficulty is kept to the eighth-grade level. Nevertheless you must be familiar with medical terms used in this country. If you do not understand what a question is asking, you will certainly have trouble answering it. For this reason you should buy or borrow a good medical dictionary, and form the habit of looking up and learning any unfamiliar nursing or medical terms that you encounter.

5. *Obtain whatever special help you need.* As you study this book and take the sample examinations, you may realize that you will have difficulty on the licensure examination. The first step is to identify the problem(s): lack of proficiency in English, and/or insufficient practical nursing education to meet U.S. standards. The next step is to seek competent help. Consider adult-education courses in English, tutoring by U.S.-educated teachers or nurses, or a commercial review course recommended by a nursing school.

BIBLIOGRAPHY

Alspach, JoAnn G., and Susan M. Williams, eds. *Core Curriculum for Critical Care Nursing.* Philadelphia: W.B. Saunders, 1985.

Brunner, Lillian S., and Doris S. Suddarth. *Manual of Nursing Practice.* Philadelphia: J.B. Lippincott, 1986.

Dorland's Illustrated Medical Dictionary. Philadelphia: W.B. Saunders, 1988.

Goodman, Louis S., and Alfred Gilman. *The Pharmacological Basis of Therapeutics.* New York: Macmillan Publishing Co., 1980.

Haber, Judith, et. al. *Comprehensive Psychiatric Nursing.* New York: McGraw-Hill Publishing Co., 1987.

Hamilton, Helen, and Minnie B. Rose. *Diseases* (Nurse's Reference Library). Springhouse, Pennsylvania: Springhouse Publishing Co., 1987.

Hoffman, Claire P., et al. *Simplified Nursing.* Philadelphia: J.B. Lippincott, 1981.

Kempe, C. Henry, et al. *Current Pediatric Diagnosis and Treatment.* East Norwalk, Connecticut: Appleton & Lange, 1987.

Skidmore, Linda. *Nursing Drug Reference.* Saint Louis, Missouri: C.V. Mosby & Co., 1990.

LIST OF DATA SUMMARIES

STATE AND TERRITORIAL BOARDS OF NURSING

Admission to the NCLEX-PN must be obtained by applying to the Board of Nursing in the state or territory where you wish to practice. Each state has its own application procedures and cut-off dates. A complete list of addresses and telephone numbers for the Boards of Nursing in the 50 states, the District of Columbia, the U.S. Virgin Islands, and Guam is provided below.

ALABAMA . . . . Executive Director
Alabama Board of
    Nursing
500 Eastern Boulevard,
    Suite 203
Montgomery, Alabama
    36117
Tel: (205) 242-4060

ALASKA . . . . Executive Secretary
Alaska State Board of
    Nursing
Dept. of Commerce and
    Economic Development
Division of Occupational
    Licensing
3601 C Street, Suite 722
Anchorage, Alaska 99503
Tel: (907) 561-2878

ARIZONA . . . . Executive Director
Arizona State Board of
    Nursing
2001 W. Camelback
    Road, Suite 35
Phoenix, Arizona 85015
Tel: (602) 255-5092

ARKANSAS . . . . State Board of Nursing
1123 S. University
University Tower Building,
    Suite 800
Little Rock, Arkansas
    72204
Tel: (501) 371-2751

CALIFORNIA . . . . . . Executive Officer
California Board of
    Registered Nursing
P.O. Box 944210
Sacramento, California
    94244-2100
Tel: (916) 322-3350

COLORADO . . . . . . Program Administrator
Colorado Board of
    Nursing
1560 Broadway,
    Suite 670
Denver, Colorado 80202
Tel: (303) 894-2430

CONNECTICUT . . . Executive Officer
Connecticut Board of
    Examiners for Nursing
150 Washington Street
Hartford, Connecticut
    06106
Tel: (203) 566-1041

DELAWARE . . . . . . Executive Director
Delaware Board of
    Nursing
Margaret O'Neill Building
P.O. Box 1401
Dover, Delaware 19903
Tel: (302) 736-4522

**DISTRICT OF
COLUMBIA** . . . . Program Administrator
District of Columbia Board
    of Nursing
614 H Street, N.W.
Washington, D.C. 20001
Tel: (202) 727-7468

FLORIDA . . . . Executive Director
Florida Board of Nursing
111 Coastline Drive East
Jacksonville, Florida
    32202
Tel: (904) 359-6331

GEORGIA . . . . Executive Director
Georgia Board of Nursing
166 Pryor Street, S.W.
Atlanta, Georgia 30303
Tel: (404) 656-3943

GUAM . . . . Nurse Examiner
    Administrator
Guam Board of Nurse
    Examiners
P.O. Box 2816
Algana, Guam 96910
Tel: (671) 734-2950

HAWAII . . . . Executive Secretary
Hawaii Board of Nursing
P.O. Box 3469
Honolulu, Hawaii 96801
Tel: (808) 548-5086

IDAHO . . . . Executive Director
Idaho Board of Nursing
280 N. 8th Street,
Suite 210
Boise, Idaho 83720
Tel: (208) 334-3110

ILLINOIS . . . . Nursing Education
Coordinator
Illinois Department of
Professional Regulation
320 W. Washington Street
Springfield, Illinois 62786
Tel: (217) 782-0458

INDIANA . . . . Board Administrator
Indiana State Board of
Nursing
Health Professions
Bureau
One American Square,
Suite 1020
Box 82067
Indianapolis, Indiana
46282-0004
Tel: (317) 232-2960

IOWA . . . . Executive Director
Iowa Board of Nursing
Executive Hills
1223 East Court
Des Moines, Iowa 50319
Tel: (515) 281-3256

KANSAS . . . . Executive Administrator
Kansas Board of Nursing
Landon State Office
Building
900 S.W. Jackson,
Suite 5515
Topeka, Kansas 66612
Tel: (913) 296-4929

KENTUCKY . . . . Executive Director
Kentucky Board of
Nursing
4010 Dupont Circle,
Suite 430
Louisville, Kentucky
40207
Tel: (502) 897-5143

LOUISIANA . . . . Executive Director
Louisiana State Board of
Nursing
907 Pere Marquette
Building
150 Baronne Street

New Orleans, Louisiana
70112
Tel: (504) 568-5464

MAINE . . . . Executive Director
Maine State Board of
Nursing
295 Water Street
Augusta, Maine 04333
Tel: (207) 289-5324

MARYLAND . . . . . . Executive Director
Maryland Board of
Examiners of Nurses
201 W. Preston Street
Baltimore, Maryland
21201
Tel: (301) 764-4747

MASSACHUSETTS Executive Secretary
Massachusetts Board of
Registration in Nursing
Leverett Saltonstall
Building
100 Cambridge Street,
Room 1519
Boston, Massachusetts
02202
Tel: (617) 727-7393

MICHIGAN . . . . Nurse Consultant
Michigan Board of
Nursing
Department of Licensing
and Regulation
Ottawa Towers North
611 West Ottawa
P.O. Box 30018
Lansing, Michigan 48909
Tel: (517) 373-1600

MINNESOTA . . . . . . Executive Director
Minnesota Board of
Nursing
2700 University Avenue
W., #108
St. Paul, Minnesota
55114
Tel: (612) 642-0567

MISSISSIPPI . . . . . . Executive Director
Mississippi Board of
Nursing
239 N. Lamar, Suite 401
Jackson, Mississippi
39201
Tel: (601) 359-6170

INTRODUCTION

MISSOURI . . . . Executive Director
Missouri State Board of
Nursing
3523 N. Ten Mile Drive
P.O. Box 656
Jefferson City, Missouri
65102
Tel: (314) 751-0681

MONTANA . . . . Executive Secretary
Montana State Board of
Nursing
Department of Commerce
Division of Business and
Professional Licensing
Arcade Building-Lower
Level
111 N. Jackson
Helena, Montana 59620-
0407
Tel: (406) 444-4279

NEBRASKA . . . . Associate Director
Bureau of Examining
Boards
Nebraska Department of
Health
P.O. Box 95007
Lincoln, Nebraska 68509
Tel: (402) 471-2115

NEVADA . . . . Executive Director
Nevada State Board of
Nursing
1281 Terminal Way,
Suite 116
Reno, Nevada 89502
Tel: (702) 786-2778

NEW HAMPSHIRE . Executive Director
New Hampshire Board of
Nursing
Health and Welfare
Building
6 Hazen Drive
Concord, New Hampshire
03301
Tel: (603) 271-2323

NEW JERSEY . . . . . Executive Director
New Jersey Board of
Nursing
1100 Raymond
Boulevard, Room 508
Newark, New Jersey
07102
Tel: (201) 648-2570

NEW MEXICO . . . . . Executive Director
New Mexico Board of
Nursing
4253 Montgomery
Boulevard, Suite 130
Albuquerque, New Mexico
87109
Tel: (505) 841-8340

NEW YORK . . . . Executive Secretary
New York State Board for
Nursing
State Education
Department
Cultural Education Center,
Room 3013
Albany, New York 12230
Tel: (518) 474-3843

NORTH CAROLINA Executive Director
North Carolina Board of
Nursing
P.O. Box 2129
Raleigh, North Carolina
27602
Tel: (919) 828-0740

NORTH DAKOTA . . Executive Director
North Dakota Board of
Nursing
919 S. Seventh Street,
Suite 504
Bismarck, North Dakota
58504
Tel: (701) 224-2974

OHIO . . . . Executive Secretary
Ohio Board of Nursing
Education and Nursing
Registration
65 S. Front Street,
Suite 509
Columbus, Ohio 43266-
0316
Tel: (614) 466-3947

OKLAHOMA . . . . . . Executive Director
Oklahoma Board of Nurse
Registration and
Nursing Education
2915 N. Classen
Boulevard, Suite 524
Oklahoma City, Oklahoma
73106
Tel: (405) 525-2076

INTRODUCTION

OREGON . . . . Executive Director
Oregon Board of Nursing
1400 S. W. Fifth Avenue,
Room 904
Portland, Oregon 97201
Tel: (503) 229-5653

PENNSYLVANIA . . Executive Secretary
Pennsylvania Board of
Nursing
Department of State
P.O. Box 2649
Harrisburg, Pennsylvania
17105
Tel: (717) 787-8503

RHODE ISLAND . . . Executive Secretary
Rhode Island Board of
Nurse Registration and
Nurse Education
Cannon Health Building
75 Davis Street, Room
104
Providence, Rhode Island
02908-2488
Tel: (401) 277-2827

SOUTH CAROLINA Executive Director
South Carolina State
Board of Nursing
1777 St. Julian Place,
Suite 102
Columbia, South Carolina
29204-2488
Tel: (803) 737-6594

SOUTH DAKOTA . . Executive Secretary
South Dakota Board of
Nursing
304 S. Phillips Avenue,
Suite 205
Sioux Falls, South Dakota
57102
Tel: (605) 335-4973

TENNESSEE . . . . . . Executive Director
Tennessee State Board of
Nursing
283 Plus Park Boulevard
Nashville, Tennessee
37217
Tel: (615) 367-6232

TEXAS . . . . Executive Secretary
Texas Board of Nurse
Examiners
P.O. Box 140466
Austin, Texas 78714
Tel: (512) 835-4880

UTAH . . . . Executive Secretary
Utah State Board of
Nursing
Division of Occupational
and Professional
Licensing
Heber M. Wells Building,
4th Floor
160 East 300 South
P.O. Box 45802
Salt Lake City, Utah
84145
Tel: (801) 530-6628

VERMONT . . . . Executive Director
Vermont State Board of
Nursing
Redstone Building
26 Terrace Street
Montpelier, Vermont
05602
Tel: (802) 828-2396

VIRGINIA . . . . Executive Director
Virginia State Board of
Nursing
1601 Rolling Hills Drive
Richmond, Virginia
23229-5005
Tel: (804) 662-9909

**VIRGIN ISLANDS
(U.S.)** . . . . Chairman
Virgin Islands Board of
Nursing
Knud Hansen Complex
Charlotte Amalie
St. Thomas, Virgin Islands
00801
Tel: (809) 776-7397

WASHINGTON . . . . Executive Secretary
Washington State Board
of Nursing
Department of Licensing
P.O. Box 9012
Olympia, Washington
98504
Tel: (206) 586-1923

WEST VIRGINIA . . . Executive Secretary
West Virginia Board of
Examiners for
Registered Nurses
Embleton Building,
Suite 309
922 Quarrier Street

Charleston, West Virginia 25301
Tel: (304) 348-3596

WISCONSIN ...... Director
Wisconsin Bureau of
   Health Professions
1400 East Washington
   Avenue
P.O. Box 8935
Madison, Wisconsin
   53708-8935
Tel: (608) 266-3735

WYOMING .... Executive Director
Wyoming State Board of
   Nursing
Barrett Building, 4th Floor
2301 Central Avenue
Cheyenne, Wyoming
   82002
Tel: (307) 777-7601

Diagnostic Test

Set aside a day to take the diagnostic test. Allow 2 consecutive hours in the morning for Part I, have your lunch and a break, and then take Part II in 2 consecutive hours in the afternoon. Take the examination in a quiet room, without interruption, and do not use aids such as notes or textbooks.

This diagnostic test, unlike the actual NCLEX-PN, uses an answer sheet and designates answer choices by letters—A, B, C, D. This is necessary in order to provide an answer key.

As you take the test, remember to:

1. Read each question and the four answer choices carefully.
2. Answer first the questions you are sure of, and then go back to the others.
3. Using a #2 pencil, indicate each answer by blackening completely the circle that corresponds to your choice:
    ⒶⒷⒸⒹ, not ⒶⒷⒸⒹ or ⒶⓍⒸⒹ.
4. Answer every question. Eliminate one or two choices if you can, and then select from the remaining answers.

ANSWER SHEET FOR DIAGNOSTIC TEST

Part I

1 Ⓐ Ⓑ Ⓒ Ⓓ	26 Ⓐ Ⓑ Ⓒ Ⓓ	51 Ⓐ Ⓑ Ⓒ Ⓓ	76 Ⓐ Ⓑ Ⓒ Ⓓ	101 Ⓐ Ⓑ Ⓒ Ⓓ
2 Ⓐ Ⓑ Ⓒ Ⓓ	27 Ⓐ Ⓑ Ⓒ Ⓓ	52 Ⓐ Ⓑ Ⓒ Ⓓ	77 Ⓐ Ⓑ Ⓒ Ⓓ	102 Ⓐ Ⓑ Ⓒ Ⓓ
3 Ⓐ Ⓑ Ⓒ Ⓓ	28 Ⓐ Ⓑ Ⓒ Ⓓ	53 Ⓐ Ⓑ Ⓒ Ⓓ	78 Ⓐ Ⓑ Ⓒ Ⓓ	103 Ⓐ Ⓑ Ⓒ Ⓓ
4 Ⓐ Ⓑ Ⓒ Ⓓ	29 Ⓐ Ⓑ Ⓒ Ⓓ	54 Ⓐ Ⓑ Ⓒ Ⓓ	79 Ⓐ Ⓑ Ⓒ Ⓓ	104 Ⓐ Ⓑ Ⓒ Ⓓ
5 Ⓐ Ⓑ Ⓒ Ⓓ	30 Ⓐ Ⓑ Ⓒ Ⓓ	55 Ⓐ Ⓑ Ⓒ Ⓓ	80 Ⓐ Ⓑ Ⓒ Ⓓ	105 Ⓐ Ⓑ Ⓒ Ⓓ
6 Ⓐ Ⓑ Ⓒ Ⓓ	31 Ⓐ Ⓑ Ⓒ Ⓓ	56 Ⓐ Ⓑ Ⓒ Ⓓ	81 Ⓐ Ⓑ Ⓒ Ⓓ	106 Ⓐ Ⓑ Ⓒ Ⓓ
7 Ⓐ Ⓑ Ⓒ Ⓓ	32 Ⓐ Ⓑ Ⓒ Ⓓ	57 Ⓐ Ⓑ Ⓒ Ⓓ	82 Ⓐ Ⓑ Ⓒ Ⓓ	107 Ⓐ Ⓑ Ⓒ Ⓓ
8 Ⓐ Ⓑ Ⓒ Ⓓ	33 Ⓐ Ⓑ Ⓒ Ⓓ	58 Ⓐ Ⓑ Ⓒ Ⓓ	83 Ⓐ Ⓑ Ⓒ Ⓓ	108 Ⓐ Ⓑ Ⓒ Ⓓ
9 Ⓐ Ⓑ Ⓒ Ⓓ	34 Ⓐ Ⓑ Ⓒ Ⓓ	59 Ⓐ Ⓑ Ⓒ Ⓓ	84 Ⓐ Ⓑ Ⓒ Ⓓ	109 Ⓐ Ⓑ Ⓒ Ⓓ
10 Ⓐ Ⓑ Ⓒ Ⓓ	35 Ⓐ Ⓑ Ⓒ Ⓓ	60 Ⓐ Ⓑ Ⓒ Ⓓ	85 Ⓐ Ⓑ Ⓒ Ⓓ	110 Ⓐ Ⓑ Ⓒ Ⓓ
11 Ⓐ Ⓑ Ⓒ Ⓓ	36 Ⓐ Ⓑ Ⓒ Ⓓ	61 Ⓐ Ⓑ Ⓒ Ⓓ	86 Ⓐ Ⓑ Ⓒ Ⓓ	111 Ⓐ Ⓑ Ⓒ Ⓓ
12 Ⓐ Ⓑ Ⓒ Ⓓ	37 Ⓐ Ⓑ Ⓒ Ⓓ	62 Ⓐ Ⓑ Ⓒ Ⓓ	87 Ⓐ Ⓑ Ⓒ Ⓓ	112 Ⓐ Ⓑ Ⓒ Ⓓ
13 Ⓐ Ⓑ Ⓒ Ⓓ	38 Ⓐ Ⓑ Ⓒ Ⓓ	63 Ⓐ Ⓑ Ⓒ Ⓓ	88 Ⓐ Ⓑ Ⓒ Ⓓ	113 Ⓐ Ⓑ Ⓒ Ⓓ
14 Ⓐ Ⓑ Ⓒ Ⓓ	39 Ⓐ Ⓑ Ⓒ Ⓓ	64 Ⓐ Ⓑ Ⓒ Ⓓ	89 Ⓐ Ⓑ Ⓒ Ⓓ	114 Ⓐ Ⓑ Ⓒ Ⓓ
15 Ⓐ Ⓑ Ⓒ Ⓓ	40 Ⓐ Ⓑ Ⓒ Ⓓ	65 Ⓐ Ⓑ Ⓒ Ⓓ	90 Ⓐ Ⓑ Ⓒ Ⓓ	115 Ⓐ Ⓑ Ⓒ Ⓓ
16 Ⓐ Ⓑ Ⓒ Ⓓ	41 Ⓐ Ⓑ Ⓒ Ⓓ	66 Ⓐ Ⓑ Ⓒ Ⓓ	91 Ⓐ Ⓑ Ⓒ Ⓓ	116 Ⓐ Ⓑ Ⓒ Ⓓ
17 Ⓐ Ⓑ Ⓒ Ⓓ	42 Ⓐ Ⓑ Ⓒ Ⓓ	67 Ⓐ Ⓑ Ⓒ Ⓓ	92 Ⓐ Ⓑ Ⓒ Ⓓ	117 Ⓐ Ⓑ Ⓒ Ⓓ
18 Ⓐ Ⓑ Ⓒ Ⓓ	43 Ⓐ Ⓑ Ⓒ Ⓓ	68 Ⓐ Ⓑ Ⓒ Ⓓ	93 Ⓐ Ⓑ Ⓒ Ⓓ	118 Ⓐ Ⓑ Ⓒ Ⓓ
19 Ⓐ Ⓑ Ⓒ Ⓓ	44 Ⓐ Ⓑ Ⓒ Ⓓ	69 Ⓐ Ⓑ Ⓒ Ⓓ	94 Ⓐ Ⓑ Ⓒ Ⓓ	119 Ⓐ Ⓑ Ⓒ Ⓓ
20 Ⓐ Ⓑ Ⓒ Ⓓ	45 Ⓐ Ⓑ Ⓒ Ⓓ	70 Ⓐ Ⓑ Ⓒ Ⓓ	95 Ⓐ Ⓑ Ⓒ Ⓓ	120 Ⓐ Ⓑ Ⓒ Ⓓ
21 Ⓐ Ⓑ Ⓒ Ⓓ	46 Ⓐ Ⓑ Ⓒ Ⓓ	71 Ⓐ Ⓑ Ⓒ Ⓓ	96 Ⓐ Ⓑ Ⓒ Ⓓ	121 Ⓐ Ⓑ Ⓒ Ⓓ
22 Ⓐ Ⓑ Ⓒ Ⓓ	47 Ⓐ Ⓑ Ⓒ Ⓓ	72 Ⓐ Ⓑ Ⓒ Ⓓ	97 Ⓐ Ⓑ Ⓒ Ⓓ	122 Ⓐ Ⓑ Ⓒ Ⓓ
23 Ⓐ Ⓑ Ⓒ Ⓓ	48 Ⓐ Ⓑ Ⓒ Ⓓ	73 Ⓐ Ⓑ Ⓒ Ⓓ	98 Ⓐ Ⓑ Ⓒ Ⓓ	123 Ⓐ Ⓑ Ⓒ Ⓓ
24 Ⓐ Ⓑ Ⓒ Ⓓ	49 Ⓐ Ⓑ Ⓒ Ⓓ	74 Ⓐ Ⓑ Ⓒ Ⓓ	99 Ⓐ Ⓑ Ⓒ Ⓓ	124 Ⓐ Ⓑ Ⓒ Ⓓ
25 Ⓐ Ⓑ Ⓒ Ⓓ	50 Ⓐ Ⓑ Ⓒ Ⓓ	75 Ⓐ Ⓑ Ⓒ Ⓓ	100 Ⓐ Ⓑ Ⓒ Ⓓ	125 Ⓐ Ⓑ Ⓒ Ⓓ

Part II

1	Ⓐ Ⓑ Ⓒ Ⓓ	26	Ⓐ Ⓑ Ⓒ Ⓓ	51	Ⓐ Ⓑ Ⓒ Ⓓ	76	Ⓐ Ⓑ Ⓒ Ⓓ	101	Ⓐ Ⓑ Ⓒ Ⓓ
2	Ⓐ Ⓑ Ⓒ Ⓓ	27	Ⓐ Ⓑ Ⓒ Ⓓ	52	Ⓐ Ⓑ Ⓒ Ⓓ	77	Ⓐ Ⓑ Ⓒ Ⓓ	102	Ⓐ Ⓑ Ⓒ Ⓓ
3	Ⓐ Ⓑ Ⓒ Ⓓ	28	Ⓐ Ⓑ Ⓒ Ⓓ	53	Ⓐ Ⓑ Ⓒ Ⓓ	78	Ⓐ Ⓑ Ⓒ Ⓓ	103	Ⓐ Ⓑ Ⓒ Ⓓ
4	Ⓐ Ⓑ Ⓒ Ⓓ	29	Ⓐ Ⓑ Ⓒ Ⓓ	54	Ⓐ Ⓑ Ⓒ Ⓓ	79	Ⓐ Ⓑ Ⓒ Ⓓ	104	Ⓐ Ⓑ Ⓒ Ⓓ
5	Ⓐ Ⓑ Ⓒ Ⓓ	30	Ⓐ Ⓑ Ⓒ Ⓓ	55	Ⓐ Ⓑ Ⓒ Ⓓ	80	Ⓐ Ⓑ Ⓒ Ⓓ	105	Ⓐ Ⓑ Ⓒ Ⓓ
6	Ⓐ Ⓑ Ⓒ Ⓓ	31	Ⓐ Ⓑ Ⓒ Ⓓ	56	Ⓐ Ⓑ Ⓒ Ⓓ	81	Ⓐ Ⓑ Ⓒ Ⓓ	106	Ⓐ Ⓑ Ⓒ Ⓓ
7	Ⓐ Ⓑ Ⓒ Ⓓ	32	Ⓐ Ⓑ Ⓒ Ⓓ	57	Ⓐ Ⓑ Ⓒ Ⓓ	82	Ⓐ Ⓑ Ⓒ Ⓓ	107	Ⓐ Ⓑ Ⓒ Ⓓ
8	Ⓐ Ⓑ Ⓒ Ⓓ	33	Ⓐ Ⓑ Ⓒ Ⓓ	58	Ⓐ Ⓑ Ⓒ Ⓓ	83	Ⓐ Ⓑ Ⓒ Ⓓ	108	Ⓐ Ⓑ Ⓒ Ⓓ
9	Ⓐ Ⓑ Ⓒ Ⓓ	34	Ⓐ Ⓑ Ⓒ Ⓓ	59	Ⓐ Ⓑ Ⓒ Ⓓ	84	Ⓐ Ⓑ Ⓒ Ⓓ	109	Ⓐ Ⓑ Ⓒ Ⓓ
10	Ⓐ Ⓑ Ⓒ Ⓓ	35	Ⓐ Ⓑ Ⓒ Ⓓ	60	Ⓐ Ⓑ Ⓒ Ⓓ	85	Ⓐ Ⓑ Ⓒ Ⓓ	110	Ⓐ Ⓑ Ⓒ Ⓓ
11	Ⓐ Ⓑ Ⓒ Ⓓ	36	Ⓐ Ⓑ Ⓒ Ⓓ	61	Ⓐ Ⓑ Ⓒ Ⓓ	86	Ⓐ Ⓑ Ⓒ Ⓓ	111	Ⓐ Ⓑ Ⓒ Ⓓ
12	Ⓐ Ⓑ Ⓒ Ⓓ	37	Ⓐ Ⓑ Ⓒ Ⓓ	62	Ⓐ Ⓑ Ⓒ Ⓓ	87	Ⓐ Ⓑ Ⓒ Ⓓ	112	Ⓐ Ⓑ Ⓒ Ⓓ
13	Ⓐ Ⓑ Ⓒ Ⓓ	38	Ⓐ Ⓑ Ⓒ Ⓓ	63	Ⓐ Ⓑ Ⓒ Ⓓ	88	Ⓐ Ⓑ Ⓒ Ⓓ	113	Ⓐ Ⓑ Ⓒ Ⓓ
14	Ⓐ Ⓑ Ⓒ Ⓓ	39	Ⓐ Ⓑ Ⓒ Ⓓ	64	Ⓐ Ⓑ Ⓒ Ⓓ	89	Ⓐ Ⓑ Ⓒ Ⓓ	114	Ⓐ Ⓑ Ⓒ Ⓓ
15	Ⓐ Ⓑ Ⓒ Ⓓ	40	Ⓐ Ⓑ Ⓒ Ⓓ	65	Ⓐ Ⓑ Ⓒ Ⓓ	90	Ⓐ Ⓑ Ⓒ Ⓓ	115	Ⓐ Ⓑ Ⓒ Ⓓ
16	Ⓐ Ⓑ Ⓒ Ⓓ	41	Ⓐ Ⓑ Ⓒ Ⓓ	66	Ⓐ Ⓑ Ⓒ Ⓓ	91	Ⓐ Ⓑ Ⓒ Ⓓ	116	Ⓐ Ⓑ Ⓒ Ⓓ
17	Ⓐ Ⓑ Ⓒ Ⓓ	42	Ⓐ Ⓑ Ⓒ Ⓓ	67	Ⓐ Ⓑ Ⓒ Ⓓ	92	Ⓐ Ⓑ Ⓒ Ⓓ	117	Ⓐ Ⓑ Ⓒ Ⓓ
18	Ⓐ Ⓑ Ⓒ Ⓓ	43	Ⓐ Ⓑ Ⓒ Ⓓ	68	Ⓐ Ⓑ Ⓒ Ⓓ	93	Ⓐ Ⓑ Ⓒ Ⓓ	118	Ⓐ Ⓑ Ⓒ Ⓓ
19	Ⓐ Ⓑ Ⓒ Ⓓ	44	Ⓐ Ⓑ Ⓒ Ⓓ	69	Ⓐ Ⓑ Ⓒ Ⓓ	94	Ⓐ Ⓑ Ⓒ Ⓓ	119	Ⓐ Ⓑ Ⓒ Ⓓ
20	Ⓐ Ⓑ Ⓒ Ⓓ	45	Ⓐ Ⓑ Ⓒ Ⓓ	70	Ⓐ Ⓑ Ⓒ Ⓓ	95	Ⓐ Ⓑ Ⓒ Ⓓ	120	Ⓐ Ⓑ Ⓒ Ⓓ
21	Ⓐ Ⓑ Ⓒ Ⓓ	46	Ⓐ Ⓑ Ⓒ Ⓓ	71	Ⓐ Ⓑ Ⓒ Ⓓ	96	Ⓐ Ⓑ Ⓒ Ⓓ	121	Ⓐ Ⓑ Ⓒ Ⓓ
22	Ⓐ Ⓑ Ⓒ Ⓓ	47	Ⓐ Ⓑ Ⓒ Ⓓ	72	Ⓐ Ⓑ Ⓒ Ⓓ	97	Ⓐ Ⓑ Ⓒ Ⓓ	122	Ⓐ Ⓑ Ⓒ Ⓓ
23	Ⓐ Ⓑ Ⓒ Ⓓ	48	Ⓐ Ⓑ Ⓒ Ⓓ	73	Ⓐ Ⓑ Ⓒ Ⓓ	98	Ⓐ Ⓑ Ⓒ Ⓓ	123	Ⓐ Ⓑ Ⓒ Ⓓ
24	Ⓐ Ⓑ Ⓒ Ⓓ	49	Ⓐ Ⓑ Ⓒ Ⓓ	74	Ⓐ Ⓑ Ⓒ Ⓓ	99	Ⓐ Ⓑ Ⓒ Ⓓ	124	Ⓐ Ⓑ Ⓒ Ⓓ
25	Ⓐ Ⓑ Ⓒ Ⓓ	50	Ⓐ Ⓑ Ⓒ Ⓓ	75	Ⓐ Ⓑ Ⓒ Ⓓ	100	Ⓐ Ⓑ Ⓒ Ⓓ	125	Ⓐ Ⓑ Ⓒ Ⓓ

DIAGNOSTIC TEST, PART I

Mr. Reynolds, 69 years of age, is found unconscious by his wife at 7:00 A.M. An ambulance is summoned by the physician, and Mr. Reynolds is admitted to the medical unit, where you work as a practical nurse, with a diagnosis of cerebral vascular accident (CVA). As you assist the team leader with the admission process, you note a previous history of hypertension. His wife has also revealed that Mr. Reynolds complained of a headache before retiring the night before.

1. In addition to the headache and hypertension, which of the following symptoms would you expect Mr. Reynolds to exhibit?
   A. Labored respirations.
   B. Dysphagia and hemiplegia.
   C. Aphasia.
   D. All of the above.

2. The team leader instructs you to remove Mr. Reynolds's dentures. You do so because
   A. the team leader will report you if you do not follow directions.
   B. the dentures need to be cleaned.
   C. the dentures might obstruct the respiratory passages.
   D. Mr. Reynolds usually removes them for sleep anyway.

3. Unresponsive patients like Mr. Reynolds may develop a drying of the cornea, which is usually caused by
   A. paralysis of the eyelid.
   B. absence of the blinking reflex and reduction in tear formation.
   C. lack of humidity in the room.
   D. bulging of the eyeballs.

4. The MAIN objective in the nursing care of the stroke patient is to
   A. prevent infection.
   B. prevent complications that will delay rehabilitation.
   C. provide good nutrition.
   D. provide relief of pain.

5. In the nursing assessment you note that Mr. Reynolds has left-side paralysis. When Mr. Reynolds is turned on his side, it is important to
   A. elevate the head and knee gatch.
   B. elevate the foot of the bed.
   C. support the affected arm and leg with pillows.
   D. support the unaffected arm and leg with pillows.

6. Mr. Reynolds regains consciousness, but is unable to speak. This disorder is known as
   A. aphonia.
   B. atresia.
   C. aphasia.
   D. aphagia.

7. Mr. Reynolds's program of rehabilitation should begin
   A. when he is ready to go home.
   B. when he is able to understand directions.
   C. when he regains consciousness.
   D. on the day he is admitted to the hospital.

8. Mr. Reynolds develops cyanosis. This may occur because
   A. he has hypertension.
   B. secretions have accumulated in his respiratory passages and he is unable to breathe well.
   C. he has developed emphysema.
   D. he is anemic.

9. Mr. Reynolds's physician has ordered that intravenous fluids be administered slowly in order to
   A. stimulate diuresis.
   B. stimulate peristalsis.
   C. prevent overloading the circulatory system.
   D. prevent respiratory secretions from accumulating.

10. Proper positioning of Mr. Reynolds is very important in order to:
    1. prevent dependent edema.
    2. prevent contractures.
    3. improve circulation.
    4. prevent aspiration.
    A. 4, only.
    B. 1, 2, and 3.
    C. 2, 3, and 4.
    D. 1, 2, 3, and 4.

> *You are employed as a practical nurse in an obstetrician's office. You have just greeted Mrs. Frank and escorted her to the examining room. Mrs. Frank is 26 years old and has missed two menstrual periods. She is eagerly anticipating confirmation of a hoped-for first pregnancy.*

11. A woman who, like Mrs. Frank, is pregnant for the first time is called a
    A. primipara.
    B. primigravida.
    C. multipara.
    D. multigravida.

12. Before the end of the 3rd month of pregnancy, the products of conception are known as the
    A. fetus.
    B. embryo.
    C. zygote.
    D. placenta.

13. Mrs. Frank's amenorrhea is classified as which type of sign of pregnancy?
    A. A positive sign.
    B. A probable sign.
    C. A presumptive sign.
    D. A negative sign.

14. Mrs. Frank's estimated date of delivery is determined by counting
    A. 300 days from the first day of the last menstruation.
    B. back 7 months from the first day of the last menstrual period and adding 3 days.
    C. back 3 months from the first day of the last menstrual period and adding 7 days.
    D. 200 days from the first day of the last menstruation.

15. Mrs. Frank's prenatal examination includes all of the following EXCEPT
    A. a routine physical, including past medical history.
    B. urinalysis for sugar and albumin.
    C. a gallbladder series.
    D. temperature, pulse, respiration, and blood pressure.

16. Mrs. Frank confides to you that she has to urinate at frequent intervals. You explain that this frequency of urination usually subsides when the
    A. placenta is fully developed.
    B. fetal kidneys begin to function.
    C. uterus rises into the abdominal cavity.
    D. mother's kidneys enlarge to accommodate the extra waste.

17. During the first half of her pregnancy, the physician will most probably wish to see Mrs. Frank every
    A. 1 to 2 weeks.
    B. 2 to 3 weeks.
    C. 3 to 4 weeks.
    D. 6 to 8 weeks.

18. Mrs. Frank complains of nausea and vomiting as well as heartburn. You recommend that she alter her diet by reducing the intake of
    A. fats.
    B. proteins.
    C. minerals.
    D. carbohydrates.

19. You also advise Mrs. Frank that her nausea and vomiting can be relieved if, one-half hour before rising in the morning, she
    A. drinks a glass of milk.
    B. drinks a cup of hot tea.
    C. eats a piece of fruit.
    D. eats a piece of dry toast or a plain cracker.

20. The most probable cause of Mrs. Frank's heartburn is
    A. an increase in the production of bile.
    B. an increase in the production of stomach acid.
    C. a rising of the uterine fundus.
    D. a decrease in digestive enzymes.

21. To prevent or control constipation, you encourage Mrs. Frank to increase all of the following EXCEPT her
    A. fluid intake.
    B. roughage.
    C. exercise.
    D. rest periods.

22. The physician prescribes mineral oil to relieve occasional constipation. You instruct Mrs. Frank not to take it at or near mealtimes because mineral oil interferes with the absorption of vitamin
    A. C.

B. B_{12}.
C. A.
D. B_2.

23. As Mrs. Frank's pregnancy progresses, the physician uses a fetoscope to check for the fetal heart sounds. The nurse first expects to hear fetal heart sounds when the woman has been pregnant
   A. 8 to 10 weeks.
   B. 10 to 12 weeks.
   C. 13 to 15 weeks.
   D. 18 to 20 weeks.

24. Mrs. Frank has chloasma, which is best described as
   A. stretch marks on the abdomen.
   B. brown spots on the face.
   C. dark rings around the nipples.
   D. a dark vertical line on the abdomen.

25. Mrs. Frank has been experiencing leg cramps. To relieve these spasms, you advise her to place the ankle in a position of
   A. rotation, by moving the foot in circles.
   B. dorsiflexion, by moving the toes up toward the knees.
   C. extension, by moving the foot so the toes point up to the ceiling.
   D. plantar flexion, by moving the foot so the toe points down to the floor.

26. For which of the following discomforts of pregnancy that Mrs. Frank may experience is the pelvic rock most often recommended?
   A. Backaches.
   B. Heartburn.
   C. Constipation.
   D. Nausea.

27. Mrs. Frank should eat which of the following foods to increase her iron intake?
   A. Cheese.
   B. Citrus fruits.
   C. Lean meat or dried beans.
   D. Green or yellow vegetables.

28. To help ensure an adequate calcium intake, you encourage Mrs. Frank to increase her daily milk intake to
   A. 2 cups.
   B. 4 cups.
   C. 6 cups.
   D. 8 cups.

Mr. Skully is an 80-year-old resident in a health-related facility. He suffers from arteriosclerotic heart disease but is ambulatory. His medications are Digoxin 0.25 mg OD daily and Lasix 40 mg BID and he is on a salt-poor diet. He has been known to sneak out and wander around the neighborhood. He is unfriendly to the other residents and considers himself superior to them.

29. The nurse discovers that Mr. Skully, who complains constantly about the "tasteless" food, has gone out and bought salt and hot, pickled peppers to put on his food. Which of the following actions should the nurse take?
   A. Call Mr. Skully's doctor and report this action.
   B. Chart the action and report it to the supervisor.
   C. Take the condiments away from Mr. Skully.
   D. Scold Mr. Skully and tell him that he is undoing all the staff's good work.

30. When planning nursing care for Mr. Skully, to which of the following behaviors is it MOST important that the staff be alerted?
   A. His constant complaints.
   B. His wandering around the neighborhood.
   C. His refusal of meals.
   D. His hiding of condiments in his room.

Mrs. Cox has an ulcer on her lower leg. Continuous warm, moist compresses have been ordered.

31. When administering these compresses, it is important to
   A. explain the procedure to Mrs. Cox carefully so that she can learn to prepare the compresses for herself.
   B. warm at least one quart of solution each time because these are continuous compresses.
   C. put Mrs. Cox in a wheelchair so that the compresses can be applied more easily.
   D. check the moisture of the compresses frequently so that they are never dry.

32. After Mrs. Cox's ulcer has healed, her physician recommends elastic stockings. The purpose of these stockings is to
   A. increase circulation in the legs.
   B. protect the legs from injury.
   C. provide warmth for the lower legs.
   D. support the blood vessels in the leg.

33. When instructing Mrs. Cox in the proper use of these stockings, the nurse should tell her that the stockings should be
   A. worn 20 hours a day.
   B. applied early in the morning before arising from bed.
   C. held up with circular garters.
   D. worn only when she anticipates standing for long periods of time.

Mrs. Rivera has been confined to bed for several weeks but refuses to change position or perform the exercises ordered by her doctor to maintain adequate circulation in her legs. One day she tells the doctor her legs hurt, and he diagnoses her condition as thrombophlebitis.

34. Thrombophlebitis is
   A. inflammation of the vein caused by a blood clot in the blood vessel.
   B. a traumatic inflammation of a blood vessel.
   C. a bulging of the wall of an artery.
   D. an ulceration within the blood vessels.

35. The most common symptom of thrombophlebitis is
   A. cyanosis of the affected leg.
   B. pain in the calf of the leg.
   C. severe swelling of the ankles.
   D. bulging of the affected blood vessels.

36. A nursing procedure that is CONTRAINDICATED in thrombophlebitis is
   A. turning the patient from side to side.
   B. elevating the head of the bed.
   C. massaging the legs.
   D. rubbing the back.

37. Thrombophlebitis is a complication of a variety of illnesses and can best be avoided by
   A. early ambulation and exercises to increase circulation.
   B. the administration of antibiotics.

C. giving the patient daily doses of vitamin K.
   D. restricting physical activity of any kind after surgery.

38. The doctor tells Mrs. Rivera to stop smoking. She cannot understand why and says, "It's my legs that are bothering me, not my lungs." As a practical nurse, your best reply to her would be
   A. "Your doctor is afraid your condition will spread to your lungs."
   B. "Nicotine, which is present in cigarettes, narrows the blood vessels in your body and makes your condition worse."
   C. "Smoking dulls your appetite, and poor nutrition makes your condition worse."
   D. "There is no connection between smoking and your condition, but you would feel better if you stopped smoking."

39. The aim of nursing care for patients with thrombophlebitis is to
   A. prevent breakdown of tissues.
   B. provide proper nutrition.
   C. provide proper rest.
   D. prevent an embolism.

Mr. Green, aged 62, is assigned to you for morning care. His diagnosis is congestive heart failure.

40. Congestive heart failure is best described as a cardiac condition in which there is
   A. an abnormality in the structure of the heart.
   B. a decreased flow of blood through the heart and great vessels, resulting from failure of the heart to function as a pump.
   C. a blood clot within one of the heart chambers.
   D. a sudden spasm of the heart muscle due to a decreased blood supply.

41. Mr. Green's doctor orders complete bedrest for him. This means that Mr. Green
   A. is encouraged to rest as much as possible.
   B. is confined to bed but can assume responsibility for much of his personal care.

C. is confined to bed but is allowed to get up to go to the bathroom as necessary.

D. must remain as quiet as possible and everything involving the slightest physical effort must be done for him.

42. Mr. Green is suffering from severe dyspnea. The position in which he will be most comfortable is
A. Sims' left lateral position.
B. Fowler's position.
C. the Trendelenburg position.
D. the supine position.

43. Back care for Mr. Green is
A. not indicated because a cardiac patient must have absolute rest.
B. less important than for most patients because the edema "pads" the bony prominences of the body.
C. more important than for most patients because a cardiac patient often has edematous tissue, which readily breaks down.
D. important when the patient's skin shows signs of developing ulcerations.

44. Cardiac patients like Mr. Green are sometimes not permitted to have cold drinks or iced foods because
A. they act as a stimulant to the heart.
B. extreme cold has a constricting effect on blood vessels and may increase the workload of the heart.
C. cold decreases circulation and overburdens the heart.
D. cold drinks cause the formation of gas and lead to stomach cramps.

45. Mr. Green is given a low-sodium diet. When edema is present, the intake of sodium is restricted because it
A. slows the heartbeat.
B. causes hardening of the arteries.
C. decreases the urinary output.
D. holds fluid in the tissues.

46. One food substance that contains sodium and is commonly part of the average person's diet is
A. fruit.
B. sugar.
C. table salt.
D. coffee.

47. Which of the following foods is LOWEST in sodium content?
A. Citrus fruits.
B. Canned meats and fish.
C. Milk and milk products.
D. Bacon.

48. Because there may be "hidden" sources of sodium, which of the following should be carefully checked by reading the label to see if sodium is present?
1. Canned or processed foods.
2. Toothpastes and mouthwashes.
3. Packaged bakery products.
4. Patent medicines.
A. 1, 2, 3, and 4.
B. 2 and 4.
C. 1 and 3.
D. 1, 3, and 4.

49. To prevent depletion of potassium by the diuretics Mr. Green is taking, the nurse advised him to eat
A. potatoes.
B. bananas.
C. chocolate chip cookies.
D. spinach.

50. Mr. Green's doctor places him on digitalis. This drug is classified as a
A. heart stimulant.
B. cerebral stimulant.
C. coagulant.
D. respiratory stimulant.

51. The chief action of digitalis is to
A. lower the blood pressure.
B. prevent the formation of blood clots.
C. increase the pulse rate.
D. slow and strengthen the heartbeat.

52. Before each dose of digitalis is administered to Mr. Green, you must remember to
A. check his pulse.
B. check his respiration.
C. take his blood pressure.
D. check with the lab to see whether a test of bleeding time has been done.

53. Digitalis must not be given without the specific direction of the doctor whenever
A. the systolic B/P is above 100.
B. the rectal temperature is subnormal.
C. the pulse is 60 or below.
D. the patient is flushed and perspiring.

54. Drugs that are sometimes given to increase the urinary output and relieve edema are called
A. urinary stimulants.
B. heart stimulants.
C. diuretics.
D. urinary disinfectants.

55. The doctor has ordered a daily weight check for Mr. Green. The reason for this is to determine the loss of
A. body fat.
B. appetite.
C. tissue fluid.
D. blood volume.

56. When weighing Mr. Green, you should
A. use the treatment-room scales, which are accurate.
B. weigh him in the late afternoon each day.
C. weigh him at the same time every day, on the same scales, and with the same amount of clothing.
D. ask the orderly to weigh him because it is difficult to get the patient out of bed.

57. Nitroglycerin tablets, which are often prescribed for cardiac patients like Mr. Green, are given sublingually. This means that the tablets are
A. dissolved and given under the skin.
B. held under the tongue until dissolved.
C. taken by mouth with a small amount of water.
D. injected into the gluteal muscle.

Mrs. Russo, a 45-year-old mother of three, has experienced bleeding between her menstrual periods for several months. She makes an appointment for an examination by a gynecologist.

58. The office nurse confirming the appointment for Mrs. Russo should caution her against
A. choosing a date on which she expects to have vaginal bleeding.
B. taking a douche immediately before coming to the doctor's office.
C. taking a tub bath immediately before coming to the office.
D. taking any foods or fluids for 8 hours before coming to the office.

59. Before Mrs. Russo is given a pelvic examination in the gynecologist's office, it is most important for the nurse to
A. direct the patient to the bathroom to empty her bladder.
B. administer a low enema.
C. catheterize the patient for a specimen.
D. scrub the perineal area with pHisohex for 5 minutes.

60. The main reason for this nursing intervention is to
A. obtain a stool specimen.
B. remove flatus and feces from the intestinal tract.
C. sterilize the skin around the vagina.
D. prevent discomfort for the patient and enable the physician to palpate the pelvic organs more easily.

61. Mrs. Russo will be more relaxed and cooperative during the gynecological examination if the nurse will
A. leave the room during the examination.
B. inform the patient that all the instruments have been sterilized.
C. explain the procedure to the patient if she does not know what to expect.
D. remind the patient that modesty is not important during any type of physical examination.

62. The physician explains to Mrs. Russo that he will do a Papanicolaou (Pap) smear of the cervical secretions. The purpose of this test is to
A. determine the presence of microorganisms that may be the cause of a disease.
B. rule out the possibility of a venereal disease.
C. rule out or confirm pregnancy.
D. determine the presence of malignant cells in the cervical secretions.

63. After the examination Mrs. Russo's gynecologist recommends that she be admitted to the hospital for further diagnostic tests. After her admission she is scheduled for a dilatation and curettage. This procedure involves
A. dilatation of the cervix and scraping of the uterus.

B. removal of several samples of cervical tissue.
C. X-ray examination of the reproductive tract.
D. visual examination of the interior of the uterus.

64. Mrs. Russo's condition is diagnosed as non-invasive carcinoma of the cervix. She is immediately scheduled for a vaginal hysterectomy. This procedure involves surgical removal of the
A. uterus and vagina through an abdominal incision.
B. uterus by way of the vagina.
C. uterus, tubes, and ovaries through an abdominal incision.
D. cervix and tubes by way of the vagina.

65. The evening before surgery Mrs. Russo receives a zephiran douche. The purpose of this procedure is to
A. help minimize vaginal bleeding.
B. cleanse the vaginal canal.
C. remove malignant cells from the vaginal canal.
D. sterilize the operative area.

66. During the immediate postoperative period it is most important for the nurse to
A. observe Mrs. Russo carefully for hemorrhage, which is a common complication of vaginal surgery.
B. keep Mrs. Russo in the Trendelenburg position to avoid strain on the sutures.
C. irrigate the operative area with normal saline to prevent infection.
D. catheterize Mrs. Russo every 4 hours to prevent overexpansion of the bladder.

67. Mrs. Russo is to receive perineal irrigations beginning the first postoperative day. Before administering the irrigations, the nurse should
A. warm the solution to room temperature.
B. assist the patient onto the commode for the procedure.
C. position the patient on her abdomen.
D. remove any soiled pads or dressings and discard them in the patient's wastebasket.

68. During the perineal irrigation the nurse must remember to

1. use one cotton ball for each stroke when cleansing the area.
2. hold the irrigating can at least 18 inches above the patient.
3. wipe toward the rectal area so as to avoid contamination of the operative area.
4. instruct the patient to void as soon after the procedure as possible.
A. 1, 2, 3, and 4.
B. 1 and 3.
C. 2 and 4.
D. 1, 3, and 4.

69. Mrs. Russo seems worried about the after-effects of her surgery and asks whether she will continue to have menstrual periods. The practical nurse knows that for menstruation to take place the organ(s) that must be present and functioning is (are)
A. the uterus and fallopian tubes.
B. the uterus only.
C. the uterus and at least part of one ovary.
D. the fallopian tubes and one or both ovaries.

70. Mrs. Russo tells the nurse that the surgeon informed her he had not removed her ovaries. His reason for leaving the ovaries intact was to
A. allow for future pregnancies.
B. provide for continuing secretion of the ovarian hormones.
C. make the surgical procedure less difficult and prolonged.
D. lessen the danger of hemorrhage in the postoperative period.

You are assigned to care for Miss Yu, aged 39, who has just returned from surgery. She has had a radical mastectomy for treatment of a malignant tumor of the breast.

71. A radical mastectomy involves removal of
A. a fibroid tumor and its capsule.
B. the entire breast, the adjacent lymph nodes under the arm, and the pectoralis major and minor.
C. both breasts.
D. the tumor and adjacent fatty tissue.

72. Miss Yu has a pressure dressing over the surgical area. When checking the dressing

for hemorrhage, it will be necessary for you to
A. remove the uppermost layers of the dressing each hour.
B. turn the patient frequently in order to check the dressings.
C. remove the entire dressing to observe the operative site.
D. always keep the patient turned onto the side opposite the operative side so that bleeding can be observed readily.

73. If, during the first 24 hours after surgery, Miss Yu complains of numbness and swelling of the lower arm on the operative side, you should know that

A. this is most unusual for patients who have had a radical mastectomy.

B. this is usual for patients who have had a radical mastectomy.

C. this is one of the first signs of hemorrhage from the operative area.

D. there has probably been some damage to the nerves in the arm and paralysis is inevitable.

74. One of the simplest ways for Miss Yu to obtain necessary exercise after a mastectomy is
A. weight lifting.
B. brushing her hair.
C. mopping the floor.
D. dusting furniture.

75. There are times during the postoperative period when Miss Yu becomes depressed and withdrawn. As a practical nurse, you realize that
A. Miss Yu is probably showing the early symptoms of a psychosis.
B. this is a difficult time of adjustment for most patients who have had a mastectomy.
C. Miss Yu is very vain and needs flattery to get her out of this mood.
D. it will be best to leave Miss Yu alone at this time and let her solve her own personal problems.

76. Miss Yu asks you when she will be able to obtain a prosthesis and begin wearing it. The best answer to this question would be
A. "When you can afford one."

B. "This will depend on the amount of scar tissue you will have."
C. "The physician must decide when healing is sufficient and the prosthesis can be worn comfortably."
D. "Some people can never adjust to a prosthesis after a mastectomy."

Mr. O'Brien, aged 72, has been experiencing difficulty in urinating for the past several months. He is examined by his family physician and found to have an enlarged prostate gland.

---

77. An enlarged prostate gland interferes with urination because the gland
A. is located near the kidneys and presses against them.
B. encircles the urethra just below the neck of the bladder.
C. secretes a substance important in the formation of urine.
D. controls the sphincter muscle at the end of the urethra.

78. Mr. O'Brien is admitted to the hospital and scheduled for a transurethral prostatic resection. In this procedure
A. an incision is made into the perineum and the entire gland is removed.
B. the prostate gland is removed through an incision.
C. a low abdominal incision is made and the prostate is removed.
D. part of the prostate gland is removed by way of the urethra.

79. Which of the following should be reported promptly if noticed during Mr. O'Brien's immediate postoperative period?
A. A pinkish drainage from the operative site.
B. Bits of clots and tissue passing through the catheter and into the drainage bottle.
C. Large amounts of urine passing through the catheter.
D. Bright red blood in the catheter and drainage bottle.

80. If Mr. O'Brien complains of severe pain in the bladder region, the nurse's first action should be to

A. check to see whether the catheter is open and draining freely.
B. administer another dose of an analgesic medication because elderly patients require large amounts of sedation.
C. clamp the catheter and gently massage the bladder region.
D. call the physician immediately.

81. Frequent irrigations of the bladder are usually ordered following a prostatectomy. The chief purpose of these irrigations is to
A. prevent infection in the bladder by destroying most bacteria.
B. keep the urinary tract free of scar tissue.
C. control hemorrhage from the bladder.
D. remove blood clots and shreds of tissue that may obstruct the catheter.

Questions 82–89 deal with the various phases of the nursing process.

---

82. Assessment is BEST defined as
A. looking at the patient's physical needs.
B. discussing the case with the physician.
C. discussing the patient with the supervising nurse.
D. observing the patient's health needs.

83. Planning is BEST defined as
A. documenting observations in the patient's chart.
B. establishing goals for nursing interventions.
C. making plans with the registered nurse for necessary treatment, and scheduling the various procedures.
D. asking the doctor what sort of treatment he/she plans.

84. Implementation is BEST defined as
A. following the doctor's orders.
B. establishing a nursing diagnosis.
C. orderly collection of the patient's symptoms.
D. administration of the nursing care plan.

85. Administration of the nursing care plan involves

A. being responsible for the nursing care of every assigned patient.
B. delegating some parts of the care to others.
C. making friends with the patient.
D. documenting all symptoms.

86. Documentation is necessary because it
A. shows what skills the practical nurse has.
B. provides a record of the medications, procedures, and other treatment the patient has had.
C. helps in the assessment of the patient.
D. establishes outcome criteria.

87. When developing the nursing plan for a patient, the nurse should take into consideration the fact that
A. most patients are difficult to manage.
B. each patient has his own unique problems irrespective of the diagnosis.
C. the needs of a patient depend solely on the diagnosis.
D. most patients feel entirely helpless and very depressed.

88. An excellent nursing care plan
A. assigns priorities to the nursing diagnoses.
B. adheres to hospital policies.
C. organizes the work efficiently.
D. considers the staff available.

89. The first thing that the practical nurse should do before carrying out a nursing procedure is
A. review in her/his mind how the procedure should be carried out.
B. explain the procedure to the patient.
C. check with the supervisor to be sure the procedure has not been canceled.
D. assemble the necessary equipment.

Nineteen-year-old Stanley Brodsky is taken to the emergency room of a hospital after being hit by a car and thrown about 20 feet. He has many bleeding lacerations and abrasions on his body, as well as a broken arm, and is unconscious upon arrival. He also has a head injury and shows signs of increasing intracranial pressure. He is accompanied by his roommate and another friend.

---

90. Which of the following can legally permit the doctor to treat him?
    A. A signed consent from his room-mate.
    B. A signed consent from his other friend.
    C. A court order.
    D. The written opinion of the hospital director that treatment is necessary.

91. When Stanley arrives in the emergency room, the HIGHEST priority is given to
    A. taking and recording his vital signs.
    B. determining whether he has a broken neck.
    C. establishing an airway.
    D. controlling the bleeding from lacerations and abrasions.

92. A very important nursing function for patients like Stanley with head injuries is
    A. careful observation.
    B. checking the pulse.
    C. forcing fluids.
    D. positioning the patient correctly.

93. Which of the following observations by the nurse does NOT indicate that Stanley is experiencing increasing intracranial pressure?
    A. The patient is increasingly restless.
    B. The pulse pressure is increasing.
    C. The pupils react unequally to light.
    D. The deep tendon reflexes are decreasing.

94. Of what possible additional injuries must the nurse be aware in making her/his assessment in head injury cases?
    A. Pulmonary atelectasis.
    B. Retinal detachment.
    C. Spinal cord injuries.
    D. Splenic contusion.

95. Postcraniotomy nursing care for Stanley will include
    A. placing him in a jacket restraint.
    B. placing him on his right side in a lying position.
    C. checking his temperature at frequent intervals.
    D. administering Demerol for pain and sedation.

Eighteen-year-old Jennifer Kelly comes to the clinic with symptoms of painful urination, vaginal itching, and a greenish-yellow discharge. She states that she has been sexually active for some time. A tentative diagnosis of gonorrhea is made.

96. A definite diagnosis of gonorrhea in Jennifer will be obtained by
    A. culturing the gonoccoccus from a specimen of vaginal discharge.
    B. noting the symptoms of profuse vaginal discharge and painful urination.
    C. testing the patient's blood for gonococci.
    D. X-ray examination of the pelvic organs.

97. Gonorrhea is a venereal disease that
    A. is incurable once it reaches the fallopian tubes.
    B. can be treated successfully with penicillin or streptomycin.
    C. can be caught only once, after which an individual becomes immune to the disease.
    D. is not classified as an infectious disease.

98. When caring for Jennifer or other patients with gonorrhea, the nurse must be especially careful to avoid
    A. contact with the patient's nasal secretions.
    B. contact with the vaginal discharge.
    C. handling syringes and needles used for injections for the patient.
    D. contact with the skin lesion of the patient.

Sarah Jensen, 2 years old, is admitted to the pediatric unit with a fractured femur. She is placed in Bryant's traction. While completing the nursing admission assessment, the practical nurse notes multiple bruises scattered over the child's body. The nurse also notes that the mother is guarded in relating the child's previous medical history. In concluding, the mother states that Sarah is a clumsy child who is always falling.

99. On the basis of the admission history, the practical nurse suspects that Sarah may suffer from
   A. osteoporosis.
   B. idiopathic thrombocytopenia.
   C. battered child syndrome.
   D. astrocytoma.

100. The practical nurse would take her findings to the charge nurse. Which of the following recommendations would the charge nurse be expected to make?
   1. Continue to assess Sarah for further evidence of abuse and to record specifics in the medical record.
   2. Avoid drawing premature conclusions.
   3. Observe and record the parent-child interaction.
   4. Question the child extensively to find out how the fracture occurred.
   A. 1 and 2.
   B. 2, 3, and 4.
   C. 1, 2, 3, and 4.
   D. 1, 2, and 3.

101. The practical nurse's PRIMARY goal in managing Sarah's care will be to
   A. notify the appropriate authorities that the Jensens are child abusers.
   B. maintain Sarah's Bryant traction in appropriate position.
   C. arrange for a CAT scan to ascertain Sarah's neurologic integrity.
   D. send laboratory slips for a platelet count on Sarah.

102. Which of the following interactions between the child and her parents would the practical nurse caring for Sarah expect to observe?
   A. Child will not seek comfort from, or contact with, parents.
   B. Child will only allow parents to feed her.
   C. Child will have a temper tantrum when parents go home.
   D. Child will demonstrate a trustful relationship with parents.

103. Children who suffer from battered child syndrome are children with special characteristics. Which of the following would the practical nurse expect to be true of Sarah?
   A. Child is viewed as different or difficult.
   B. Child is physically unattractive.
   C. Child is normal in achieving developmental goals.
   D. Child responds to strangers in an age-appropriate manner.

> Karen Aronsky, a 34-year-old epileptic, is brought to the emergency room following a motor vehicle accident. She is alert and responsive.

104. As the practical nurse enters Ms. Aronsky's room, the nurse observes that the patient is having a seizure. The IMMEDIATE nursing action would be to
   A. establish an airway.
   B. call a physician.
   C. hold the patient's arms and legs to prevent injury.
   D. force the patient onto her back.

105. During the seizure, the practical nurse would be responsible for monitoring all of the following EXCEPT
   A. the duration of seizure.
   B. respirations.
   C. incontinence.
   D. an aura.

106. Ms. Aronsky is admitted to a medical unit and placed on Dilantin (phenytoin sodium) 300 mg po OD. The pharmacy dispenses four 150-mg capsules into Ms. Aronsky's medication drawer. How many capsules would the nurse administer daily?
   A. ½.
   B. 1.
   C. 2.
   D. 4.

107. For which of the following side effects of Dilantin therapy would the practical nurse monitor Ms. Aronsky?
   1. Agranulocytosis.
   2. Aplastic anemia.
   3. Gum hypertrophy.
   4. Leukopenia.
   A. 1, 2, and 3.
   B. 1, 2, 3, and 4.
   C. 1 and 4.
   D. 3 only.

108. When preparing for Ms. Aronsky's discharge, the practical nurse would include which of the following in the patient's discharge plan?
  A. Tell her that regular hours of sleep are unimportant.
  B. Encourage daily compliance with the medication regime.
  C. Inform her that there is no need for follow-up blood studies.
  D. Instruct her to limit activity.

> Ms. Benita Gomez, 48 years old, is admitted to the hospital with a diagnosis of hyperthyroidism. She is scheduled the next day for a subtotal thyroidectomy.

109. During the admitting assessment, the practical nurse would expect Ms. Gomez to complain of which of the following clinical symptoms?
  A. Nervousness, weight loss, heat intolerance.
  B. Alopecia, weight gain, intolerance to cold.
  C. Polyuria, exophthalmus, tachycardia.
  D. Glycosuria, puffy tongue, scaly skin.

110. In picking up the preop orders, the practical nurse would expect to see which of the following diet orders for Ms. Gomez?
  A. Low-calorie, high-protein, regular diet.
  B. High-calorie, high-carbohydrate, soft diet.
  C. Low-calorie, high-carbohydrate, regular diet.
  D. High-calorie, high-protein, soft diet.

111. After surgery, Ms. Gomez is returned to the surgical unit. The practical nurse will place her in which of the following positions?
  A. Semi-Fowler's.
  B. High Fowler's.
  C. Trendelenburg.
  D. Supine.

112. Which of the following items of equipment will the practical nurse make sure is kept at Ms. Gomez's bedside?
  A. Blood pressure cuff and stethescope.
  B. Vaporizer and suction equipment.
  C. Rectal thermometer and dressing change kit.
  D. Tracheostomy set and suction equipment.

113. Ms. Gomez is receiving intravenous fluids. The doctor orders 1000 cc lactated Ringer's solution every 8 hours. The solution administration set delivers 15 gtts per cc. To ensure that Ms. Gomez will get the correct amount of solution, her I.V. should be regulated at
  A. 55 gtts per minute.
  B. 28 gtts per minute.
  C. 31 gtts per minute.
  D. 41 gtts per minute.

114. The practical nurse cannot regulate Ms. Gomez's I.V. at the desired rate. It appears to be clogged. Which of the following actions should the practical nurse take?
  1. Check the site of the I.V. infusion.
  2. Place 2 cc of sterile saline into the I.V. site.
  3. Notify the charge nurse.
  4. Pull the I.V.
  A. 1 and 4.
  B. 1 and 2.
  C. 1 and 3.
  D. None of the above.

115. Ms. Gomez is being discharged. Her discharge plan will include instructions for
  A. planned rest periods.
  B. small, frequent feedings.
  C. testing her urine for sugar and acetone.
  D. increase her oral intake to 1500 cc per day.

The rest of the text consists of unrelated questions.

116. A tilt table is most useful in increasing skin and vascular tone. In which of the following conditions would it NOT be useful?
  A. Spinal cord injuries.
  B. Brain damage.
  C. Diabetic acidosis.
  D. Orthostatic hypotension.

117. Upon receiving a patient in the recovery room from the anesthesiologist and the circulating nurse, the FIRST action that the nurse must take is to
  A. determine the patient's vital signs.
  B. appraise the patient's air-exchange

status.
C. verify the patient's identity.
D. check the patient's dressing for bleed-ing.

118. A complication that often occurs after lower abdominal operation is
A. shock.
B. hemorrhage.
C. phlebitis.
D. apprehension.

119. A patient with cirrhosis of the liver requires good skin care to
A. relieve the itching caused by jaun-dice.
B. minimize the danger of infection.
C. prevent complications.
D. prevent hemorrhaging.

120. The behavior pattern in which a person avoids accepting full responsibility for his/her own actions by blaming someone else is called
A. rationalization.
B. compensation.
C. projection.
D. repression.

121. Avoiding unpleasant past experiences by "forgetting" them and pretending they nev-er happened is an example of
A. identification.
B. repression.
C. regression.
D. compensation.

122. Psychotherapy is a form of treatment in which the patient is

A. given dosages of medication to induce sleep and rest.
B. given occupational therapy.
C. encouraged to talk about him-/herself and his/her problems and therefore face reality.
D. placed in isolation.

123. Psychotherapy is possible only if the pa-tient is
A. willing to listen to advice from others.
B. sedated and restrained so he/she will cooperate.
C. admitted to a mental hospital.
D. able to communicate with others and express his/her true feelings.

124. The acute communicable disease that can cause serious deformities in the develop-ing fetus is
A. chickenpox.
B. pneumonia.
C. rubella.
D. tuberculosis.

125. A 94-year-old man has been hospitalized and treated for pneumonia. At the end of his hospitalization, his family decide that they can no longer care for him because he is completely dependent in all activities of daily living and has become incontinent. To meet this patient's needs, Social Services will apply for
A. institutional room and board.
B. intermediate supervised personal care.
C. intermediate nursing care.
D. skilled nursing care.

ANSWER KEY—PART I

1. D	26. A	51. D	76. C	101. B
2. C	27. C	52. A	77. B	102. A
3. B	28. B	53. C	78. D	103. A
4. B	29. B	54. C	79. D	104. A
5. C	30. B	55. C	80. A	105. D
6. C	31. D	56. C	81. D	106. C
7. D	32. D	57. B	82. D	107. B
8. B	33. B	58. B	83. B	108. B
9. C	34. A	59. A	84. D	109. A
10. D	35. B	60. D	85. B	110. B
11. B	36. C	61. C	86. B	111. A
12. B	37. A	62. D	87. B	112. D
13. C	38. B	63. A	88. A	113. C
14. C	39. D	64. B	89. A	114. C
15. C	40. B	65. B	90. C	115. A
16. C	41. B	66. A	91. C	116. C
17. C	42. B	67. A	92. A	117. B
18. A	43. D	68. B	93. D	118. C
19. D	44. B	69. C	94. C	119. A
20. C	45. D	70. B	95. C	120. C
21. D	46. C	71. B	96. A	121. B
22. C	47. A	72. D	97. B	122. C
23. D	48. D	73. A	98. B	123. D
24. B	49. B	74. B	99. C	124. C
25. B	50. A	75. B	100. D	125. B

EXPLANATIONS FOR ANSWERS—PART I

1. **D** CVA is a neurologic disorder due to a pathologic process in a blood vessel, causing damage to the brain. All of the listed symptoms may occur, depending on what area of the brain is affected.
2. **C** The patient's airway must be maintained. Therefore it is essential to remove anything, such as dentures, that may obstruct the airway.
3. **B** Absence of the blinking reflex is due to neurologic impairment. Tear formation will return when the cerebral blood flow improves.
4. **B** In the case of stroke, the main purpose of nursing intervention is to prevent deformities, physical deterioration, and loss of range of motion. Proper positioning and support are therefore necessary.
5. **C** Providing proper support of the affected arm and leg will help to prevent deformities.
6. **C** Aphasia is inability to speak, write, or comprehend spoken or written language because of a brain lesion. Aphonia is loss of voice. Atresia is congenital absence of a normal body orifice. Aphagia is refusal to eat.
7. **D** Rehabilitation includes monitoring and preserving vital functions, stimulating the patient, ensuring hydration and nutrition, and preventing physical deterioration. All these should begin on the day the patient is admitted to the hospital.
8. **B** Cyanosis (bluish discoloration of the skin and mucous membranes) indicates insufficient oxygen in the blood. To maintain the airway, secretions must be suctioned from the respiratory passages.
9. **C** Blood pressure and cardiac output must be maintained. However, the rate of flow of intravenous fluids must not be so great as to overload the circulatory system or, in cases of cerebral hemorrhage, to restart the hemorrhage.

10. **D** Proper positioning of a stroke victim will help to prevent complications (dependent edema, contractures, poor circulation, and aspiration) that will delay rehabilitation.

11. **B** A primipara has given birth to one child. A multipara has given birth to more than one child. A multigravida has been pregnant more than once.

12. **B** After the third month, the term *fetus* is used. A zygote is a fertilized ovum. The placenta is the spongy structure in the uterus through which the fetus derives its nourishment.

13. **C** Absence of menstruation is a presumptive but not diagnostic sign of pregnancy.

14. **C** This is Naegele's rule.

15. **C** A gallbladder series is not part of a routine prenatal examination.

16. **C** When the uterus rises into the abdominal cavity, there is less pressure on the bladder.

17. **C** The interval between visits grows less as the pregnancy continues.

18. **A** Fats are very hard to digest.

19. **D** Dry food such as unbuttered toast or a plain cracker is tolerated most readily in any type of nausea, including that due to pregnancy.

20. **C** As the uterine fundus rises, it pushes the stomach and diaphragm up, thereby causing some regurgitation.

21. **D** Choices A, B, and C are essential to the patient's good health.

22. **C** Vitamin A is an oil-soluble vitamin. If mineral oil is taken at or near mealtimes, any vitamin A in the food is excreted with the oil rather than absorbed.

23. **D** Fetal heart tones are heard with a fetoscope (De Lee-Hillis stethoscope) beginning in the 18th to 20th week of pregnancy.

24. **B** Chloasma ("mask of pregnancy") usually disappears after delivery.

25. **B** The cause of leg cramp is unknown. Dorsiflexion gives immediate relief, probably by stretching the dorsal leg muscles.

26. **A** Backaches are caused by the change in the center of gravity, which causes lordosis and backache. Late in pregnancy, relaxation of pelvic joints aggravates the problem.

27. **C** Lean meat and dried beans are high in iron content.

28. **B** Skim or low-fat milk (1 quart daily) may be used if excessive weight gain is a problem.

29. **B** It would do no good to take the condiments from Mr. Skully, who would buy more. The supervisor can alert the staff to watch Mr. Skully and prevent him from wandering away.

30. **B** This wandering is a hazard to Mr. Skully's safety and should be the primary concern. His complaints can be ignored. Many elderly persons hide condiments and other foods, and the staff should search his room for these substances.

31. **D** Checking the compresses for moisture frequently is good nursing practice. Dry compresses are not therapeutic.

32. **D** The stockings should be put on with the legs elevated so that the veins are drained of blood. The stockings act as accessory valves.

33. **B** See the answer to question 32.

34. **A** Thrombophlebitis is partial or complete occlusion of a vein by a thrombus (blood clot) with secondary inflammatory reaction in the wall of the vein. The condition may be postsurgical, postpartum, or posttraumatic and occurs also in persons with heart disease or cancer.

35. **B** Choices A, C, and D are not symptomatic of thrombophlebitis.

36. **C** Massaging the legs may dislodge the thrombus, causing a pulmonary embolism.

37. **A** Increasing the circulation by early ambulation and exercise will reduce stasis of the blood.

38. **B** Narrowing of the blood vessels caused by nicotine increases stasis of the blood and may lead to formation of a clot.

39. **D** Long-term pressure on the calves of hospitalized patients with thrombophlebitis should be avoided. Pulmonary emboli can be fatal.

40. **B** Congestive heart failure is a disorder of the cardiovascular system characterized by circulatory congestion due to failure of the heart as a pump.

41. **B** It is important that the patient on complete bedrest assume as much responsibility for personal care as possible. Such a patient should be expected to take care of much of his/her own personal hygiene. However, frequent rest periods are indicated so as not to overtax the individual.

42. **B** Semi-Fowler's and Fowler's positions are indicated in dyspnea from any cause.

43. **D** Massages and other types of care are important to restore circulation to the skin of the back.

44. **B** Because cold food and drinks constrict blood vessels, they are often contraindicated for cardiac patients.

45. **D** Neglect of sodium restriction is a major cause of failure in the treatment of cardiac patients. The result is fluid accumulation in the tissues.

46. **C** The chemical name for table salt is sodium chloride (NaCl).

47. **A** Canned foods are frequently processed with salt. Of the four choices, citrus fruits are lowest in sodium content.

48. **D** Toothpastes and mouthwashes, unlike items 1, 3, and 4, are not swallowed.

49. **B** Bananas are an excellent source of potassium.

50. **A** Digitalis increases the force of contraction of the myocardium and the efficiency of the heart.

51. **D** See the answer to question 50. Digitalis does not act on the vascular system.

52. **A** If the pulse is 60 or below, the supervising nurse must be notified.

53. **C** See the answer to question 52. Digitalis slows the ventricular rate and increases the force of myocardial contraction.

54. **C** By definition, a diuretic is a drug that promotes the production and excretion of urine.

55. **C** Weight will decrease as fluid is eliminated. If edema increases, however, weight will also increase.

56. **C** If a record of the patient's weight is to be meaningful, the weighing conditions must be the same each day.

57. **B** *Sublingual* means "under the tongue."

58. **B** A vaginal douche may wash away cells important for diagnosis.

59. **A** The patient will be more comfortable with an empty bladder, and the physician will be able to palpate the structures more easily.

60. **D** See the answer to question 59.

61. **C** An explanation of what to expect will make the patient less anxious.

62. **D** The Pap test, in which stained cells shed by mucous membranes of the cervix are examined microscopically, is used for the diagnosis of cancer and of precancerous changes in cells.

63. **A** Dilatation and curettage (D & C) is used to obtain uterine tissue for examination and diagnosis.

64. **B** Choices A and C refer to an abdominal hysterectomy.

65. **B** The douche will not sterilize the vagina but will remove any extraneous secretions.

66. **A** Such observation is good nursing procedure and is necessary after a vaginal hysterectomy.

67. **A** The solution should feel comfortable to the patient.

68. **B** Items 1 and 3 represent good nursing procedure.

69. **C** Hormones from at least one *ovary* are needed to produce menstruation, which is the flow of blood and other material from the *uterus*.

70. **B** Removal of the ovaries would have resulted in a surgical menopause.

71. **B** Other possibilities are *lumpectomy*—tumor and area around it are removed; *total mastectomy*—breast is removed, but pectoralis muscles and lymph nodes are left intact; *modified radical mastectomy*—entire breast, pectoralis minor, and lymph nodes are removed.

72. **D** With a mastectomy patient, a fresh surgical wound may bleed downward. Keeping the patient off the operative side allows easy visualization of the dressing. Additionally, the nurse may feel under the patient's back for overt bleeding.

73. **C** The increasing hemorrhage under the pressure dressing causes swelling, which in turn causes the dressing to become tighter and block the circulation of blood to the arm.

74. **B** Brushing the hair raises the arm and necessitates a motion that can exercise the muscles on that side.

75. **B** Depression and withdrawal are common reactions to this type of surgery and do not indicate psychosis or vanity.

76. **C** Choice A is flip, choice B is less informative than choice C, and choice D may cause the patient to worry needlessly.

77. **B** The prostate gland is not located near the kidneys, has no role in the production of urine, and does not control the sphincter muscles.

78. **D** This procedure may be defined as removal of part or all of the prostrate gland via the urethra.

79. **D** Bright red blood may indicate frank hemorrhage and requires prompt action.

80. **A** With this procedure it is not uncommon for blood clots to clog the catheter and prevent drainage. This causes bladder spasms and concurrent pain.

81. **D** The irrigation will not prevent infection or scar tissue or control hemorrhage.

82. **D** Assessment, the first phase of the nursing process, involves the collection of a data base about the patient by observation, and the use of the information gathered to form a nursing diagnosis.

83. **B** In the planning phase, goals are established for appropriate nursing interventions.

84. **D** Implementation is administration of the nursing care plan to achieve the desired goals.

85. **B** The other members of the health care team must be taken into consideration. It is not possible or even desirable for one person to be responsible for all the health care needs of a patient.

86. **B** Documentation is a most important part of patient care. It serves as a record of medications, procedures and other treatments for the medical care team and is also a legal necessity.

87. **B** Both the patient's problems AND the diagnosis have to be considered in making the plan.

88. **A** This will take the patient into consideration and facilitate the establishment of goals.

89. **A** If this is done, then the explanation to the patient and the assembling of the equipment can follow. The supervisor is there to answer any questions.

90. **C** When no legally responsible relative is available, a court order is necessary for permission to treat an unconscious person. This can be obtained very quickly.

91. **C** It is important in trauma cases to be sure that the patient can breathe.

92. **A** Careful observation is essential to detect changing signs, which are very important in head injuries as indicators of the patient's condition.

93. **D** Choices, A, B, and C are symptomatic of increasing intracranial pressure.

94. **C** In all head injury cases, the nurse must be aware that there may be some injury also to the spinal cord. This can easily be overlooked, especially when the patient has been under the influence of alcohol, which may mask the symptoms.

95. **C** Hyperthermia or hypothermia is a complication of brain surgery. The goal is to keep the patient normothermic. It is therefore necessary to check the patient's temperature frequently in order to correctly assess his condition.

96. **A** This laboratory procedure is the only way to obtain a definite diagnosis of gonorrhea.

97. **B** Other antibiotics can be used as well. None of the other choices is true.

98. **B** If the patient's vaginal discharge gets on the nurse's hands, the disease may be spread not only to the nurse but also to others.

99. **C** Physical, sexual, or emotional abuse of children by parents or others is described as battered child syndrome. When assessing for battered child syndrome, the practical nurse would expect all or some of the following clinical manifestations: child is usually under the age of 3; child shows neglected health status; child presents with various skeletal fractures; child presents with multiple abrasions, bruises, or burns.

100. **D** The nursing care plan and interventions should include a further, more detailed assessment than an admission assessment, the avoidance of hasty conclusions, and observation of the parent-child interaction. It is necessary for the nurse to develop a trusting relationship with

both child and parents so appropriate interventions and discharge planning can be provided.

101. **B** Though the nurse may eventually notify child protective services or arrange for a CAT scan or a platelet count, the primary goal is to maintain the child's traction in appropriate position, that is, with the legs extended at right angles to the body, the hips and buttocks elevated off the bed, and the heels and ankles free from pressure. The child lies flat on the bed, unable to move from side to side. This position is essential in order for the femur to heal.

102. **A** A child suffering from battered child syndrome may be either withdrawn or hyperactive. In either case, the nurse will notice that this child will not trust his/her parents and will not seek contact with them or comfort from them. One of the goals in nursing care for the battered child is to develop a nonthreatening, nurturing relationship between parent and child.

103. **A** The special characteristics a battered child may exhibit include the following: the child is seriously or chronically ill, the child was premature, and the child is viewed as different or difficult. The parents view these characteristics within the context of their own psychosocial problems that lead to child abuse.

104. **A** The immediate nursing action is to establish a patent airway and thus preserve respiratory integrity. However, it is important to note that the practical nurse would never force an airway into the mouth of a seizing patient as it may damage the teeth or jaw. The patient would be positioned on his/her side, not the back, to prevent aspiration. Restraining the arms and legs is not indicated as this may damage the extremities.

105. **D** An aura may precede a seizure but cannot be monitored by the nurse. An aura is a peculiar sensation that is recognized by the patient as a warning of an impending convulsion. Observing the duration of a seizure, changes in the rate of respirations, and the occurrence of incontinence is important in nursing management.

106. **C** The formula for computation the practical nurse would use is as follows:

$$\frac{\text{desired dosage}}{\text{available dosage}} = \text{number of capsules}$$

$$\frac{300 \text{ mg}}{150 \text{ mg}} = 2 \text{ capsules}$$

107. **B** Agranulocytosis (a marked reduction or complete absence of granulocytes), aplastic anemia (inability to form new red blood cells), gum hypertrophy (an increase in the bulk of tissues in the gums) and leukopenia (a subnormal white blood count) are all serious side effects of prolonged use of Dilantin therapy.

108. **B** The patient must take medication daily to maintain the blood level of medication needed to prevent seizures. Medication may have to be adjusted because of changes in the patient's health status. Blood studies are necessary to regulate serum blood levels of medication as well as to monitor possible hematologic side effects. Maintaining normal activity and normal sleeping patterns is encouraged as it is useful in controlling or eliminating seizures.

109. **A** In hyperthyroidism an increased secretion of thyroxin results in a higher metabolic rate, which causes the patient to experience symptoms of nervousness, weight loss, and heat intolerance.

110. **B** The thyroid gland is located in front of the trachea. When a patient experiences hyperthyroidism, enlargement of the gland causes difficulty in swallowing. A soft diet is less difficult to swallow. Hyperthyroidism increases the metabolic demands on the body, and the need for readily available energy can be provided by an increase in calories and carbohydrates.

111. **A** Semi-Fowler's position will maintain patient comfort, as well as maintaining a patent airway and decreasing the stress on the suture line.

112. **D** Postoperatively, Ms. Gomez is at high risk for increased laryngeal edema, which may compromise her airway, thereby necessitating an emergency tracheostomy. Suction equipment

will be needed if Ms. Gomez is unable to clear her airway of increased secretions—a potential problem with this type of surgery.

113. **C** 31 gtts per minute is the correct answer. To compute the flow rate in number of drops per minute, the following formula may be used:

$$\frac{\text{number of cc/hr}}{60 \text{ min}} \times \frac{\text{administration set drop factor}}{1} = \text{number of drops/minute}$$

$$\frac{1000 \text{ cc}}{8 \text{ hr}} = 125 \text{ cc/hour}$$

$$\frac{125}{\cancel{60}\atop 4} \times \frac{\cancel{15} \text{ gttc/cc}}{1} = 31\frac{1}{4} \text{ gtts/minute}$$

114. **C** The practical nurse should check the I.V. site and assess whether the intravenous infusion is infiltrated. If the site is red, swollen, and painful, infiltration is apparent and the charge nurse should be made aware of this finding.

115. **A** Postoperatively, Ms. Gomez may feel fatigued. This is a common postop complication that can be minimized with planned rest periods. None of the other choices is indicated for this patient.

116. **C** The tilt table would not be of any value in diabetic acidosis. This equipment has two MAIN purposes: to condition the vascular system, and to help the patient adjust to an upright position. Its other uses are all related to these two main functions.

117. **B** The most important thing is for the nurse to establish that the patient can breathe. The remaining actions are secondary to appraising the air status.

118. **C** Phlebitis is a not-uncommon complication after lower abdominal surgery. Injury to veins resulting from leg straps applied during surgery, concentration of blood due to fluid loss, or circulatory depression leading to slower blood flow may cause phlebitis.

119. **A** Good skin care is most important to relieve itching due to jaundice. Nursing interventions include applying soothing lotions and assisting the patient to overcome the tendency to scratch. Soothing massages at bedtime also help.

120. **C** Projection, in which a person attributes his/her own unacceptable behavior to another person, is an unconscious defense mechanism.

121. **B** The act of repression is not voluntary. The unpleasant experience is so painful that the mind automatically blocks it out.

122. **C** This choice is a definition of psychotherapy.

123. **D** Communication with others is essential to psychotherapy. The other choices are not.

124. **C** Rubella (German measles), if contracted in early pregnancy, may cause serious damage to the fetus.

125. **B** This patient needs only custodial, not nursing, care.

DIAGNOSTIC TEST, PART II

Mrs. Irene Burton, an 85-year-old widow, is taken to the local multiservice center by her neighbors. She has been wandering around the grounds of her cooperative apartment and appears confused and disoriented.

1. Mrs. Burton is malnourished. In developing a nursing plan for her, the nurse will
   A. plan small, frequent nutritious meals.
   B. order two slices of bread with each meal.
   C. order a soft diet.
   D. allow her two desserts.

2. Each time anyone enters Mrs. Burton's room, she asks that person what place she is in. The nurse recognizes that this repeated questioning is typical of
   A. poor memory.
   B. confusion.
   C. disorientation.
   D. faulty judgment.

3. Mrs. Burton wets herself before she can get to the bathroom. She is very upset and starts to cry. The nurse should
   A. tell Mrs. Burton that she must start sooner hereafter.
   B. tell her not to worry, that incontinence happens frequently.
   C. tell her to go into her room and change her clothes.
   D. help Mrs. Burton wash up and change her clothes.

4. While collecting Mrs. Burton's wet clothes, the nurse notes fecal staining on the patient's underwear. When questioned Mrs. Burton complains of rectal pain and states that she has been unable to move her bowels. The practical nurse assesses the problem as
   A. mild constipation.
   B. diarrhea.
   C. rectal sphincter spasm.
   D. fecal impaction.

5. The practical nurse reports her observation to the supervisor, who orders her to
   A. prepare the patient for a low saline enema.
   B. prepare the patient for a fecal disimpaction.
   C. prepare the patient for an oil enema.
   D. insert a glycerin suppository into the patient's rectum.

Daniel Sweeney, aged 3 years, is taken to the clinic by his mother. He has a cold, is irritable, and has had a temperature of 102°F for a few hours. A purulent discharge is draining from his left ear. A diagnosis of otitis media, acute, is made.

6. The nurse knows that otitis media is
   A. an inflammation of the left nasal sinuses.
   B. an inflammation of the middle ear.
   C. an inflammation of the tonsils and adenoids.
   D. an upper respiratory infection.

7. Otitis media occurs in infants and toddlers like Daniel because
   A. the eustachian tube is shorter and straighter in these children than in an adult.
   B. the sinuses of small children are not fully developed.
   C. the eustachian tube is not fully developed in small children.
   D. small children are unable to cough up sufficient mucus to clear out the nasal passages.

While in the clinic, Daniel's temperature goes to 104°F, and the child begins to vomit and is very restless. He is admitted to the hospital. The morning after admission his temperature rises to 105°F. After examination, a diagnosis of meningitis is made. The physician orders I.V. fluids and I.V. antibiotics.

8. Which of the following nursing interventions is NOT indicated?
   A. Watching for side effects of I.V. antibiotics.
   B. Positioning Daniel carefully to lessen neck pain.
   C. Giving Daniel tepid water sponge baths.
   D. Encouraging family visits.

9. What sign should the practical nurse recognize as indicating a complication in Daniel's condition?
   A. Complaints that the light hurts his eyes.
   B. Headache.
   C. Altered respirations.
   D. Irritability.

10. Daniel's mother becomes hysterical, crying to the nurse, "I know that my child is going to die." Which of the following should be the nurse's answer?
    A. "Be calm. Daniel is being given appropriate treatment."
    B. "Daniel needs a quiet, relaxing atmosphere, and you are upsetting him by your crying."
    C. "You are getting yourself upset unnecessarily."
    D. "Daniel will get worse before he gets better."

11. In developing a nursing plan for the treatment of Daniel, the nurse tentatively lists the following:
    1. Control temperature.
    2. Prevent seizures.
    3. Control pain.
    4. Treat infection.
    Which of the items listed should be included in the final plan?
    A. 1, 2, and 3.
    B. 1, 3, and 4.
    C. 2, 3, and 4.
    D. 1, 2, 3, and 4.

12. Daniel's aunt comes to the pediatric unit to visit. The nurse notices that she has a loose cough and constantly wipes her nose. What should the nurse say?
    A. "You may see Daniel but don't cough around him."
    B. "You may go in to see Daniel, but you must put on a mask and gown."
    C. "You may not go in to see Daniel."
    D. "Daniel needs a quiet, relaxing atmosphere, preferably without visitors. Also, with your cold, it is better for you that you wait until he is discharged."

13. The pediatrician orders a pill for Daniel that the child refuses to take. The nurse should then
    A. tell Daniel to chew up the pill.
    B. crush the pill and mix it with applesauce, which Daniel likes.
    C. dissolve the pill in water.
    D. push the pill between his lips.

14. Daniel improves with treatment and is discharged from the hospital. His mother is instructed to keep him home for a few weeks and to provide periodic rest for him. In providing rest for Daniel, his mother is advised to
    A. keep him in a darkened room.
    B. provide a quiet atmosphere in the home and avoid noise and confusion.
    C. allow him to watch TV several hours during the day.
    D. allow three of his friends to come to visit every day.

Angel Cruz, a heavy smoker aged 55, has had a harsh, productive cough with scanty sputum for several years. Recently he has been troubled by intermittent wheezing. His wife persuades him to go to the chest clinic for an examination.

15. The first tests ordered for Mr. Cruz are blood chemistries, CBC, and urinalysis. "It is my throat that hurts. Why must blood be taken?" he complains to the nurse. Her BEST answer is
    A. "It is clinic policy."
    B. "You may have a serious infection that will show up in the blood examination."
    C. "The doctor ordered it."
    D. "There could be many reasons for your cough and wheezing. In order for you to have a complete examination, we must have the blood count done."

16. After the blood is drawn, the nurse takes Mr. Cruz to the radiology department for a chest X-ray. For this examination, Mr. Cruz
    A. has a dye injected into an arm vein.
    B. has to remove his shirt and undershirt.
    C. is given a barium solution to drink.
    D. is told to lie on the X-ray table.

17. Mr. Cruz is told to return to the clinic the next day for a bronchoscopy. His instructions are to eat nothing after midnight. When Mr. Cruz

returns to his room after the bronchoscopy, the nurse will
A. give him sips of cool water.
B. watch for the return of the gag reflex.
C. urge him to eat a soft diet.
D. take him into the sitting room.

18. When Mr. Cruz is discharged, the nurse will tell him that
A. he may continue to smoke.
B. he should smoke only one half a package of cigarettes daily.
C. he should stop smoking.
D. he should stop smoking and chew tobacco instead.

Mrs. Anna Miles, 59 years old, visits her physician because of prolonged, unusual fatigue, intermittent constipation and diarrhea, and burning of her tongue. During the course of examinations, a gastric analysis is done and an absence of hydrochloric acid reported. A diagnosis of pernicious anemia is made.

19. Which of the following symptoms that usually accompany the acute stage of pernicious anemia requires special nursing interventions?
A. Unusual fatigue.
B. Intermittent constipation and diarrhea.
C. Burning of the tongue and sore mouth.
D. Pallor.

20. The treatment prescribed for Mrs. Miles is vitamin B_{12} by intramuscular injection. Mrs. Miles asks when she can stop taking injections of the vitamin. The nurse's answer is
A. "When the disease is cured."
B. "In 2 months."
C. "Between remissions."
D. "Never; you will need them for the rest of your life."

21. During the discussion about the medication, Mrs. Miles states that she would rather take the vitamin B_{12} by pill than by injection. The nurse explains that this will not be possible because
A. oral preparations destroy the effectiveness of the vitamin.
B. resistance to vitamin B_{12} can develop if oral preparations are used.

C. oral preparations of vitamin B_{12} are rapidly excreted from the body.
D. oral preparations of vitamin B_{12} cannot be absorbed from the small intestine.

22. In discussing the proper diet for Mrs. Miles, the nurse will indicate that the foods from which the body normally can extract the most vitamin B_{12} are
A. multigrain breads and bakery products.
B. green and yellow vegetables.
C. fresh fruits.
D. meats and dairy products.

You have accepted a position in a nursing home as a licensed practical nurse. Since you have chosen geriatric nursing, you review the physiologic aspects of aging and the general nursing care of the aged.

23. Aging can best be defined as a
A. gradual onset of senility.
B. degenerative disease.
C. normal, gradual slowing of body functions.
D. decrease in the will to live.

24. The basic needs of the aged include
1. a clean, safe place to live.
2. recreation.
3. good nutrition.
4. someone to care about them.
A. 1 and 3.
B. 1, 3, and 4.
C. 1, 2, and 3.
D. 1, 2, 3, and 4.

25. Complete daily bed baths are considered unnecessary for the elderly because
A. they are much less active than younger persons.
B. their oil and sweat glands are no longer as active.
C. the elderly do not like to bathe.
D. the elderly do not have body odor.

26. Physiologic changes related to the normal aging process include
1. sluggish bowel functions.
2. arteriosclerosis.
3. reduced circulation.
4. obesity.
A. 1, 2, and 4.

B. 1 and 3.
C. 2, 3, and 4.
D. 1, 2, 3, and 4.

> *Ms. Ruth O'Malley, 32 years old, has a high fever and persistent, harsh, dry cough. In the clinic a diagnosis of acute bronchitis is made. Medication is ordered for her, and the doctor advises her to rest in bed at home and to use a vaporizer in her bedroom.*

27. Ms. O'Malley asks the nurse why the vaporizer was advised. The best reply by the nurse is
   A. "It helps to kill the germs in the respiratory tract."
   B. "It provides moist air for the patient to breathe."
   C. "It reduces the inflammation in the sinuses."
   D. "It helps the action of the antibiotics."

28. Ms. O'Malley's harsh, dry cough can be described as
   A. productive.
   B. nonproductive.
   C. persistent.
   D. loose.

29. In addition to antibiotics, cough syrup is prescribed for Ms. O'Malley. The kind of cough syrup prescribed is
   A. antitussive.
   B. expectorant.
   C. mucolytic.
   D. sedative.

30. An expectorant cough syrup
   A. lessens the desire to cough.
   B. depresses the central nervous system.
   C. increases the respiratory tract secretions by loosening the mucus.
   D. increases the sputum.

> *Mrs. Jane Thompson has a normal vaginal delivery of her third child, a girl. The Apgar score is 9. A routine examination of the cord blood reveals a low T 3 and a low T4 with a high serum level of TSH (thyroid-stimulating hormone). A diagnosis of congenital cretinism is made.*

31. The nurse knows that cretinism is
   A. hyperthyroidism.
   B. hypothyroidism.
   C. thyroiditis.
   D. hypoparathyroidism.

32. In talking to the nurse, Mrs. Thompson states, "The doctor told me that my baby needs treatment, but I am not sure why. The other two did not need any medication. Suppose I wait for a few months." The nurse's best reply is
   A. "The sooner, the better."
   B. "If she does not receive treatment before 3 months, her skeleton will not develop normally."
   C. "If she does not receive treatment before 3 months, she will be mentally retarded."
   D. "Without treatment she will develop diabetes."

> *Nine-year-old Julia Weinberg is taken to the clinic by her mother because of symptoms of fever and joint pain. After a diagnosis of rheumatic fever is made, it is decided to admit her to the hospital. Included in the physician's orders are complete bedrest, antibiotics I.M., and aspirin for pain.*

33. An important nursing intervention in this case is to
   A. tell the family that Julia must have complete bedrest.
   B. tell the family that with the treatment Julia will recover without complications.
   C. teach the family the specific symptoms of streptococcal infection.
   D. teach the mother how to count Julia's pulse.

> *After 10 days Julia is discharged home on bedrest and a maintenance daily dose of penicillin. The instructions of the discharge nurse to the family include*
> *1. the signs of allergy to penicillin.*
> *2. the early signs of congestive heart failure.*
> *3. the need for bedrest.*
> *4. the need to minimize boredom.*

34. The important instructions are
  A. 1 and 2
  B. 1, 2, and 3
  C. 2, 3, and 4
  D. 1, 2, 3, and 4

35. Bedrest and restricted activity are necessary in order to
  A. reduce the swelling and pain of the joints.
  B. reduce the work of the heart.
  C. keep the fever down.
  D. reduce the chance of further infection.

36. Penicillin acts by
  A. reducing symptoms.
  B. eradicating the streptococcal infection.
  C. decreasing the pathogenicity of streptococci.
  D. decreasing the swelling.

37. For which of the following symptoms will the nurse tell the parents to watch while Julia is taking large doses of aspirin for pain?
  A. Headache.
  B. Brownish urine.
  C. Ringing in the ears.
  D. Inflamed eyes.

38. In her instructions to the parents, the nurse stresses that the reason for the strict regimen is to
  A. prevent contractures of Julia's joints.
  B. prevent heart disease.
  C. encourage Julia's continued growth.
  D. help Julia to return to school sooner.

Carl Martin, aged 65, a two-pack-a-day cigarette smoker, has intermittent claudication of both legs. When the cramping in his left leg becomes unbearable, he goes to the clinic.

39. When the doctor tells him to stop smoking, he asks the nurse, "What does my smoking have to do with my leg? My lungs are not bothering me." The BEST answer that the nurse can make is
  A. "The doctor told you to stop smoking because she doesn't want your lungs to become affected."
  B. "The nicotine in tobacco is a drug that causes constriction of the blood vessels. You have pain because not

enough blood is supplying your leg muscles."
  C. "Because of your age, you have severe arteriosclerosis of your legs. Your other arteries are probably affected also."
  D. "Even though your smoking has no effect on your present complaints, you would be wise to stop smoking."

After several weeks of clinic treatment, Mr. Martin's leg does not improve and a by-pass operation is performed on his left leg. This is unsuccessful, and an above-the-knee amputation is scheduled.

40. An amputation is defined as
  A. a vein stripping.
  B. surgical removal of a limb or appendage.
  C. a venotomy.
  D. a venesection.

41. The nurse must be aware of what possible serious complication after amputation?
  A. "Ghost pains" suffered by the patient.
  B. Hemorrhage.
  C. Urinary suppression.
  D. Intestinal obstruction.

42. Which of the following should the nurse do to avoid flexion contraction of Mr. Martin's hip?
  A. Elevate the stump on a pillow.
  B. Encourage the patient to move the stump.
  C. Place a pillow under the patient's hip.
  D. Place a pillow between the patient's legs.

43. All of the following are important nursing interventions for Mr. Martin EXCEPT
  A. monitoring for symptoms of excessive blood loss.
  b. maintaining an accurate record of bloody drainage.
  C. reinforcing dressings as necessary, using aseptic technique.
  D. encouraging the patient not to move the stump.

44. In teaching Mr. Martin self-care of the stump, the nurse instructs him in all of the following procedures EXCEPT

A. washing the healed stump daily and rinsing well.
B. soaking the healed stump daily.
C. inspecting the stump daily for skin breakdown.
D. Rewrapping the stump daily in a smooth tension wrapping.

Carol King, age 14 years, is admitted to the hospital with a diagnosis of sickle-cell anemia in crisis.

45. The nurse knows that sickle-cell anemia is a
A. severe iron-deficiency anemia.
B. severe chronic hemolytic anemia.
C. severe acute hemolytic anemia.
D. form of hemophilia.

46. A very prominent symptom of crisis is
A. headache.
B. abdominal pain.
C. hypoxia.
D. fatigue.

47. An important sign exhibited by Carol upon admission is jaundice. Which of the following is responsible for this jaundice?
A. Liver necrosis.
B. Enlarged spleen.
C. Red blood cell destruction.
D. Iron deficiency.

48. The MOST important nursing intervention in Carol's case is to
A. institute passive exercises.
B. administer an iron compound.
C. alleviate pain.
D. encourage the child to eat.

49. Sickle-cell anemia is an autosomal recessive disease. What is the LOWEST possible percentage of Mr. and Mrs. King's children who can have the disease, assuming that both parents carry the trait?
A. 25%
B. 50%
C. 0%
D. 100%

50. Sickle-cell anemia has a very high incidence among
A. African Americans.
B. Polish Americans.
C. Asian Americans.
D. Irish Americans.

Mrs. Mary Nickolakis, aged 85 years, has come to the arthritis clinic complaining, "This arthritis is killing me." The nurse notices that she is obese, her legs appear bowed, and she is obviously in pain. A diagnosis of osteoarthritis is made by the examining team.

51. Which of the following treatments does the nurse advise Mrs. Nickolakis to use at night?
A. Apply cold packs to her knees.
B. Apply hot, moist compresses to her knees.
C. Use a soft pillow under her knees.
D. Bandage her knees tightly with an Ace bandage.

52. The nurse understands that osteoarthritis
A. is primarily a disease of the elderly.
B. is caused by a virus.
C. affects only the lower extremities.
D. is of sudden onset.

53. Mrs. Nickolakis's doctor decides to do a total right-knee replacement. This procedure is known as
A. osteotomy.
B. arthroplasty.
C. arthrotomy.
D. osteoplasty.

54. The postoperative nursing management for Mrs. Nickolakis will include all of the following EXCEPT
A. evaluating the patient's vital signs and chart.
B. assessing changes in the patient's color.
C. watching the patient's toes for healthy color.
D. checking urinary intake and output.

55. All of the following are postoperative nursing interventions for Mrs. Nickolakis EXCEPT
A. evaluating the patient's position in bed for compliance with the orthopedist's orders.
B. monitoring the patient for the development of complications.
C. keeping the patient on complete bedrest for 3 days.
D. monitoring the patient for possible joint dislocation.

Mrs. Elizabeth Grant, 80 years old, is admitted to the hospital with a diagnosis of bacterial bronchopneumonia. She has a fever of 102°F, a harsh cough, chest pain, and difficulty in breathing. In addition to the laboratory work already performed, the physician orders a sputum culture and smear.

56. Mrs. Grant's chest pain is due to
A. difficulty in breathing.
B. friction rub between pleural layers.
C. inadequate intake of oxygen.
D. cardiac involvement.

57. In taking Mrs. Grant's temperature, the nurse will preferably use which area?
A. axillary.
B. rectal.
C. oral.
D. groin.

58. Rust-colored sputum, which is frequent in bacterial bronchopneumonia, is colored by blood. The medical term for expectorating blood-tinged sputum is
A. hematemesis.
B. hemoptysis.
C. hemobilia.
D. hemophthalmia.

59. Fluids are very important in Mrs. Grant's diet at this time because they
A. cool her fever.
B. ease her scratchy throat.
C. help liquefy the sputum.
D. disguise the taste of the cough syrup she is taking.

60. In the treatment of patients with bacterial bronchopneumonia, which of the following medications is likely to be prescribed to combat the pneumococcus?
A. Aspirin.
B. Penicillin.
C. Codeine sulfate.
D. Phenobarbital.

61. During the night, Mrs. Grant rings for the nurse and says, "I'm so tired, but I can't sleep. I'm short of breath from the coughing. Would a sleeping pill help me?" Which of the following answers is correct for the nurse to give to Mrs. Grant?

A. "Your doctor did not order a sleeping pill for you."
B. "Let me crank up the head of your bed and raise your knees a little. You will breathe easier and will go to sleep."
C. "I'll give you another dose of your cough medicine."
D. "You are just nervous. Close your eyes and count sheep."

After Mrs. Grant recovers from the pneumonia, she discovers that she has developed a small umbilical hernia from the severe coughing. After 2 months it has become very large, and her doctor advises surgery.

62. Which of the following positions will be BEST for assessment of Mrs. Grant's hernia?
A. The recumbent position.
B. The sitting position.
C. The left-side lying position.
D. The right-side lying position.

63. If the surgeon decides to have Mrs. Grant's bowel cleansed before surgery, the nurse will expect that he will order
A. a colonic irrigation.
B. a suppository.
C. a cathartic.
D. a cleansing enema.

64. The basic goal of preoperative skin preparation for Mrs. Grant is to
A. render the operative area sterile.
B. improve the skin's natural defenses against infection.
C. decrease the number of organisms on the skin.
D. enhance the action of the anesthetic.

Mrs. Kidd is having her second baby and is at term. She is in the first stage of labor when she is admitted to the hospital. Her contractions are regular and are occurring at 10-minute intervals. Mrs. Kidd reports having had a "show" several hours before the onset of labor.

65. The "show" mentioned by Mrs. Kidd refers to

A. the presence of the fetal head in the vagina.
B. a pinkish vaginal discharge.
C. an urge to bear down.
D. the enlargement of the abdomen.

66. The admission record about Mrs. Kidd should contain all of the following information EXCEPT
A. the time when the contractions started.
B. the duration and frequency of the contractions.
C. the time of the impending delivery.
D. the expected date of confinement.

67. Mrs. Kidd's labor and delivery experience will be influenced by
A. the structure of her pelvis and the size and position of the fetus's head.
B. the acceptance, skill, and assistance of the nurse.
C. her previous delivery experience.
D. all of the above.

68. As part of Mrs. Kidd's preparation for delivery, her genital area is shaved. The purpose of this procedure is to
A. allow for easier delivery.
B. provide a clean area for delivery.
C. allow easier viewing of the presenting part.
D. provide a smoother area for the episiotomy.

69. Most obstetricians order an enema on admission. Under what circumstances would an enema NOT be ordered?
A. Excessive vaginal bleeding.
B. Advanced labor.
C. Evidence of a prolapsed cord.
D. All of the above.

70. Mrs. Kidd's doctor wishes to determine how much her cervix has dilated. Which of the following should the nurse have ready?
A. A fetoscope.
B. A speculum and lubricant.
C. A rubber glove and lubricant.
D. A maternal monitor.

71. You are timing Mrs. Kidd's contractions. The term used to describe the period from the beginning to the end of a contraction is
A. duration.
B. interval.

C. intensity.
D. frequency.

72. You check the fetal heart rate every 30 minutes. The normal expected rate per minute is between
A. 80 and 100 beats.
B. 100 and 120 beats.
C. 120 and 160 beats.
D. 160 and 200 beats.

> *Seventy-year-old Mr. Jared Smith is under the care of a physician who has prescribed digoxin 0.25 mg daily for congestive heart failure. Mr. Smith becomes tired of taking the medication and stops. Ten days later he is admitted to the hospital with a diagnosis of congestive heart failure with acute pulmonary edema. Complete bedrest, oxygen by nasal prongs, a low-sodium diet, and morphine sulfate q. 4 h. p.r.n. are prescribed for him. He is digitalized with digoxin I.V. and given Lasix 40 mg.*

73. The practical nurse places a caution sign at the door of Mr. Smith's room because oxygen
A. is combustible.
B. promotes lung damage when breathed in concentrated form.
C. depresses respiration.
D. must not be used in concentrations greater than 30%.

74. Because Mr. Smith is receiving digoxin, the nurse must be observant for evidence of
A. diaphoresis.
B. slow pulse.
C. dyspnea.
D. restlessness.

75. Because Mr. Smith is on a low-sodium diet, the nurse will urge him to select all of the following foods EXCEPT
A. canned vegetable soup.
B. fresh fruits and vegetables.
C. cottage cheese.
D. Jello-O.

76. When Mrs. Smith asks the nurse why her husband is weighed every day, the MOST logical answer is
A. "The doctor wants to be sure that Mr. Smith is eating enough."

B. "That is the way we can check his fluid loss."

C. "It is a routine of the hospital."

D. "We have to check whether he is losing weight."

77. One week later, Mr. Smith reports to the nurse that the palpitations of his heart are very annoying. The practical nurse notes that his heart has become irregular and reports this fact to the supervising nurse. The physician then orders that Mr. Smith's blood be evaluated for electrolytes. The rationale for this order is that
A. the sodium may have increased.
B. the chlorides may be low.
C. the potassium may be low.
D. the sodium may be low.

78. While Mr. Smith is on bedrest, the nurse knows that she must observe his skin carefully each day and record her findings in his chart. The primary reason for this is that an edematous patient is prone to develop
A. itchy skin.
B. jaundice.
C. decubitus ulcers.
D. distended veins.

79. Mr. Smith complains to his wife that his meals are tasteless and requests that she bring some condiments to the hospital to season his food. Which of the following substances would be CONTRAINDICATED on his rigid low-sodium diet?
A. Chili sauce.
B. Herbs.
C. Lemon juice.
D. Sugar.

80. The practical nurse tells Mrs. Smith that for a snack Mr. Smith may have which of the following foods that is high in potassium?
A. Apples.
B. Grapes.
C. Bananas.
D. Plums.

81. The practical nurse asks Mr. Smith how he knew that he was in congestive failure. He replies that he
A. started to lose weight.
B. had to get up to void at night.
C. became very short of breath.
D. discovered that his pulse was quite slow.

82. The practical nurse knows that one of the following diagnostic procedures used to determine cardiac function is invasive and requires sterile technique. Of which procedure is this true?
A. Chest X-ray.
B. Electrocardiogram.
C. Angiocardiography.
D. Echocardiography.

William Tedesco, a 20-year-old college student, is brought to the emergency room by his roommate. He is complaining of severe precordial pain, is perspiring profusely and breathing rapidly, and has heart palpitations; his hands are ice cold. After history and appropriate physical and laboratory examinations are done, a diagnosis of acute anxiety reaction is made.

83. Which of the physiological reactions suffered by William could give the nurse a clue as to the diagnosis?
A. Heart palpitations.
B. Severe precordial pain.
C. Ice-cold hands.
D. Hyperventilation.

84. To relieve the symptoms of hyperventilation, the nurse advises William to
A. lower his head between his knees.
B. rebreathe into a brown paper bag.
C. breathe 100% oxygen.
D. lie flat on his back with his legs extended.

85. Which of these medications is generally used in the treatment of acute anxiety reaction?
A. Codeine sulfate.
B. Meprobamate.
C. Aspirin.
D. Benadryl.

86. The practical nurse on duty learns that William is worried about his math exam and has had nightmares about it. Which of the following feelings in regard to his examination relate to his diagnosis of acute anxiety reaction?
A. Alienation.
B. Inadequacy.
C. Distrust.
D. Superiority.

Mrs. Clark brings her 4-year-old daughter, Susan, to the pediatric clinic because for 10 days the child has been running a fever and has had a hacking cough. This morning the mother noticed a reddish rash behind Susan's ears. When the nurse asks whether Susan has been in contact with other children with a rash, Mrs. Clark reveals that her family is homeless and has been living in an armory shelter. Another child in the shelter developed measles the week before. Mrs. Clark is vague about Susan's immunizations and has no written record.

87. The practical nurse in the clinic should
    A. order Mrs. Clark to move from the armory immediately, as her family's health is jeopardized.
    B. tell Mrs. Clark to keep Susan in bed for one week.
    C. notify Social Service so that a visit can be made to the armory to assess the situation.
    D. tell Mrs. Clark that the rash will spread and then peel away.

88. When Mrs. Clark asks, she is told by the nurse that measles is spread by
    A. contaminated food.
    B. droplet infection from respiratory secretions.
    C. rats and mice.
    D. communal toilets.

89. Which of the following signs is diagnostic of measles?
    A. Coryza and a dry, hacking cough.
    B. Enlarged lymph nodes in the neck.
    C. Red spots with white centers visible on the buccal mucosa.
    D. Intolerance to light.

90. A major complication of measles is
    A. chickenpox.
    B. sore throat.
    C. pneumonia.
    D. acute glomeruonephritis.

91. After the pediatrician prescribes bedrest for Susan, Mrs. Clark asks the nurse how long she should keep the child in bed, considering the difficulties of her situation. The best response of the nurse would be

A. "Until Susan is eating normally."
B. "Until Susan's temperature returns to normal."
C. "Until the rash disappears."
D. "Through the third day of the rash."

92. Mrs. Clark states that she is also unsure about measles vaccination for her other children. The nurse explains that, in order to make the disease less severe, the pediatrician will probably order
    A. an antibiotic.
    B. a vaccine.
    C. a toxoid.
    D. an immunoglobulin.

93. The organism that causes measles is a
    A. pneumococcus
    B. staphylococcus.
    C. virus.
    D. streptococcus.

Marie Torres, 26 years old, is admitted to the hospital with a diagnosis of hepatitis B (serum hepatitis).

94. The nursing care plan for Ms. Torres will include all of the following EXCEPT
    A. wearing gloves when giving care.
    B. using disposable needles and syringes.
    C. placing the patient in complete isolation.
    D. encouraging an adequate diet.

95. Ms. Torres complains to the nurse, "Why did the doctor say that I have hepatitis? I haven't eaten any raw seafood for years." The BEST answer from the nurse would be "Your type of hepatitis is spread by
    A. infected insect bites."
    B. contaminated toilet seats."
    C. contaminated needles."
    D. contaminated clothing."

96. Ms. Torres states, "I had my ears pierced in a jewelry store about 6 weeks ago. Do you think that's how I became infected?" The nurse's BEST answer is
    A. "Probably not."
    B. "Maybe. One has to be careful about sanitation."
    C. "Yes, if there was no other instance of needle puncture."

D. "Who knows?"

97. In which organ of Ms. Torres did the viruses causing the hepatitis grow?
A. Brain.
B. Liver.
C. Intestinal tract.
D. Blood.

98. Ms. Torres's doctor prescribes a prophylactic preparation to protect other members of her family. This preparation is
A. an antitoxin.
B. gamma globulin.
C. an antibiotic.
D. a vaccine.

99. In the nursing plan for Ms. Torres, what sort of diet should be called for?
A. High-carbohydrate.
B. Low-fat.
C. Low-protein.
D. Normally balanced.

100. The virus causing the hepatitis B will be excreted from Ms. Torres's body primarily through
A. feces.
B. blood.
C. skin.
D. urine.

Mrs. Helen Hirsch, 80 years old, is admitted to the hospital after a fall in her home. She suffers pain in her left hip and is unable to move her left leg. After examination and X-rays, a diagnosis of intracapsular fracture of her left hip is made.

---

101. The surgeon decides to correct the fracture with the insertion of a pin (surgical internal fixation). The nurse knows that this procedure is the treatment of choice for Mrs. Hirsch because
A. the fracture will heal more rapidly.
B. her bones are very brittle.
C. this procedure makes it possible to walk earlier.
D. this procedure carries less danger of infection.

102. Flexion contraction is an undesirable complication of hip fracture. Which procedure should be included in the nursing plan to help guard against this?
A. Using a flotation mattress.
B. Having Mrs. Hirsch's feet rest against a footboard.
C. Having an overhead trapeze.
D. Encouraging Mrs. Hirsch to move by herself.

103. Upon getting Mrs. Hirsch out of bed, what kind of chair does the nurse choose to give her proper support?
A. A recliner with elevated footrest.
B. A swivel chair.
C. A padded, upholstered chair.
D. A high, straight-backed chair with arm rests.

Jimmy Bruce, 2 years old, is hospitalized with extensive atopic dermatitis. A CBC, blood chemistry, and urinalysis are ordered by the doctor.

---

104. The nurse notes that the CBC reveals
A. elevated lymphocytes.
B. elevated eosinophils.
C. elevated neutrophils.
D. increased sodium.

105. The MOST obvious characteristic of Jimmy's rash is
A. erythema.
B. burning.
C. itching.
D. swelling.

106. Nursing interventions for Jimmy include which of the following?
1. Elbow restraints.
2. Gloves.
3. Soft toys.
4. Trimming his fingernails.
A. 1 and 4.
B. 2, 3, and 4.
C. 1, 2, and 3.
D. 1, 2, 3, and 4.

Your next-door neighbor, aged 62, has started to have trouble reading. Also, her eyes tear easily and she has frequent headaches. She asks you to recommend an optometrist so that she can get some reading glasses.

---

107. As a practical nurse, you know that an optometrist is
- A. a physician who examines the eyes and prescribes reading glasses.
- B. a medical specialist in the diagnosis and treatment of diseases of the eyes and visual defects.
- C. a person who is trained only in the examination of eyes for the purpose of prescribing glasses.
- D. an individual who is trained to make eye glasses and optical instruments.

108. You persuade your neighbor to consult an ophthalmologist. During the examination by the ophthalmologist, the neighbor is discovered to have glaucoma. As a nurse, you know that glaucoma is caused by
- A. increased intraocular pressure.
- B. nearsightedness.
- C. farsightedness.
- D. weak eye muscles.

Mrs. Jeanne Jacobs, a 50-year-old mother of four, suddenly develops vaginal bleeding and goes to her gynecologist for an examination.

---

109. Before the examination, the nurse
- A. gives Mrs. Jacobs an enema.
- B. tells Mrs. Jacobs to void and to give a urine sample.
- C. advises Mrs. Jacobs to douche with a solution of white vinegar.
- D. catheterizes Mrs. Jacobs

110. During the examination the physician takes a Papanicolaou smear in order to
- A. screen for ovarian cancer.
- B. screen for cervical cancer.
- C. screen for Fallopian-tube patency.
- D. screen for fibroid tumors.

Mr. Gary Hanlon, a 32-year-old, married hemophiliac, is admitted to the hospital complaining of a nonproductive cough, weight loss, fatigue, and skin rash. He is tentatively diagnosed as having AIDS.

---

111. The practical nurse who is assigned to care for Mr. Hanlon will be expected to

- A. wash her hands before and after direct patient care.
- B. wear gloves when giving Mr. Hanlon a bath.
- C. wear a mask and gown when changing Mr. Hanlon's bed.
- D. double-bag Mr. Hanlon's dinner tray when he has finished with it.

112. Mr. Hanlon confides to his nurse that he is fearful that he may have given AIDS to his wife. The BEST response for the nurse to make is
- A. "Don't worry. AIDS is not contagious."
- B. "I don't blame you for being afraid. You wife probably did catch it from you."
- C. "Is your wife sick too?"
- D. "This must be a difficult time for you. Tell me how you are feeling."

113. Mr. Hanlon's doctor comes in to see the patient. The doctor plans to do a blood test to confirm that Mr. Hanlon has HIV infection. In preparing for this test, the nurse needs to know that
- A. the blood specimen will be drawn by a representative from the health department.
- B. the physician needs to obtain a written consent from the patient before the blood can be drawn.
- C. the nurse will need to send a hospital laboratory slip to the lab to draw the blood sample.
- D. the patient must be taken to the county laboratory to have his blood drawn.

114. Mr. Hanlon is ready to be discharged. The diagnosis of AIDS has been confirmed. Mrs. Hanlon asks the practical nurse whether she can safely have sexual intercourse with her husband. The nurse's BEST reply is
- A. "You better ask your doctor."
- B. "Sure; AIDS is transmitted only through blood transfusions."
- C. "The AIDS virus is transmitted by exchanging body fluids, such as his semen with your partner."
- D. "You can have sexual intercourse with your husband as long as you use a diaphragm."

115. AIDS is characterized as a sexually transmitted disease. Which of the following diseases is also included in this category?
    A. Condylomata.
    B. Varicella.
    C. Toxoplasmosis.
    D. Dysmenorrhea.

The rest of the test consists of unrelated questions.

116. A persistent, irresistible urge to do something, such as washing one's hands, despite an intellectual disinclination to carry out the act, is
    A. an obsession.
    B. an hallucination.
    C. a phobia.
    D. a compulsion.

117. An autistic child is totally concerned with
    A. him-/herself.
    B. material things.
    C. his friends.
    D. the opinions of others.

118. Hearing voices that are not really present is an example of
    A. an obsession.
    B. an hallucination.
    C. a phobia.
    D. a compulsion.

119. A very serious mental breakdown with severe personality changes is termed
    A. a neurosis.
    B. an emotional disturbance.
    C. hypochondria.
    D. a psychosis.

120. In the female, the urinary meatus is located
    A. about ½ inch below the neck of the bladder.
    B. between the vaginal orifice and the rectum.
    C. about 6 inches below the neck of the bladder.
    D. between the clitoris and vaginal orifice.

121. Materials for the production of urine come from the
    A. kidney.
    B. bloodstream.
    C. lymph nodes.
    D. bladder.

122. All of the following responsibilities should be included in general postoperative care EXCEPT
    A. maintaining the patient flat in bed.
    B. inspecting dressings for drainage.
    C. observing and recording vital signs as ordered.
    D. recording intake and output daily.

123. One of the most common disturbances following surgery is abdominal distension, due primarily to
    A. inability of the patient to eat.
    B. depressed respiration.
    C. reaction to a blood transfusion.
    D. absence of peristalsis.

124. All of the following are symptoms of abdominal distension EXCEPT
    A. swollen abdomen.
    B. difficult breathing.
    C. pains in the abdomen.
    D. vomiting blood.

125. A patient with a blood pressure of 180/90 has a pulse pressure of
    A. 135.
    B. 80.
    C. 90.
    D. 270.

DIAGNOSTIC TEST

ANSWER KEY—PART II

1.	A	26.	A	51.	B	76.	B	101.	C
2.	C	27.	B	52.	A	77.	C	102.	D
3.	D	28.	B	53.	B	78.	C	103.	D
4.	D	29.	B	54.	D	79.	A	104.	B
5.	B	30.	C	55.	C	80.	C	105.	C
6.	B	31.	B	56.	B	81.	C	106.	D
7.	A	32.	C	57.	B	82.	C	107.	C
8.	D	33.	D	58.	B	83.	C	108.	A
9.	C	34.	D	59.	C	84.	B	109.	B
10.	B	35.	B	60.	B	85.	B	110.	B
11.	D	36.	B	61.	B	86.	B	111.	A
12.	D	37.	C	62.	B	87.	C	112.	D
13.	B	38.	B	63.	D	88.	B	113.	B
14.	B	39.	B	64.	C	89.	C	114.	C
15.	D	40.	B	65.	B	90.	C	115.	A
16.	B	41.	B	66.	C	91.	D	116.	D
17.	B	42.	B	67.	D	92.	D	117.	A
18.	C	43.	D	68.	B	93.	C	118.	B
19.	C	44.	B	69.	D	94.	C	119.	D
20.	D	45.	B	70.	C	95.	C	120.	D
21.	B	46.	B	71.	A	96.	C	121.	B
22.	D	47.	C	72.	C	97.	B	122.	A
23.	C	48.	C	73.	A	98.	D	123.	D
24.	D	49.	A	74.	B	99.	D	124.	D
25.	B	50.	A	75.	A	100.	B	125.	C

EXPLANATIONS FOR ANSWERS—PART II

1. **A** Malnourished elderly patients have become accustomed to eating irregularly. They generally do better with small, frequent meals rather than three large ones. It is important to increase Mrs. Burton's nutrition but at her own pace.

2. **C** Mrs. Burton is not oriented to person, place, or time.

3. **D** The nurse must continue to help the patient increase her self-esteem and not ridicule or scold her. It is important to help her in a kindly way.

4. **D** In severe constipation leading to fecal impaction, there can be liquid fecal leakage around the impaction.

5. **B** The impaction must be removed in order for the patient to establish bowel regularity.

6. **B** Otitis media, an inflammation of the middle ear, is a common disorder in children.

7. **A** The short, straight eustachian tube lends itself to the spread of infections from the upper respiratory tract.

8. **D** Family visits are not encouraged because the patient needs a relaxed, quiet atmosphere. In addition, there is no way to monitor infections that members of the family may be harboring.

9. **C** Altered respirations are the only sign that a complication may be present. Choices A, B, and D are generally seen in meningitis, rather than otitis media, cases.

10. **B** This answer is the best of those listed. It explains to the mother the kind of atmosphere needed by her son, which choices A, C, and D do not. In addition, choice D is hardly likely to calm the mother.

11. **D** All of the items listed should be included in the nursing plan for Daniel's treatment.

12. **D** This answer makes clear to the aunt that Daniel needs quiet and should be isolated from additional infections.

13. **B** This method is frequently used in giving medication to children.

14. **B** It is better to keep Daniel quiet for a short time, although there is no reason to keep him in a darkened room. Visits from his friends may be too taxing. Television watching should be limited (several hours is too much) and the programs monitored so that nothing too exciting is shown.

15. **D** This is the best answer because it states exactly why blood must be taken and the tests done. Choices A and C are unhelpful, and "serious infection" in choice B may frighten the patient.

16. **B** A chest X-ray is a noninvasive test for which the patient removes his/her upper garments and jewelry and dons a hospital gown. Contrast media (choices A and C) are not necessary for chest X-rays. The patient stands upright, does not lie down on the table (choice D), for this procedure.

17. **B** After a bronchoscopy nothing can be given by mouth until the gag reflex returns and the patient indicates that he can cough.

18. **C** Mr. Cruz's symptoms indicate that he should stop smoking.

19. **C** A sore mouth with beefy, red, burning tongue (glossitis) is a typical symptom of pernicious anemia that requires the nurse to focus on good oral hygiene. Additionally, the nurse may offer ice chips or fluids to keep the mouth well lubricated.

20. **D** Vitamin B_{12} therapy must be a lifetime procedure because the intrinsic factor lacking in pernicious anemia does not return to the gastric secretions. Symptoms will recur without this therapy, which should be given every 4 weeks.

21. **B** It has been found that patients taking vitamin B_{12} by mouth develop a resistance to the vitamin. None of the other choices is true.

22. **D** Meats and dairy products are the best sources of vitamin B_{12}. The other foods listed are good sources of vitamin C and of other vitamins of the B complex.

23. **C** This is an excellent definition of aging.

24. **D** All of the items describe human needs.

25. **B** A decrease in the activity of oil and sweat glands is an aspect of aging.

26. **A** Circulation is not reduced because of aging. If circulation is reduced, it is due to disease process.

27. **B** Vaporizers are indicated whenever moist air can be helpful to the patient. A vaporizer does not kill germs, reduce inflammation, or enhance antibiotic action.

28. **B** A nonproductive cough is harsh and dry.

29. **B** An expectorant cough syrup loosens the mucus and thus decreases the cough.

30. **C** See the answer to question 29.

31. **B** Hypothyroidism (decreased activity of the thyroid gland) in children is known as cretinism.

32. **C** Treatment must be started before 3 months to prevent mental retardation in children. Choice A is uninformative, and choices B and D are untrue.

33. **D** The treatment will be continued at home after hospital discharge. Tachycardia is a clinical manifestation of rheumatic fever. The mother must be taught to monitor the child's pulse and report an increase to the physician.

34. **C** All of the instructions are important. Allergy to penicillin may appear at any time, and the family must be alert to signs of heart failure. The other two items are important parts of the treatment.

35. **B** In rheumatic fever the heart must always be protected.

36. **B** Maintenance doses of penicillin are necessary for several years.

37. **C** Ringing in the ears, or tinnitus, is a sign of salicylate toxicity.

38. **B** See the answer to question 35.

39. **B** This informative answer explains the action of nicotine, an addictive drug.

40. **B** Vein stripping is ligation of the greater or lesser saphenous vein, done to correct leg varicosities. Venotomy is surgical incision of a vein. Venesection is phlebotomy, incision of a vein for the letting of blood.

41. **B** Because large blood vessels have been separated, hemorrhage is a possible complication that must be monitored.

42. **B** Flexion contractures occur easily in lower limb amputations if the muscles are not exercised and stretched.
43. **D** See the answer to question 42. The other choices are important measures.
44. **B** Soaking the stump increases edema and must be avoided.
45. **B** Sickle-cell anemia is chronic, that is, lifelong and never cured.
46. **B** The pain is the result of the occlusion of small blood vessels by the sickle-shaped cells, causing infarction.
47. **C** The sickled red cells are fragile and are rapidly destroyed in the circulation. Hypoxia also contributes to the destruction of the red blood cells, and their rapid breakdown causes an overabundance of bilirubin in the blood, resulting in yellowing of the skin. Bilirubin is a waste product from the breakdown of hemoglobin.
48. **C** The alleviation of pain is most important in the crisis.
49. **A** If both parents have the trait, 25% of their children will be normal, 50% will have the trait, and 25% will inherit the disease.
50. **A** Sickle-cell anemia occurs mainly in blacks.
51. **B** Heat and moistness help relieve the pain and stiffness of osteoarthritis.
52. **A** This disease is generally found in the obese, aging population and can affect any joint, although the weight-bearing joints do suffer the most. Osteoarthritis is not known to be caused by a virus, nor is it of sudden onset.
53. **B** Arthroplasty restores motion to a joint and function to the structures that control it. Osteotomy is surgical division or cutting of bone. Arthrotomy is an incision into a joint. Osteoplasty is any plastic operation on bone.
54. **D** It is not necessary to check urinary input/output after arthroplasty unless there has been some renal involvement.
55. **C** An arthroplasty patient is not kept on complete bedrest for 3 days, but rather is ambulatory with a walker on the second day.
56. **B** Friction rub is common in bronchopneumonia.
57. **B** Since Mrs. Grant is breathing through her mouth, the oral method will not give a true reading. A rectal reading is more accurate than choices A and D.
58. **B** Hematemesis is the vomiting of blood. Hemobilia is bleeding into biliary passages. Hemophthalmia is bleeding into the eye.
59. **C** Liquefaction of the sputum will reduce the cough.
60. **B** Penicillin is the antibiotic of choice. If the patient is allergic to penicillin, a broad-spectrum antibiotic can be used.
61. **B** The nurse will place the patient in Fowler's position, which always eases breathing when a patient is dyspneic.
62. **B** In the sitting position, the hernia will protrude.
63. **D** The enema will cleanse the lower bowel sufficiently.
64. **C** The skin can never be completely sterilized.
65. **B** The "show" consists of a plug of cervical mucus mixed with blood, and its appearance is evidence of cervical dilatation and effacement and of the descent of the presenting part.
66. **C** The time of the delivery is not known at admission. The record should contain all of the other information in choices A, B, and D.
67. **D** All three of the factors listed as choices A, B, and C will influence labor and delivery.
68. **B** Shaving the genital area promotes cleanliness and reduces the likelihood of postpartum infection.
69. **D** Excessive vaginal bleeding is a true emergency; no procedures should be attempted that may increase the bleeding. If labor is far advanced, an enema is contraindicated. Prolapse of the cord puts the fetus in danger, and nothing should be done to increase pressure on the cord.
70. **C** The doctor will do a vaginal examination to measure the dilatation.
71. **A** The interval is the time between contractions. The intensity is the strength of the contraction. The frequency is the number of contractions that occur within a specific interval of time.

72. **C** A persistent fetal heart rate below 120 or above 160 indicates some fetal abnormality and needs investigation.
73. **A** Fire is escalated by the presence of oxygen.
74. **B** A pulse rate below 60 is evidence of toxicity.
75. **A** Canned vegetable soups are processed with a sodium compound as a preservative.
76. **B** Fluid gain or loss can be monitored by recording the patient's weight every day.
77. **C** Diuretics remove potassium, and too little potassium causes cardiac arrhythmias and potential death.
78. **C** In edema the circulation of the skin is compromised, and decubitus ulcers will develop unless proper precautions are taken.
79. **A** Chili sauce has too much sodium.
80. **C** Bananas contain large amounts of potassium.
81. **C** Dyspnea is one of the first symptoms of congestive heart failure.
82. **C** Angiocardiography is an invasive procedure that will reveal internal cardiac pressures in the left ventricle and the aorta. A chest X-ray is used to determine left ventricular enlargement. An electrocardiogram determines the myocardial function. An echocardiogram determines pericardial effusion in a noninvasive way.
83. **C** The other signs are seen in cardiac disease also.
84. **B** Rebreathing into a bag will increase the carbon dioxide that William has been losing through hyperventilation.
85. **B** The minor tranquilizers are used in treatment of anxieties.
86. **B** Inadequacy feelings cause the anxiety reaction. William probably feels that he does not understand math well enough to pass the exam.
87. **C** Social Service must examine the situation in the shelter and decide whether the Health Department should be notified to send in its team.
88. **B** A highly contagious disease, measles is spread by direct contact with droplets from the nose, mouth, or throat of infected persons, often in the earliest stages.
89. **C** Koplik's spots are diagnostic of measles (rubeola).
90. **C** Pneumonia. There are additional complications, but pneumonia is the major one.
91. **D** After the rash has been present for at least 3 days, the patient is no longer infectious.
92. **D** Immunoglobulin will ameliorate the symptoms if the other children contract the disease.
93. **C** The causative organism is a virus.
94. **C** Complete isolation of the patient is not necessary in serum hepatitis.
95. **C** Hepatitis B is transmitted orally via saliva or through blood transfusion, skin prick, sexual intercourse, or contaminated equipment.
96. **C** The sterility of the needle used in ear piercing cannot be guaranteed. The other answers are completely unhelpful.
97. **B** The virus grows in the liver but circulates in the blood.
98. **D** Hepatitis B vaccine is recommended for individuals at high risk for hepatitis B.
99. **D** No special diet is required. A normally balanced diet will provide adequate nutrition.
100. **B** Hepatitis B is a virus transmitted through the blood. Transmission can occur in a number of ways, for example, through parenteral contamination, intimate sexual contact, or contaminated instruments such as syringes or renal dialysis machines. Universal precautions need to be in effect with hepatitis B patients to prevent cross-infection.
101. **C** Long periods of immobilization should be avoided in the elderly. Mrs. Hirsch will walk more quickly with a pin than with a cast.
102. **D** Exercising the muscles by moving around will reduce the chance of flexion contractions.
103. **D** A straight, high-back chair with arms allows for proper body alignment of the elderly patient.
104. **B** Elevated eosinophils are diagnostic of allergy.
105. **C** Atopic dermatitis causes severe itching.
106. **D** All of the listed interventions will help reduce the ability to scratch. Scratching will lead to infection.

107. **C** An ophthalmologist is a physician who specializes in the care and treatment of eyes. An optician it trained to make eye glasses and optical instruments.

108. **A** There are two kinds of glaucoma: open angle and closed angle. Closed-angle glaucoma generally is an emergency that needs immediate surgery.

109. **B** It is necessary to have the bladder empty for the examination, but catheterization is not required. Douching is contraindicated because some of the cervical cells may be washed away. There is no reason to give an enema.

110. **B** The Papanicolaou test is a cytological test of secretions and cells from the cervix or vagina for early detection of the presence of cancer cells.

111. **A** Hands should be washed before and after direct patient care and after contact with the blood, body fluids, or other body secretions of all patients, not only those who have been diagnosed as having AIDS. Wearing gloves and a gown are not indicated unless the nurse expects to be in contact with the AIDS patient's body fluids. A mask is needed only if the AIDS patient has a productive cough. Double bagging of the AIDS patient's dinner tray is not indicated because contact with saliva does not result in transmission of infection.

112. **D** This answer reflects the nurse's support of the patient's feelings. Additionally, the nurse is attempting to elicit more information about the patient's feelings so that a nursing care plan addressing these issues can be developed. Choice A is too reassuring; choice B is callous, and C serves no particular purpose.

113. **B** The physician must obtain a written consent from the patient before his blood is drawn. This is done to preserve the patient's right to informed treatment, and to maintain his confidentality, particularly because of the societal implications of a positive AIDS blood test. Additionally, in most areas, a kit is prepared by the county health department indicating how the sample is to be drawn. The blood is usually drawn by the physician, and the sample is transported to the county health department for testing.

114. **C** This is a direct, open, and honest reply. Hopefully, it would encourage the wife to seek sexual counseling and would serve as a suggestion that she might benefit from having a blood test performed to determine whether she too has the HIV infection.

115. **A** Condylomata is a sexually transmitted disease characterized by pointed dry warts, which are highly infectious, under the prepuce on the male or on the vulva of the female. Varicella is better known as chicken pox, a communicable disease usually contracted in childhood. Toxo-plasmosis is an infection caused by the toxoplasma parasites that occur in birds and may infect human beings. Dysmenorrhea is painful menstruation.

116. **D** A compulsion is an irresistable urge to perform some act, usually against one's better judgment or moral standards.

117. **A** An autistic child fails to relate in the ordinary way to people and situations. He has a marked inability to adjust socially.

118. **B** An hallucination is a perception of something that is not really present. Hallucinations are common in severe mental illness and may also occur after head injury, in delirium, and from the use of certain drugs.

119. **D** Psychosis is a general term to describe a major mental disorder in which contact with reality is lost. A neurosis is an emotional disorder. Hypochondria is morbid anxiety about one's health.

120. **D** This is an anatomical fact.

121. **B** Waste products from the bloodstream are secreted into urine by the kidneys. The urine is then transported through the ureters to the bladder, where it is stored until excreted.

122. **A** The patient's recovery from surgery can be enhanced by proper positioning in bed, frequent changes of position, exercise, and progressive ambulation.

123. **D** After surgery, peristalsis is absent or ineffective because of disturbance to the nerves supplying the intestine.

124. **D** Vomiting blood is a serious symptom not indicative of abdominal distension.

125. **C** The pulse pressure is obtained by subtracting the diastolic pressure from the systolic pressure; $180 - 90 = 90$.

I

Basic Sciences

UNIT 1: CHEMISTRY

VOCABULARY

acid	compound yielding hydrogen ions (H+) and no other positive ions in solution
adhesion	molecular force between masses of different substances that holds them together
base	compound yielding hydroxyl ions (OH−) in solution
biology	science of life
electrolyte	substance that conducts electric current
enzyme	chemical substance made by plants and animals that speeds up certain chemical reactions in cells without itself being changed
hypertonic	having a concentration of salts in a solution greater than concentration in body fluids
hypotonic	having a concentration of salts in a solution less than concentration of body fluids
ion	atom carrying positive or negative charge
isotonic	having a concentration of salts in a solution in the same proportion as in the blood
mass	a quantity of material, such as cells, that adheres together by molecular force
pH	expression of degree of acidity or alkalinity of a solution (pH 7 is neutral, i.e., water)
physiology	science of functions of living cells, tissues, and organs
solute	dissolved substance in a solution
solution	homogeneous molecular dispersion
solvent	substance in which solute is dissolved

I. **Foundations of Chemistry**

　A. Definition of **Chemistry**: Science that deals with (1) the composition, structure, and properties of *matter*, and (2) the *energy* changes that accompany changes in matter. Called *biological chemistry* when it deals with body functions:
　　1. Respiration
　　2. Digestion
　　3. Acid-base balance of the body
　　4. Kidney function
　　5. Action of hormones

　B. Matter and Energy
　　1. Matter
　　　a) Is anything that occupies space and has mass
　　　b) May be liquid, gas, or solid depending upon temperature, pressure, and type of matter

        (1)   Gas—e.g., steam, which has no form or limits

        (2)   Liquid—e.g., water, which has no definite form but takes the form of its container

        (3)   Solid—e.g., ice, which does have an identifiable form

   c)   Exists in three classifications

        (1)   Element—simple substance that cannot be broken down by ordinary chemical means (atoms)

        (2)   Compound—chemical combination of two or more elements in definite proportions by weight

        (3)   Mixture—consists of two or more substances, each of which retains its own characteristics and properties

   d)   Has two distinguishing characteristics

        (1)   Physical properties—those that involve no change in the composition of the substance, e.g., grinding ice

        (2)   Chemical properties—those that are the result of chemical actions between molecules or elements that yield new substances, e.g., chemical combining of H and O to form water

2.   Energy

   a)   Is the ability to do work

   b)   Can be neither created nor destroyed

   c)   Occurs in two forms

        (1)   Potential energy—inactive or stored energy (available for use because of its relative position, configuration, or chemical composition, e.g., ball at the top of a hill)

        (2)   Kinetic energy—energy resulting from actively moving particles, e.g., child on a swing

             Heat

            (a)   Accompanies chemical change

            (b)   Can be used to diagnose disease (body temperature)

            (c)   Can be used in treatment (applications of heat)

C.   The atom

   1.   Characteristics (see Figure 1)

      a)   Has mass and occupies space

      b)   Is composed of protons, electrons, and neutrons

      c)   Has a nucleus that always has a positive charge (protons)

      d)   Has as its major portion, "empty space" that contains nearly weightless electrons

      e)   Comprises a particular element in which all atoms have the same nuclear charge

      f)   Has its chemical and physical characteristics determined by the charge of its nucleus

      g)   Has a total charge of zero, since the number of protons (+) is always equal to the number of electrons (−)

      h)   Has nearly its entire mass centered in the nucleus

   2.   Basic principles of atomic structure

      a)   Atomic number—whole number representing the number of units of positive charge on the nucleus of an atom (identifies each element)

      b)   Isotopes—atoms of the same element that have the same atomic number but different numbers of neutrons

      c)   Nucleons—the particles making up the nucleus (protons and neutrons)

      d)   Atomic weight—average weight of the atom's isotopes compared to the weight of carbon-12

BASIC SCIENCES

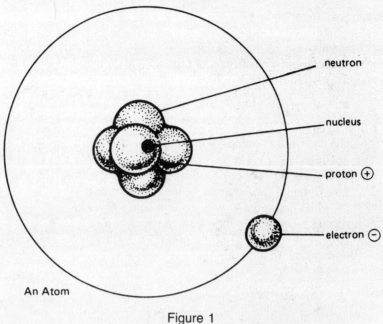

Figure 1

D. Radioactivity
  1. Principles concerning nuclear reactions
    a) The nucleus of an atom does not change in an *ordinary* chemical reaction.
    b) A nuclear reaction is a reaction in which the nucleus undergoes change, as in the giving off of particles and energy.
    c) A nuclear change will influence the atomic number and mass number of any atoms undergoing such a change.
    d) All elements above atomic number 83 are unstable.
    e) Isotopes are different forms of the same element that have similar chemical properties but differ in atomic weight.
    f) Characteristic products are emitted from unstable nuclei: alpha particles, beta rays, and gamma rays.
  2. Uses in medicine
    a) Radioactive elements are called *radioisotopes* and give off alpha particles, gamma rays, and beta rays.
    b) ^{131}I is one of the most useful radioisotopes (one of its uses is to destroy cancerous thyroid cells).
    c) Radioactive chromate, ^{51}Cr, is used to investigate red blood cells
  3. Uses in research
    a) Radioisotopes are used to study how drugs act.
    b) Radioisotopes used as tracers have aided in research on cancer, blood-forming systems, iron metabolism, hormone activity, and liver and kidney function.

II. Gases Important in Medical Therapeutics and Physiology

A. Oxygen
  1. Importance
    a) Abundant in air, water, all vegetable matter, and in our bodies
    b) Necessary for conversion of chemical energy of foods and tissues into heat and energy

    2. Physiological importance
      a) Respiration
        (1) Combines with hemoglobin to circulate throughout the body
        (2) Is important in oxidation of organic substances (sugars, fats)
      b) Hypoxia—oxygen lack
      c) Asphyxia—decrease in the amount of O_2 and increase in the amount of CO_2 in the body due to interference with respiration
    3. Uses in medicine
      a) Anesthesia—mixed with anesthetic gases to prevent asphyxia
      b) Therapeutics
        (1) Administered in hypoxia caused by any impediment to respiration, as in bronchial asthma, pneumonia, emphysema, etc.
        (2) Used as high-pressure oxygen in some illnesses
      c) Diagnostics—computing the basal metabolic rate

B. Nitrogen—physiological importance
    1. Essential to life for rebuilding tissue
    2. Generally found only in compounds that are transformed into protein and that, after being consumed, are metabolized into animal protein; the waste products are eliminated from the body in the form of urea, creatinine, and ammonia

C. Carbon Dioxide—physiological importance
    1. Is mainly a waste product, as the end product of carbon combustion
    2. Is useful as an indicator of the state of acidosis or of alkalosis of the body, i.e., CO_2-combining power
    3. In tiny amounts, stimulates respiration

III. Water

A. Occurrence
    1. Most abundant compound
    2. Universal solvent

B. Physiological importance
    1. Constituent of all tissues and protoplasm
    2. Constituent of every body fluid
    3. Lubricant
    4. Temperature regulator
    5. Aid in digestion

IV. Solutions

A. Composition
    1. Solute, the dissolved substance, which may be either
      a) Solid
      b) Gas
      c) Liquid
    2. Solvent, the dissolving substance, which may be either
      a) Solid
      b) Gas
      c) Liquid

Note: Water is often called the "universal solvent" because many things dissolve in it. However, fats and oils will not dissolve in water but will dissolve in alcohol, ether, or carbon tetrachloride.

B. Examples of Solutions
  1. Solid in water solution—sugar dissolved in water
  2. Gas in liquid solution—ginger ale
  3. Solid in solid solution—brass

C. Concentrations of Solutions—affected by proportion of solute dissolved in solvent
  1. The greater the solute by proportion in the solvent, the more concentrated the solution.
  2. The lesser the solute by proportion, the weaker the solution.
  3. A saturated solution is a solution that holds all the solute that it can normally hold at a given temperature, e.g., saturated solution of potassium iodide.
  4. An unsaturated solution does not hold all the solute it can normally hold at a given temperature.
  5. A supersaturated solution holds more solute than it can normally hold at a given temperature.

D. Application of Physical Chemistry to Solutions
  1. Osmosis
    a) The passage of a solvent through a membrane that separates solutions of different concentrations
    b) The passage of pure solvent from the lesser to the greater concentration when two solutions are separated by a membrane that is permeable to the solvent
  2. Diffusion
    a) The movement of solutions or gases from an area of high to an area of low concentration (see Figure 2)

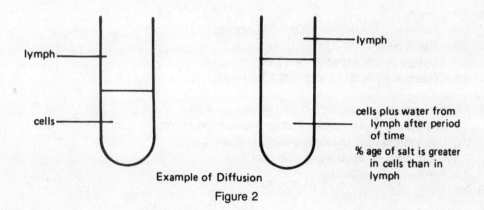

Example of Diffusion

Figure 2

  3. Filtration
    a) The passage of a solution through a membrane resulting from greater pressure on one side of the membrane
    b) The filtration of constituents of the blood through the walls of the capillaries into Bowman's capsule—glomerular fluid

E. Examples of Solutions Used Therapeutically in Medicine
  1. 5% Glucose in water—used for intravenous therapy
  2. Ringer's solution
    a) Contains the salts of the blood in exactly the same proportions that they occur in the blood
    b) Is used to combat dehydration and to replace necessary salts in the body tissues

    3. Isotonic saline
      a) Used for intravenous or intramuscular injections
      b) Used for irrigations or soaks

V. Acids

A. Properties
1. Liberate hydrogen ions (H+) in solution
2. Taste sour
3. Cause litmus paper to turn red
4. React with metals to form hydrogen gas and a salt
5. React with bases to form salts and water

B. Importance
1. Gastric juice has hydrochloric acid.
2. Acids of gastric juice must be neutralized in a patient who suffers from gastric ulcer.
3. Amino acids are the end product of protein digestion.
4. Severe acidosis is the result of untreated and uncontrolled diabetes mellitus.
5. Colostomy patients must have their skin protected against the leakage of gastric juice because of its corrosive action on skin.
6. Acidic douches are used to counteract the effect of alkalinity in certain vaginal infections.
7. Many antiseptics used in medicine are mild acids.

VI. Bases

A. Properties
1. Liberate hydroxyl ions (OH−) in solution
2. Taste bitter
3. Cause litmus paper to turn blue
4. React with acids to form salts and water

B. Importance
1. Are used in therapeutics to counteract the acidosis in diabetes mellitus
2. Include certain basic gels used in gastric ulcer
3. Are used as antidote in acid burns

VII. Salts

A. Properties
1. Have salty taste (seawater)
2. Aqueous solutions—have no effect on litmus paper or may turn it red or blue
3. React with acids, bases, or other salts to form another salt

B. Importance in Medicine
1. Isotonic sodium chloride (0.9%) is used for intravenous and/or intramuscular injections, wet compresses, etc.
2. Solutions of other salts, such as aluminum acetate (Burrow's solution), are used for compresses in skin diseases.
3. Salts help maintain the proper acid-base balance in the body.
4. Some salts are used to replace those lost during diuretic therapy.
5. Some salts are used to replace those lost during diarrhea.
6. Some salts are used to replace those lost during severe burns.

BASIC SCIENCES

VIII. Acid-Base Balance

A. Importance
1. Acid-base balance depends upon pH of blood.
2. pH expresses the degree to which a solution is acidic or basic.
3. pH of 7 is neutral (neither acidic or basic).
4. pH less than 7 is acidic.
5. pH more than 7 is basic (alkaline).
6. pH of blood plasma is 7.39.
7. pH of pancreatic juice is 10.0.
8. pH of gastric juice is 1.0-1.3.

B. Changes
1. Excessive loss of base or mineral—acidosis
    a) Diarrhea
    b) Uncontrolled diabetes
2. Excessive loss of hydrochloric acid (HCl)—alkalosis
    a) Persistent vomiting
    b) Prolonged administration of alkalies in treatment of peptic ulcer

UNIT 2: MICROBIOLOGY

VOCABULARY

aerobe	organism requiring oxygen for growth
anaerobe	organism not requiring oxygen for growth (found in deep wounds such as stab wounds)
antibiotics	organic metabolic wastes of living organisms that, in minute amounts, are destructive of certain microorganisms
antiseptic	agent that combats sepsis
bacteriocidal	capable of killing bacteria
bacteriostatic	inhibiting growth of bacteria
chlorophyll	green coloring matter in plants; important in photosynthesis
culture	growth of microorganisms on a medium
disinfectant	agent that kills bacteria
fermentation	decomposition of carbohydrates by bacterial action
filtration	removal of impurities by passing through a filter (any porous material)
fluorescent	having one color by transmitted light and another by reflected light
medium (pl. media)	substance used for cultivation of microorganisms
pathogenic	disease-producing
serology	science that studies serum reactions, diagnosis, and treatment
spore	minute, thick-walled, round or oval body containing entire cell contents in condensed form and highly resistant to heat, chemical disinfectants, sunlight, and drying, e.g., *Bacillus anthracis* (anthrax bacillus) and *Clostridium tetani* (tetanus bacillus)
sporicidal	capable of destroying spores
vacuum	space depleted of air

I. **Introduction**

A. Definition of **Microbiology:** Study of living organisms so small that they are visible only through a microscope

B. Importance
   1. Knowledge of method of transfer of microorganisms will aid in preventing spread of disease
   2. Knowledge of sterilization and disinfection will assist in protecting both nurse and patient
   3. Knowledge of immunity teaches importance of immunization for prevention of specific diseases

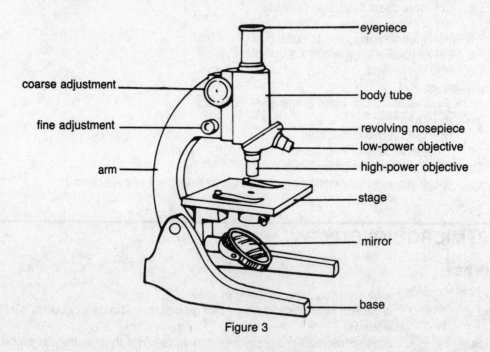

Figure 3

C. The Microscope
   1. Magnifies objects too small to be seen by naked eye
   2. Is used in medicine to study
      a) Microorganisms
      b) Blood cells
      c) Tissues
   3. Types
      a) Simple microscope—magnifying glass—magnifies 5 to 20 times
      b) Compound microscope—consists of three principal lens groups and a reflecting mirror—magnifies up to 1000 times
      c) Electron microscopic
         (1) Used to view objects too small to be seen with optical microscope
         (2) Uses beams of electrons instead of beams of light
         (3) Magnifies 200 times more than the optical microscope (over 1,000,000 times)

II. Classification of Microorganisms

A. Unicellular Microorganisms
   1. Bacteria
   2. Protozoa
   3. True fungi
   4. Rickettsiae

B. Multicellular Microorganisms
1. Flatworms (flukes, tapeworms)
2. Roundworms (pinworms, hookworms, etc.)

C. Noncellular Infective Agents (Viruses)

III. Identification of Microorganisms

A. Morphology (size and shape)

B. Staining Properties
1. Gram's method—positive or negative
2. Acid-fast stain

C. Growth on Culture Media

D. Culturing Characteristics
1. Aerobic or anaerobic
2. Fast or slow growing
3. Isolated colonies or bunched-up colonies

E. Serological Tests

F. Biochemical Tests

G. Pathogenicity—tests on laboratory animals

IV. Bacteria

A. Characteristics
1. Can be pathogenic or nonpathogenic
2. Are one-celled organisms
3. Reproduce principally by binary fission
4. Can be spore-formers or non-spore-formers
5. Are classified according to their shape
6. Can be seen only with a microscope
7. Can be identified in the laboratory by various isolation methods
   a) Gram's method
   b) Pure culture
8. Can be destroyed by chemicals and/or heat
   Spore formers resistant to heat, e.g., *Bacillus anthracis* and *Clostridium tetani*
9. Can confer immunity

B. Classifications
1. Rods—variable motility (see Figure 4)
   a) Non-spore-forming (included are organisms of typhoid, parathyphoid, dysentery, urinary tract infection and epidemic diarrhea, plague, chancroid, pertussis, influenza, and tularemia; all are gram-negative)
   b) Spore-forming (all are gram-positive and motile except *Clostridium perfringens;* of special interest are *Clostridium tetani* and *Bacillus anthracis*)

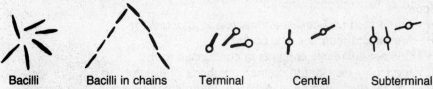

| Bacilli | Bacilli in chains | Terminal | Central | Subterminal |

Bacilli showing spores

Figure 4

2. Cocci (s. coccus)—round or spherical bacteria that have characteristic cell arrangements (see Figure 5)
   a) Diplococci—grow in pairs, e.g., pneumococci (in cause of pneumonia)
   b) Staphylococci—grow in grapelike clusters (the cause of pimples and boils)
   c) Streptococci—grow in chains (the cause of strep throat)

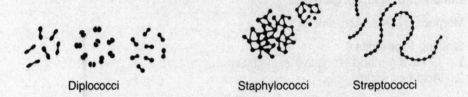

Diplococci   Staphylococci   Streptococci

Figure 5

3. Helical, flexible bacteria (spirochetes)
   a) *Treponema*
   b) *Borrelia*
   c) *Leptospira*
4. Bacteria (see Figure 6)
   (1) Mycoplasma—cause of urethritis, arthritis, etc.
   (2) Atypical pneumonia
5. Minute bacteria—obligate intracellular parasites
   a) Rickettsia
   b) *Coxiella*
   c) *Chlamydia*

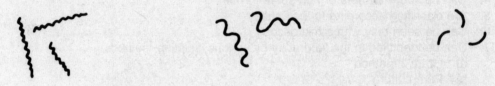

Flexible bacteria   Vibrio comma
                                                     (nonflexible)

Figure 6

C. Structure of Bacteria
   1. Capsule that surrounds bacterium
      a) Consists of gummy film made up of carbohydrates
      b) Is, in many species, toxic
      c) Gives type specificity to bacteria
      d) Increases virulence of bacteria (protects against leukocytes, drugs, antibodies, and the defense mechanisms of infected person)
   2. Spores
      a) Are formed by *Bacillus anthracis* and *Clostridium*
      b) Are minute round or oval bodies
      c) Contain entire cell contents in condensed form
      d) Are highly resistant to ordinary methods of disinfection
      e) Can be destroyed by autoclaving, intermittent sterilization, sporicidal gases (ethylene oxide)

3. Motility and flagella
   a) All spirochetes and many rod-shaped bacteria are motile.
   b) Motility is due to hairlike appendages (flagella).
   c) Flagella protein
      (1) Differs from protein of body of bacteria
      (2) Has immunological specificity
      (3) Is important in diagnosis

D. Reproduction
   1. Asexual
   2. Binary fission—results in two daughter cells

V. Rickettsia

A. Distinctive Patterns in Common
   1. Are closely related to bacteria
   2. Are minute in size as compared to bacteria
   3. Can grow only in living cells of other organisms
   4. Reproduce intracellularly (similar to viruses)
   5. Can be seen with ordinary microscope (unlike viruses)

B. Specific Diseases Caused by Rickettsia
   1. Typhoid fever—louse-borne
   2. Rocky Mountain spotted fever—tick-borne
   3. Trachoma, lymphogranuloma, parrot fever

C. Immunity—conferred by vaccine from killed rickettsia against typhus

VI. Viruses

A. Pathogenic Agents
   1. Are visible only with electron microscope
   2. Are parasitic (grow and multiply only on living cells)
   3. Are not true cells
   4. Have inclusion bodies
   5. Contain core of genetic and infective DNA *or* RNA (never both)
   6. Are filterable (pass readily through most filters that withhold ordinary bacteria)
   7. Can be retained by very-fine-pore plastic filters (membrane or molecular filters)
   8. Are not susceptible to currently known antibiotics
   9. Are susceptible *in vitro* to oxidizing agents, ultraviolet light, and heat

B. Bases for Classification
   1. Presence of RNA or DNA
   2. Resistance to heat
   3. Presence and type of inclusion bodies

C. Common Diseases Caused by Viruses
   1. Poliomyelitis
   2. Yellow fever
   3. Rabies—virus carried through infected saliva
   4. Measles (rubeola)
   5. German measles (rubella)
   6. Smallpox (low incidence due to global immunization program)

7. Mumps (infectious parotitis)
8. Influenza

VII. Fungi

A. Microorganisms
   1. Are plants without chlorophyll
   2. Reproduce sexually and asexually
      a) Some form spores
      b) Others develop daughter cells
   3. Thrive in warm, moist places
   4. Are parasitic or saprophytic
      a) Parasites
         (1) Feed on living tissue
         (2) Are usually harmful
         (3) Destroy living tissue
         (4) Cause diseases in humans
      b) Saprophytes
         (1) Feed on dead and decayed tissue
         (2) Are useful to humans

B. Uses
   1. Food
      a) Yeasts—used in baking
      b) Mushrooms—cultivated commercially (nonpoisonous)
   2. Medicine
      a) Penicillin and other antibiotics
      b) Vitamin and protein supplements

C. Pathogenic Fungi
   1. Produce lesions in mouth and vagina, on hands, nails, and face
   2. Cause lung disease resembling tuberculosis

VIII. Protozoa

A. Characteristics
   1. One-celled
   2. Larger than bacteria
   3. Found in stagnant water
   4. Identified by laboratory methods (staining, microscopic examination)

B. Pathogenic Protozoa
   1. Cause amebic dysentery
   2. Cause malaria, African sleeping sickness, and trichomoniasis (Trichomonas vaginalis)
   3. Are susceptible to tetracyclines and hydroxyquinolines

C. Prevention of Protozoal Infections
   1. Drainage of stagnant water sources
   2. Personal cleanliness (refers to carriers)
   3. Boiling of drinking water in dysentery-ridden countries
   4. Avoidance of fresh, unwashed fruits or vegetables in dysentery-ridden countries

BASIC SCIENCES

IX. **Parasitic Worms (Helminthes)**

    A. Characteristics
       1. Multicellular
       2. Macroscopic (can be seen with the naked eye)

    B. Two principal groups
       1. Flatworms (flukes and tapeworms)
         a) Are parasitic
         b) Infect specific organs, e.g., liver, intestines
         c) Infect humans either by direct penetration of skin (flukes) or through intestinal tract (tapeworms and flukes)
       2. Roundworms (hookworms, giant roundworms, whipworms, pinworms, *Trichina* worms)
         a) Are parasitic
         b) Infect specific organs, e.g., intestines, lymphatics, etc.
         c) Infect humans either by direct penetration of skin (hookworm), through ingestion, or though bite of insect (filaria)
         d) Can be controlled by
           (a) Control of insect vectors
           (b) Adequate cooking of pork
           (c) Personal cleanliness

X. **Sterilization and Disinfection**

    A. Importance
       1. Prevent infection
       2. Prevent spoilage of food and other materials
       3. Prevent contamination of pure cultures in laboratories

    B. Differences between Sterilization and Disinfection
       1. Sterilization
         a) Frees substance from all life
         b) Is accomplished by
           (1) Heat
           (2) Gases
           (3) Solutions of chemicals
           (4) Irradiation
           (5) Filtration
       2. Disinfection
         a) Kills or removes pathogenic organisms
         b) Is accomplished by
           (1) Chemicals
           (2) Heat (pasteurization)

XI. **Methods of Sterilization**

    A. Heat
       1. Moist heat (steam or boiling water)
         a) Boiling water
           (1) Destroys all living bacteria; spores are difficult to kill
           (2) Destroys cutting edges of instruments
           (3) Leaves scale deposits
           (4) Process hindered if articles not clean

        b) Steam under pressure (autoclave); air is removed to raise temperature of steam
           (1) Destroys all bacteria and spores
           (2) Is most desirable method of sterilization for most objects
           (3) Is used for saline solutions, surgical supplies, intravenous solutions, bandages, dressings, glassware
           (4) Is not used for oils, Vaseline, etc.
    2. Dry heat
        a) Hot air (dry-heat sterilizer, oven)
           (1) Is used for objects for which moist heat is inappropriate
           (2) Requires prolonged time
           (3) Is used only for small quantities of materials
        b) Cautery
           (1) Used to sterilize tissue surfaces (stump of appendix)
           (2) Not used for instruments
        c) Burning and flaming
           (1) Involves direct application of flame
           (2) Is generally used in laboratories

  B. Filtration
    1. Used to sterilize serums, toxins, antitoxins, bacterial filtrates, and viruses
    2. Used in water purification

  C. Radiant Energy
    1. Sunlight—not adequate for modern methods
    2. Ultraviolet light
        a) Extended exposure is injurious to eyes, skin, and tissues.
        b) There are limitations to this method.
    3. Infrared rays

  D. Chemical Method (more accurately called *disinfection*)
    1. Factors of importance relating to this method
        a) Cleanliness—cleansing with soap and water preliminary
        b) Concentration of solution
        c) Time—depends on type of chemical, its strength, and nature of bacteria
        d) Temperature—generally room temperature
        e) Organisms—some organisms resistant, i.e., spores, viruses, tubercle bacilli
    2. Use
        a) Is used only when heat sterilization of objects is not practical
        b) Must be used in weak solutions in wounds and on skin

XII. Destruction of Bacteria

  A. Importance
    1. Relates to sterilization, disinfection, bacteriostasis, antibiosis
    2. Prevents serious complications as result of bacteria in wounds
    3. Promotes uncomplicated healing of wounds as result of surgery and/or other causes (sterilization of materials used)

  B. Methods of Destruction (see Section XI, Methods of Sterilization)

XIII. Staining Methods

  A. Gram's Method
    1. Bacteria are distinguished by their ability to hold or lose a violet-iodine combination dye (Gram's stain) in the presence of a decolorizing agent (see Data Summary 1).

a) Gram-positive bacteria hold the violet dye.
b) Gram-negative bacteria lose the violet dye and take on the red counterstain.
2. Some bacteria are intermediate and will appear gram-positive or gram-negative.
a) Depends on age of cells
b) Depends on chemical factors such as pH and kind of medium

B. Ziehl-Neelsen Method (Acid-Fast)
1. Acid-fast bacteria absorb red carbolfuchsin dye and hold the dye against acidified alcohol solution.
2. Non-acid-fast bacteria lose the carbolfuchsin dye and take a contrasting counterstain such as yellow picric acid.
3. Organisms of tuberculosis, leprosy, and some saprophytes such as the smegma bacillus are examples of acid-fast bacteria.

DATA SUMMARY 1
Gram-Stain Reactions of Some Common Bacteria

Gram-positive	*Gram-negative*
All streptococci	Gonococcus
All staphylococci	Meningococcus
Pneumococci	Typhoid, paratyphoid, *Escherichia coli* (enteric bacilli)
Diphtheria bacilli	Organisms of influenza, pertussis
All acid-fast bacilli	Cholera, chancroid
All spore-forming anaerobes	

UNIT 3: PHARMACOLOGY

VOCABULARY

drug any substance used to prevent or cure disease
official drugs—those listed in the *United States Pharmacopeia (USP)* or in the *National Formulary (NF)*
nonofficial drugs—those not listed in *USP* or *NF*

pharmacology science that deals with actions of drugs on living systems
pharmacy science of compounding and dispensing drugs
poison substance that injures body cells
therapeutics treatment of disease
toxicology study of poisons and their actions

I. Introduction

A. Listings of Drugs
1. *United States Pharmacopeia*
a) Is compiled and periodically revised by a committee
b) Lists all official drugs
c) Describes sources, chemical properties, dosages, formulae, and methods of compounding
2. *National Formulary*
a) Is published by the American Pharmaceutical Association
b) Lists drugs not in the *USP*

3. *New Drugs*
    a) Is published annually by the American Medical Association
    b) Lists and includes new drugs acceptable to the AMA
4. *Physicians' Desk Reference (PDR)*
    a) Is published by drug manufacturers to promote their drugs
    b) Lists drugs according to action under manufacturers' names

B. Drug Legislation
    1. Federal
        a) Controlled Substances Act of 1970 regulates the use and handling of narcotics, hallucinogens, and CNS depressants.
        b) Drug Enforcement Agency controls distribution of habit-forming drugs.
        c) Food, Drug and Cosmetic Act controls distribution of drugs in interstate commerce.
    2. State—local laws in force regarding dispensing of drugs

C. Drug Standardization
    1. Purity
    2. Strength
    3. Dosage

D. Drug Terminology
    1. Chemical name identifies the chemical compound.
    2. Generic name is official name assigned by producer.
    3. Brand or trade name is copyrighted name assigned by producer.

II. Classification of Drugs

A. Origins
    1. Plants—leaves, bark, or roots (opium, digitalis, castor oil, mustard)
    2. Animal—glandular secretions (hormones, serums, gamma globulin)
    3. Minerals—iron, calcium, zinc (ferrous sulfate, calcium gluconate, zinc oxide)
    4. Synthesis—chemical compounds (sulfonamides)
    5. Microorganisms (penicillin, streptomycin)

B. Actions
    1. Local (drugs that act on skin and mucous membranes and are usually applied directly) Antiseptics, antibiotics, local anesthetics, etc. (iodine, penicillin, benzocaine)
    2. Systemic
        a) Central nervous system
            (1) Stimulants—increase activity of brain and spinal cord (caffeine)
            (2) Depressants—decrease activity of brain and spinal cord (morphine)
            (3) Hypnotics—induce sleep (chloral hydrate)
            (4) Anticonvulsants—reduce involuntary convulsive movements (Dilantin)
            (5) Anesthetics—produce loss of sensitivity to pain (Novocain)
        b) Cardiovascular system
            (1) Heart stimulants—increase action of heart (adrenaline)
            (2) Heart tonics—strengthen and slow heart beat (digitalis)
            (3) Heart depressants—decrease heart beat (quinidine)
            (4) Vasoconstrictors—produce narrowing of blood vessels, increase blood pressure (Levophed)
            (5) Vasodilators—increase size of blood vessels (nitroglycerin)

      (6)   Coagulants—increase process of coagulation (vitamin K)

      (7)   Anticoagulants—suppress formation of blood clots (Coumadin)

c)   Respiratory system

      (1)   Stimulants—increase rate and depth of respiration (carbon dioxide)

      (2)   Depressants—decrease and deepen respirations (morphine)

      (3)   Bronchodilators—relax and dilate bronchi (aminophylline)

      (4)   Sedative cough mixture—reduce irritation and lessen desire to cough (Cheracol)

      (5)   Expectorants—induce expectoration by increasing secretion of mucus in respiratory tract (potassium iodide)

      (6)   Specific antibiotics for pulmonary tuberculosis—effective in destroying tubercle bacilli (streptomycin, isoniazid hydrochloride, para-aminosalicylic acid)

d)   Gastrointestinal

      (1)   Antacids—counteract gastric acidity (Amphojel)

      (2)   Digestants—aid process of digestion; usually replace substances normally found in digestive tract (hydrochloric acid)

      (3)   Emetics—induce vomiting (apomorphine)

      (4)   Antiemetics—relieve nausea and vomiting (Dramamine)

      (5)   Cathartics—act to empty the colon (cascara sagrada)

      (6)   Antidiarrhetics—soothe intestinal tract and quiet an overactive bowel (Kaopectate)

e)   Urinary system

      (1)   Diuretics—increase flow of urine (Diuril)

      (2)   Urinary antiseptics—control minor infections of urinary tract (Mandelamine)

f)   Reproductive system

      (1)   Uterine stimulants—increase contractions of uterine muscles (ergotamine tartrate)

      (2)   Uterine sedatives—decrease uterine contractions; antiabortives (Lutrexin)

      (3)   Emmenagogues—induce or increase menstruation (progesterone)

      (4)   Local drugs to treat vaginal infections (Sporostacin)

g)   Musculoskeletal system

      (1)   Analgesics—relieve pain (aspirin)

      (2)   Muscle relaxants—diminish muscular spasms (liniments, locally; systemic relaxants—Robaxin)

h)   Blood

    Hematinics—increase the production of hemoglobin and red blood cells (ferrous sulfate)

i)   Antiinfectives

      (1)   Antibiotics—kill or inhibit growth of microorganisms; produced by molds, bacteria, or yeasts; e.g., penicillin—effective against gram-positive organisms; streptomycin—effective against gram-negative organisms; tetracyclines—have broad-spectrum activity but prolonged use can lead to development of fungal infections in intestinal tract

      (2)   Antifungal drugs—treat fungal infections (Nystatin, Griseofulvin)

j)   Chemotherapeutics (chemical reagents)

      (1)   Chemotherapeutics inhibit growth of bacteria and other microorganisms (sulfonamides).

      (2)   Cancer chemotherapeutics are used in the palliative treatment of symptoms of inoperable cancer (Fluoracil).

k)   Antiallergenics

    Antihistamines counteract the effects of histamines, thereby relieving the symptoms of simple allergic reactions; may cause drowsiness and other side effects (Benadryl, Chlor-trimeton, Dramamine, Phenergan).

l) Endocrine drugs
   (1) Secretions from the endocrine glands enter directly into blood, are carried by blood to various organs of body, and directly affect certain activities of organs.
   (2) Pituitary gland secretes trophic hormones from anterior lobe.
       (a) Thyrotrophic hormone affecting thyroid gland (Levothyroxine)
       (b) Adrenocorticotrophic hormone (ACTH) affecting cortex of adrenal gland
   (3) Pituitrin from posterior lobe of pituitary stimulates uterine contractions.
   (4) Thyroid gland secretes thyroxine.
   (5) Adrenal gland secretes cortical hormones (cortisone and hydrocortisone, used as anti-inflammatory agents) and medullary hormones (epinephrine, or adrenaline).
   (6) Pancreas secretes insulin from islands of Langerhans (small clusters of cells located on surface of pancreas).
       (a) Insulin given by subcutaneous injection only (poorly absorbed by muscle tissue—destroyed by gastric juice)
       (b) Available in strengths of U40 and U100 (U40: 40 units of insulin per ml of solution); one phamaceutical company makes a strength of U500, available in pork insulin only.

DATA SUMMARY 2
Insulin Sources and Activities

Type of Preparation	Source	Strength	Onset	Activity Peak	Duration
Rapid-acting	Beef Pork Human	U40 U100	15–30 min	2–4 hr	6–8 hr
Rapid-acting (semilente)			1–2 hr	4–9 hr	10–16 hr
Intermediate-acting (NPH and lente)	Beef Pork Human	U40 U100	1–3 hr	6–12 hr	18–26 hr
Long-acting (ultralente and PZI)	Beef Pork	U40 U100	4–8 hr	14–24 hr	28–36 hr

---

m) Tranquilizers and antidepressants
   (1) Tranquilizers—calm emotions without depressing central nervous system (Equanil, Librium)
   (2) Antidepressants—help overcome severe depression due to emotional disturbances (Ritalin, Tofranil, Lithium)
3. Therapeutic (effective in the treatment of disease)
   a) Antiseptics and disinfectants
      (1) Antiseptic—inhibits growth and development of microorganisms (70% alcohol)
      (2) Disinfectant—destroys microorganisms (Betadine)
   b) Analgesic—relieves pain without loss of consciousness (aspirin)
   c) Anesthetic—local produces loss of sensation without loss of consciousness; general produces loss of consciousness (procaine hydrochloride or ether)
   d) Stimulant—causes an increase in activity of an organ or system (caffeine)

e) Sedative, tranquilizer, hypnotic
   (1) Sedative—quiets without producing sleep except in large doses (phenobarbital)
   (2) Tranquilizer—relieves tension and anxiety without producing sleep (Librium)
   (3) Hypnotic—produces sleep (phenobarbital)
f) Anti-inflammatories—corticosteroids
g) Antifungals—Griseofulvin
h) Astringents—Burrow's solution
i) Counterirritants (mustard)
j) Emollients and protectives (mineral oil)
k) Antacids (aluminum hydroxide)
l) Antiemetics (Tigan)
m) Antipyretics (aspirin)
n) Anthelmintics (Riperzine citrate)
o) Antiparasitics (chloroquine)
p) Antiluetics (penicillin, bismuth)
q) Cancer chemotherapeutics (Fluoracil)
r) Cathartics (castor oil, Dulcolax)
s) Diuretics (Hydrodiuril, Diuril, Mercuhydrin)
t) Vasoconstrictors (Ergotamine)

III. Preparation of Drugs

A. Solids for Internal Use
   1. Pills—small, round masses that are to be swallowed whole and cannot be broken for smaller doses
   2. Tablets—small, flat masses that are scored so that they can be broken into halves or quarters
   3. Capsules—drugs placed in a gelatinous shell and swallowed whole
   4. Powders—drugs ground and used in powder form
   5. Troche—drug formed in a flat disk that is held in the mouth
   6. Suppositories—semisolid substances shaped like a cylinder or cone, made of soap, gelatin, or cocoa butter, containing a drug for introduction into vagina, rectum, or urethra (melts at body temperature)

B. Solids for External Use
   1. Ointments or salves—drugs incorporated in specific quantities in petroleum jelly, lanolin, or lard
   2. Pastes—moist, doughy substances to which medication is added in specific quantities

C. Liquids for Internal Use
   1. Solution—liquid containing dissolved drugs
   2. Elixir—drug dissolved in solution containing water, alcohol, sugar, and flavoring
   3. Spirit—alcoholic solution of volatile drug
   4. Tincture—alcoholic solution of drug
   5. Fluid extract—concentrated fluid preparation of drug
   6. Emulsion—mixture of liquids that do not dissolve in each other

D. Liquids for External Use
   1. Tinctures
   2. Lotions—soothing solutions
   3. Liniments—solutions that act as counterirritants

IV. Nursing Concepts Associated with Medication
Note: **The administration of drugs** is one of the most important duties of a nurse and must be performed with utmost accuracy.

A. General Rules
1. Give medication only on written order of physician.
2. Read physician's order carefully.
3. Measure dose ordered accurately, using measuring spoon or glass.
4. Give correct drug to correct patient.
5. Administer drug at correct time.
6. Use correct route of administration.
7. Read label three times—*before pouring, while pouring, and after pouring.*
8. Observe patient swallowing oral medication.
9. Do not use medications from unmarked or illegibly marked containers.
10. Know side effects of drug administered.
11. Do not leave medications in patient's room.
12. Do not mix drugs without an order to do so.
13. Observe medications for changes in color, odor, or texture.
14. Chart if medication is not given, or is not given at proper time.
15. Chart given medications immediately.
16. Report and chart any untoward side effects.

B. Prescriptions
1. Written order to pharmacist for dispensing drug(s) to patient signed by physician or dentist
2. Parts
    a) Name and location of patient
    b) Date on which it was written
    c) Rx symbol
    d) Names, strengths, and quantities of drugs
    e) Instructions to pharmacist
    f) Instructions to patient
    g) Signature of physician
    h) Physician's DEA number where required

V. Medication Administration in the Elderly

A. Factors Changing Drug Response
1. Body functions decline.
2. Metabolism of drugs is affected by aging.

B. Nursing Management
1. Note the following:
    a) Over-the-counter medications taken
    b) Amount of alcohol used
    c) Drugs not currently prescribed but still used
    d) Compliance with physician's orders
2. Be aware of the necessity for twice-a-year drug review.
3. Relieve patient's confusion about medications.
4. Be sure that patient can open container of oral medications.

C. Intramuscular Medications   See Section VII, Routes of Administration.

D. Intravenous Medications   See Section VII, Routes of Administration.

BASIC SCIENCES

VI. Medication Administration in Children

    A. Pediatric Dosage
        1. Clark's rule: Child's weight in pounds/150 × adult dose = child's dose
        2. Fried's rule: Child's age in months/150 = 1/10 of adult dose
        3. Young's rule: Age of child/age + 12 = 2/5 of adult dose

    B. Communication with Child
        1. Nurse must be truthful concerning medication.
        2. Medication should be explained to child.
        3. Medication can be disguised in food.
        4. Medication should not be used as punishment.

    C. Oral medications
        1. Infants—give by dropper or nipple
        2. Toddlers—give by spoon or medicine cup
        3. School age—use same techniques as for adult: pill or capsule put on back of tongue and swallowed with water or juice

    D. Intramuscular Medications   See Section VII, Routes of Administration.

    E. Intravenous Medications   See Section VII, Routes of Administration.

VII. Routes of Administration

    A. Local Administration
        1. Drug is applied directly to tissue, organ, or skin.
        2. Effect is at site of application.
        3. Forms are sprays, irrigations, wet dressings, compresses, painting, rubbing of ointment or lotion into skin.

    B. Oral Administration (P.O.)—most convenient method
        1. Drug is taken by mouth.
        2. Absorption may differ among patients.
        3. Absorption may be slow.
        4. Some drugs may be irritating and should be given with food or water.

    C. Injection
        1. Drug is introduced directly into body by various methods.
        2. In *subcutaneous* (s.c.) injection, drug is given at 45° angle into loose tissues under the skin.
            a) Small amounts of nonirritating drug given to avoid irritation and sloughing of tissues
            b) Usually given in outer aspects of upper arm or thigh or abdomen
            c) Area massaged very gently to help absorption (except with heparin)
        3. In *intradermal* injection, drug is given between layers of skin.
            a) Used for diagnostic tests
            b) Used for inoculations
            c) Used for local anesthesia
        4. In *Intramuscular* injection, drug is given at 90° angle into muscle.
            a) Used for irritating drugs or large amounts of fluid
            b) Usually given in upper, outer quadrant of gluteus maximus, deltoid, or lateral aspect of thigh (less danger of involving sensory nerves in these areas)

    5. In *intravenous* injection, drug is given directly into bloodstream through vein (given by physician).
       a) There is immediate and definite effect.
       b) Drug may be given through already-running venous drip.
       c) Medication and syringes are assembled by nurse for physician.

D. Rectal Administration
    1. Drug is administered directly into rectum.
    2. Absorption of many drugs is good.
    3. Dose is usually double amount of oral dose.
    4. Amount should be less than 4 ounces.
    5. Irritating drugs are dissolved in soothing vehicle to prevent peristalsis and to soothe rectal mucosa.

E. Sublingual Administration
    1. Drug is placed under tongue and held there until it dissolves.
    2. This method is generally used for nitroglycerin.

F. Inhalation
    1. Drug is inhaled directly through nose.
    2. Absorption is good because of large surface and excellent blood supply of lung.
    3. Action is rapid.
    4. Absorption ceases when administration is stopped.
    5. This method is used to administer gases and drugs in gaseous form.

VIII. Procedures for Preparing Drugs for Administration and for Instilling Eye and Ear Drugs

A. Oral Medications
    1. Review general rules.
    2. Check required equipment—medicine cards, tray, medicine glasses or cups, dropper, calibrated dropper or graduate, paper cups for water, drinking tubes, tongue blades, glass stirring rod, paper tissues, paper towels.
    3. Proceed as follows:
       a) Solid medications: Shake required number of pills, tablets, or capsules into container cap and transfer to medicine glass or cup.
       b) Liquid medications poured directly from bottle
         (1) Place cap upside-down on table.
         (2) Hold medicine glass so that calibration mark of prescribed amount is at eye level, and place thumbnail on mark.
         (3) Hold bottle label next to palm of hand and pour from side opposite label so that spillage will not obscure label.
       c) Liquid medications measured in drops
         (1) Draw up solution into dropper.
         (2) Count aloud correct number of drops into medicine glass.
         (3) Discard solution remaining in dropper.
         (4) Dilute measured medication with 15 cc of water.
       d) Powders or granules
         (1) Measure prescribed amount into medicine cup.
         (2) At bedside, add small amount of water and stir.
         (3) After patient takes medication, rinse medicine cup with small amount of water and give to patient.
       e) Sublingual medications
         (1) Have patient place medication under tongue.

        (2) Give no water.

        (3) Instruct patient not to swallow until taste of medication has gone.

    f) Troche

        (1) Instruct patient to hold troche in mouth and let it dissolve slowly.

        (2) Be aware that patient may swallow saliva.

    g) Medications with special requirements

        (1) Note special requirements.

        (2) Perform special requirements, such as taking patient's pulse before dispensing digitalis

        (3) Record finding next to patient's name

B. Injectable Medications
1. Review general rules.
2. Check required equipment on hypodermic tray—medicine cards, supply of germicidal wipes or a sterile container of 70% alcohol sponges, correct-size sterile syringe and correct-size sterile needle for each individual medication, ampule file, emergency drugs, waste receptacle.
3. Prepare prescribed injection.

    a) Prepare syringe and needle.

    b) Withdraw medication (protect needle by replacing sterile sheath).

    c) Put prepared syringe, alcohol sponges, and medicine card on small tray to take to bedside.

C. Instillation of Eye Drops
1. In adult

    a) Check orders and medication.

    b) Wash hands.

    c) Check eye dropper for defects.

    d) Squeeze to allow medication to come to tip.

    e) Prevent medication from flowing back into bulb end.

    f) Using forefinger, pull patient's lower lid down gently.

    g) Instruct patient to look upward.

    h) Drop medication into center of lower lid.

    i) Instruct patient to close eyes slowly.

    j) Wipe off excess solution with gauze square.

    k) Wash hands.

2. In newborn

    a) Check medication—1% silver nitrate.

    b) Place 2 drops in conjunctival sac of each eye.

D. Instillation of Ear Drops
1. In adult

    a) Pull outer ear upward and backward.

    b) Instill drops as ordered by physician.

2. In child

    a) Pull outer ear downward and backward.

    b) Instill drops as ordered by physician.

IX. Drug Measurement

A. The Apothecaries' System
1. Used in all English-speaking countries
2. Rapidly being superseded by the metric system

3. Quantities expressed in Roman numerals, except fractions of a grain, which are expressed fractionally (gr. ss or gr. 1/4)

```
TABLE OF WEIGHTS
60 grains = 1 dram
8 drams = 1 ounce
16 ounces = 1 pound

TABLE OF CAPACITIES
60 minims = 1 fluid dram
8 drams = 1 ounce
16 ounces = 1 pint
2 pints = 1 quart
4 quarts = 1 gallon
```

B. The Metric System
   1. Used generally worldwide
   2. Rapidly superseding apothecaries' system
   3. Quantities expressed as decimals

```
TABLE OF METRIC WEIGHTS
1.0 gram = unit of weight
1000.0 grams = 1 kilogram
0.001 gram = 1 milligram
```

DATA SUMMARY 3
Measuring System Equivalents

Apothecary	Metric	Household
Volume		
1 minim		1 drop
m.XV	1 cc	15 drops
m.LX	4 cc	1 teaspoon or 60 drops
1 fluid ounce	30 cc	2 tablespoons
8 fluid ounces	250 cc	1 cupful
16 fluid ounces	500 cc	1 pint
32 fluid ounces (1 qt)	1000 cc	1 quart
Weight		
1 grain (gr)	60.0 milligrams (mgm)	
15 grains	1 gram (gm)	
1 dram (dr)	4 grams	1 teaspoon
1 ounce (oz)	30 grams	2 tablespoons

UNIT 4: ANATOMICAL STRUCTURE AND FUNCTION OF THE HUMAN BODY

VOCABULARY

anatomy   science of the structure of the body and the relationships of its parts

conductivity   transmission of messages initiating from a stimulus in one part of the body to another part, thereby causing a response action

contractility   specialized ability of a cell to shorten upon receiving a voluntary or involuntary stimulus

excitability   ability to respond to any stimulus in the internal or external environment; the term **irritability** is used to describe this vital life process

excretion   process by which the body eliminates waste products

homeostasis   those processes that tend to maintain stability in the normal states of the organism

metabolism   sum total of all processes required to maintain life; the processes that build and repair are called **anabolism;** The processes that break down substance and produce heat and energy are called **catabolism**

reproduction   production or growth of new cells, including production of new beings

physiology   science of the functions of the living organism and its parts

I. Introduction

A. The Human Body
1. The body functions as an integrated whole, each part cooperating with one or more parts to carry out functions essential to the life processes of the total organism.
2. Practical nurse must be able to identify normal structure and functions of the body in order to recognize deviations.
3. Life processes and functions are carried out by one or more cells, tissues, organs, and systems in the body.

B. Anatomical Positions
1. Cranial—near the head, e.g., the cranial nerves
2. Caudal—near the end of the spine (tail region)
3. Ventral or anterior—near the front of the body
4. Dorsal or posterior—near the back of the body
5. Lateral—near the side of the body
6. Medial—near the midline or middle of the body
7. Superior—above

C. Body Cavities
1. Cranial cavity
   a) Is the space inside the skull
   b) Contains the brain
2. Spinal cavity
   a) Is the space inside the spinal column
   b) Contains the spinal cord
3. Chest or thoracic cavity
   a) Is enclosed by the ribs, sternum, and thoracic vertebrae
   b) Contains the lungs, heart, some blood vessels and nerves
   c) Is separated from the abdominal cavity by the diaphragm
4. Abdominal cavity
   a) Is below the chest cavity

   b) Contains the stomach, most of the intestines, liver, gallbladder, pancreas, appendix, spleen, aorta, venae cavae, and kidneys (lie under the lining of the cavity)
   5. Pelvic cavity
      a) Is not really separate from the abdominal cavity
      b) Contains the lowest part of the intestine, urinary bladder, and female reproductive organs

II. The Cell

A. Basic Living Microscopic Unit of the Body
   1. There are about 100 trillion cells of different sizes, shapes, and types, with a general plan of structure.
   2. Cells are composed of protoplasm.
   3. Cells are continuously bathed in extracellular fluid (the internal environment).
      a) Components of this fluid are exactly controlled.
      b) Regulation of this fluid is called *homeostasis.*
   4. Each cell is bound by a cell membrane.
   5. Each cell is capable of living as an individual unit.

Types of Cells

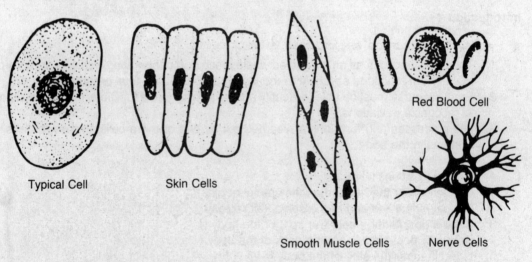

Typical Cell   Skin Cells   Smooth Muscle Cells   Nerve Cells   Red Blood Cell

Figure 7

B. Structure
   1. Two major parts (see Figure 7)
      (a) Nucleus near center of cell
         (1) Is surrounded by permeable membrane
         (2) Is filled with thick fluid containing
            (a) Proteins
            (b) Glucose
            (c) Electrolytes
         (3) Has 23 pairs of chromosomes called *genes*
         (4) Chromosomes are made up of nucleoproteins and deoxyribonucleic acid (DNA).
      b) Cytoplasm
         (1) Is surrounded by permeable membrane
         (2) Contains mitochondria, endoplasmic reticulum, and ribonucleic acid (RNA)

2. Reproduction
   a) Cell divides by mitosis to form two cells.
   b) New cells have same chromosomal content as parent cells.

C. Cell Metabolism
   1. Cell energy
      a) Energy is necessary for chemical reactions.
      b) Energy is derived from cellular respiration of carbohydrates, fats, and proteins of foods.
   2. Importance of protein in cell function
      a) All enzymes are proteins.
      b) Most of cell structure is protein.
      c) Genes control protein metabolism and cell function.
      d) Each gene is a molecule of deoxyribonucleic acid, DNA, which carries the genetic code.
   3. Formation of protein in the cytoplasm: protein is manufactured by ribonucleic acid (RNA).

D. Cell Membrane
   1. Cell membrane allows materials in solution to pass back and forth (osmosis).
   2. Oxygen and nutrients pass from blood into cell through membrane.
   3. Waste products pass from cell into blood.
   4. Cell membrane is very important to life of cell.

III. Tissues

A. Definition of Tissue: The grouping together of cells having similar structure and function

B. Classification
   1. Epithelial tissue (skin)
      a) Stratified epithelium (protection)
      b) Simple squamous epithelium (absorption)
   2. Connective tissue
      a) Types
         (1) Areolar (occupies interspaces of the body)
         (2) Fibrous (tendons, ligaments)
         (3) Cartilage (lines bones and joints), e.g., costal cartilages, knee joints
         (4) Adipose
      b) Function—connects one type of tissue to another and supports various body structures
   3. Muscular tissue
      a) Types
         (1) Skeletal or striated
            (a) Attaches to bones
            (b) Is voluntary—controlled by conscious effort
         (2) Cardiac or branching
            (a) Found only in heart
            (b) Striated but involuntary
         (3) Smooth
            (a) Forms walls of many internal organs: intestines, bladder, blood vessels
            (b) Is involuntary—not controlled by conscious effort
      b) Function—contraction

    4. Bone: hard form of connective tissue
       a) Types
          (1) Flat
          (2) Irregular
          (3) Short
          (4) Long
       b) Functions
          (1) Forms framework of the body
          (2) Serves as a storage place for mineral salts
          (3) Aids in the formation of blood cells
          (4) Surrounds and protects some vital organs
          (5) Provides points of attachment for the skeletal muscles

    5. Blood
       a) Types
          (1) Arterial or oxygenated blood—bright red
          (2) Venous or unoxygenated blood—dark red
       b) Functions
          (1) Transports nutrients and oxygen to tissues in all parts of body
          (2) Transports waste products from tissues to organs of excretion
          (3) Maintains body heat
          (4) Maintains body chemical balance
          (5) Defends against infection by action of leukocytes and antibodies

    6. Body Fluids
       a) Types
          (1) Extracellular—fluids outside the cells (tissue fluid)
          (2) Intracellular—fluids within the cell
       b) Characteristics
          (1) Contain electrolytes—maintain balance between intra- and extracellular fluids
          (2) Provide media for exchange of nutrients, oxygen, and cellular waste products by means of osmosis and/or diffusion
       c) Cerebrospinal fluid
          (1) Found in ventricles of brain and subarachnoid spaces
          (2) Cushions nervous system against blows to brain and spine
          (3) 400 ml secreted each day
          (4) Blockage of flow or excess secretion results in hydrocephalus.
       d) Ocular fluid
          (1) Fluid in eyes helps to keep normal dimensions between ocular elements.
          (2) Behind lens is vitreous humor.
          (3) In front of lens is aqueous humor.
          (4) Rate of fluid absorption determines pressure—normal is 19 mm Hg; excessive rise in pressure (30–80 mm Hg) is glaucoma.

    7. Nervous tissue
       a) Consists of nerve cells and their processes
       b) Serves as a pathway for nerve impulses
       c) Types of nerve cells
          (1) Sensory neurons—transmit impulses to brain and spinal cord
          (2) Motor neurons—transmit impulses away from brain and out to muscles and glands
          (3) Central neurons—transmit impulses from sensory neurons to motor neurons

IV. Organs

  A. Structure—different types of specialized tissues group together to form organs.

BASIC SCIENCES

B. Function
  1. Each organ has a specific function or functions.
  2. Organs do not work independently but function in conjunction with others.

V. Systems

A. Structure and Functions
  1. Systems are formed by groups of organs (see Data Summary 4).
  2. Systems perform specialized work in the body.

B. Types
  1. Skeletal—forms the body framework
  2. Muscular—makes movement of the body possible
  3. Circulatory
    a) Consists of heart, blood, and blood vessels
    b) Transports nutrients, water, oxygen, and waste products
  4. Lymphatic
    a) Minute lymphatic capillaries
      (1) Are present in almost all tissues
      (2) Lead into progressively larger lymphatic channels
      (3) Finally converge on thoracic duct
    b) Thoracic duct
      (1) Passes upward through chest
      (2) Empties into venous system at juncture of internal carotid and subclavian veins
  5. Digestive
    a) Consists of mouth, salivary glands, pharynx, esophagus, stomach, intestines, liver, gallbladder, and pancreas
    b) Liquifies and absorbs food and eliminates solid wastes
  6. Respiratory
    a) Consists of nose, pharynx, larynx, trachea, bronchi, bronchioles, lungs
    b) Takes in oxygen and eliminates carbon dioxide
  7. Urinary
    a) Consists of kidneys, ureters, urinary bladder, urethra
    b) Eliminates liquid wastes from body
  8. Reproductive
    a) Consists of ovaries, fallopian tubes, uterus, vagina, breasts, testes, accessory glands to testes, penis
    b) Functions in cooperation with the endocrine system to produce new living organisms
  9. Nervous
    a) Consists of brain, spinal cord, nerves
    b) Controls activities of muscular systems
    c) Controls functions of internal organs
    d) Enables humans to think and to regulate environment
  10. Endocrine
    a) Consists of ductless glands
    b) Secretes hormones directly into bloodstream
  11. Skin—is both organ and system
    a) Functions
      (1) Protection
      (2) Excretion

(3) Regulation of body temperature
(4) Production of vitamin D upon exposure to sunshine
b) Composition
    (1) Epidermis (outer layer)
        (a) Protects layers underneath
        (b) Contains pigment that varies among individuals
        (c) Has no blood supply
    (2) Dermis (true skin) (inner layer)
        (a) Has nerve endings that give sense of touch, pressure, pain, heat and cold
        (b) Regulates size of capillaries
    (3) Hair
    (4) Sebaceous glands
    (5) Sudoriferous glands
    (6) Nails
    (7) Hair

DATA SUMMARY 4
The Body's Systems

Skin (integumentary)	Epidermis Dermis Nails	Hair Sudoriferous glands Sebaceous glands
Skeletal system	Bones Joints	
Muscular system	Striated muscles Smooth muscles	
Nervous system	Brain Spinal cord	Special senses Nerves
Circulatory system	Heart Blood vessels	Blood
Lymphatic system	Spleen Lymph glands	Thoracic duct Lymphatic vessels
Respiratory system	Nose Larynx Trachea	Bronchi Lungs Pleura
Digestive system	Mouth Teeth Tongue Esophagus Stomach Small Intestine duodenum jejunum ileum	Large Intestine (colon) appendix ascending colon transverse colon descending colon sigmoid colon rectum anus Liver Gallbladder Pancreas (also part of endocrine system)

BASIC SCIENCES

DATA SUMMARY 4 Continued

Urinary system	Kidneys	
	Ureters	
	Urinary bladder	
	Urethra	

Reproductive system	*Male*	*Female*
	Testes	Ovaries
	Epididymis	Uterine tubes
	Vas deferens	Uterus
	Seminal ducts	Vagina
	Seminal vesicles	Bartholin glands
	Ejaculatory ducts	Vulva
	Urethra	Mammary glands
	Prostate gland	
	Scrotum	
	Penis	
	Spermatic cord	

Endocrine system	Thyroid gland	Pancreas
	Parathyroid glands (4)	Thymus gland
	Adrenal or suprarenal glands (2)	Pineal gland
	cortex	
	medulla	
	Pituitary gland	
	anterior lobe	
	posterior lobe	
	Testes (2) also in male reproductive system	
	Ovaries (2) also in female reproductive system	

UNIT 5: NUTRITION

Vocabulary

anabolism	the building up of complex substances from simpler substances, e.g., building new bone or hemoglobin or muscle tissue
catabolism	the breaking down of complex substances; breakdown of glucose to yield heat and energy
cellulose	fibrous form of carbohydrate constituting supporting framework of plants; it is not ordinarily chemically changed or absorbed in digestion
dietetics	application of the science of nutrition to the feeding of people
enzyme	protein substance that acts on specific substances without being changed itself
fiber	part of food that is indigestible
food	substance that nourishes the body
glycogen	animal starch; form in which carbohydrate is stored in the body for future conversion to glucose
hormone	substance produced by ductless glands in one part of the body and carried by the blood to act on substances in another part of the body

metabolism   sum total of all the changes that take place in the body
nutrition   sum total of all the processes in the body for making use of nutrients

I. **Nutrients**

  A. Requirements for Balanced Diet and Adequate Nutrition
     1. Has recommended daily dietary allowances
     2. Consists of basic-four food groups
        a) Milk group
           (1) Children and teenagers—equivalent of 3-4 cups daily
           (2) Adults—equivalent of 2 cups daily
              (a) Pregnant women—3 cups daily
              (b) Lactating women—4 cups daily
        b) Meat group—2 or more servings daily
        c) Vegetable-fruit group—4 or more servings daily
        d) Bread-cereal group
        e) Small amount of oil daily

  B. Importance of Balanced Diet
     1. Individual nutrients are responsible for definite vital functions.
     2. All nutrients depend on each other to perform their activities.
     3. Depletion in one nutrient will decrease the effect of the others.
     4. Balanced diet is important to the preschool child.
        a) Rate of growth is very rapid.
        b) Child is very active.
        c) Metabolism is very high.
        d) Nutritional habits are formed at this time.
     5. Balanced diet is important to the school-age child.
        a) Child is growing.
        b) "Junk foods" decrease child's appetite.
        c) Nourishing breakfast gives energy to start day.
     6. Balanced diet is important to the pubertal child.
        a) Rapid growth, both physical and emotional
        b) Concerns about weight control and developing physical strength
        c) Need to stimulate red blood cell formation in girls to replace blood lost in menstruation
     7. Balanced diet is important to the woman of childbearing years.
        a) Physical health and well-being of fetus are affected by diet of mother during pregnancy.
        b) Adequate protein is very important.
        c) Minerals such as iron, calcium, iodine are necessary.
     8. Balanced diet is important to the elderly.
        a) Decreased caloric requirements
        b) Need for high protein for repair of tissues
        c) Poor appetite due to ill-fitting dentures, loneliness, etc.
        d) Ethnicity and superstitions relating to food

  C. Carbohydrates
     1. Are composed of carbon, hydrogen, and oxygen
     2. Include starches, sugars, grains, vegetables, and fruits
     3. Provide quickest form of energy for human body
     4. Make up about 50% of the American diet and a greater percentage among the poor
     5. Yield 4 calories per gram when metabolized

6. Serve three functions:
   a) Provide energy and heat
   b) Spare protein for building and maintaining the tissues
   c) Help in the normal oxidation of fats
7. Are divided into three principal groups:
   a) Monosaccharides (single sugars)
      (1) Require no digestion
      (2) Are found abundantly in fruits and vegetables
      (3) Consist of glucose and fructose
   b) Disaccharides (double sugars)
      (1) Sucrose (table sugar)
      (2) Lactose (milk sugar—the only one of the sugars not found in plants)
         (a) Is less sweet and less soluble than the others
         (b) Encourages growth of useful bacteria in intestines
   c) Polysaccharides (compound sugars)
      (1) Starches
         (a) Are found in grains, vegetables, and some fruits
         (b) Require a longer time to digest than sugars
         (c) Must be ground or cooked to be promptly used by the body
      (2) Glycogen—found in liver and muscles
      (3) Cellulose
         (a) Has little or no food value
         (b) Is fibrous and forms framework of fruits, vegetables, and cereals
         (c) Furnishes the bulk which aids peristalsis in the large bowel
      (4) Hemicellulose (agar-agar, pectin, etc.)

D. Proteins
   1. Are composed of carbon, hydrogen, nitrogen, and oxygen
   2. Are main structural elements of every body cell
   3. Are normal constituents of all body fluids except urine and bile
   4. Yield 4 calories per gram when metabolized
   5. Yield amino acids as the end products of their metabolism
   6. Serve four functions:
      a) Build and repair body cells
      b) Regulate water balance within the body
      c) Manufacture hormones, enzymes, and antibodies
      d) Form hemoglobin
   7. Are not stored in the body as protein; in case of severe deficiency, the body will metabolize its own cellular protein
   8. Are divided into two groups:
      a) Complete proteins
         (1) Contain all of the essential amino acids
         (2) All from animal sources
         (3) Necessary for normal growth and development
      b) Incomplete proteins
         (1) Cannot maintain life or support normal growth
         (2) Lack one or more of the essential amino acids
         (3) Supplement the complete proteins and thus decrease the amounts necessary
         (4) Found in cereals, gelatin, and vegetables

E. Fats
   1. Are composed of carbon, hydrogen, and oxygen

BASIC SCIENCES

2. Are part of many foods used daily, such as egg yolk, meat, nuts, chocolate, cheese, butter
3. Supply ⅓ of the American diet which is high in carbohydrate and in fat
4. Produce 9 calories per gram when metabolized
5. Are not easily digested
   a) Remain in stomach longer
   b) Satisfy hunger longer
6. Serve five functions:
   a) Supply heat and energy
   b) Carry fat-soluble vitamins A, D, E, and K
   c) Provide padding for some vital organs
   d) Provide insulation for body heat
   e) Serve as sources of the essential fatty acids needed for growth
      (1) Linoleic
      (2) Linolenic
      (3) Arachidonic
   f) Are stored as fatty tissue
   g) Exist in a complex form known as cholesterol
      (1) Cholesterol is found in most body tissues.
      (2) Cholesterol is synthesized in the body independently of dietary intake.
      (3) High levels in the blood are unhealthy
      (4) Foods lowest in cholesterol are fruits, vegetables, cottage cheese, skim milk, buttermilk, bread, cereals.

F. Minerals
    1. Exist in the body in organic and in inorganic combinations
    2. Make up 4% of the body weight
    3. Include the following:
       a) Calcium
          (1) Most abundant mineral in the body
          (2) 99% exists in bones and teeth
          (3) Helps muscles contract
          (4) Helps to regulate the heart beat
          (5) Aids in the clotting of blood
          (6) Is found in milk, milk products, shellfish, green vegetables, oranges, and figs
       b) Phosphorus
          (1) Comprises ¼ of body minerals
          (2) 90% combines with calcium in bones and teeth
          (3) Helps maintain the acid-base balance of the body fluids
          (4) Is found in whole-grain cereals, fish, nuts, milk, milk products, poultry, and legumes
       c) Iron
          (1) Is constituent of hemoglobin and of important enzymes
          (2) Is used to manufacture new blood cells
          (3) Assimilation increased by presence of vitamin C
          (4) Need increased during periods of growth, after loss through menstrual flow, during pregnancy and lactation
          (5) Is found in great supply in liver, kidney, enriched cereals, green leafy vegetables, dried beans, and peas
          (6) Is not found in milk
       d) Sodium
          (1) Occurs mostly in the extracellular fluid
          (2) Helps maintain normal water balance

(3) Helps maintain acid-base balance
(4) Is restricted in the treatment of hypertension and in cardiac failure
 e) Potassium
  (1) Occurs mostly in the intracellular fluid
  (2) Helps maintain acid-base balance
  (3) Helps maintain water balance
  (4) Is widely distributed in foods
  (5) Is necessary for a number of enzyme functions
  (6) Deficiencies occur after long bouts of diarrhea and long administration of sodium chloride and glucose
  (7) Is found in great supply in orange juice
 f) Iodine
  (1) Essential to growth and development of the thyroid gland
  (2) Found in great supply in fish, vegetables grown on iodine-rich soils, and iodized salt

G. Vitamins
 1. Structure and functions
  a) Group of accessory organic substances
  b) Present in most foods in minute amounts
  c) Essential for regulation of body processes
  d) Needed in diet for metabolism
  e) Needed to prevent malnutrition and specific deficiency diseases
 2. Fat-soluble vitamins—A, D, E, and K
  a) Stored in the body
  b) Not destroyed by cooking
  c) Destroyed by rancidity
 3. Water-soluble vitamins—B, C, G, H, P, etc.
  a) Stored in the body to an extremely slight degree
  b) Destroyed by improper cooking
  c) Can be lost by discarding water in which food was cooked or soaked
  d) Excreted by kidneys

H. Water
 a) Importance—next to oxygen, the most important substance
 b) Functions
  (1) Supplies fluid for secretions
  (2) Serves as solvent for materials in the body
  (3) Enables digested food to pass through intestinal walls
  (4) Acts as a lubricant
  (5) Provides fluid for metabolic purposes
  (6) Aids in temperature control
  (7) Is major constituent of body cells and tissues
  (8) Is major constituent of blood, which transports nutrients to all body tissues and carries body wastes for elimination by kidneys, lungs, skin, and bowels

II. Deficiencies and Metabolic Diseases

A. Nutritional Deficiencies—due to lack of one or more nutritional factors (mineral, vitamin, protein, etc.) necessary for well-being and health
 1. Cause
  a) Congenital malformation: pyloric stenosis
   (1) It occurs more often in male than in female infants.

        (2) Symptoms generally start soon after birth with projectile vomiting after feeding, dehydration, and constipation.

        (3) Treatment is surgical.

    b) Decreased intake of nutrients due to poor eating habits or to economic or regional factors

    c) Failure of absorption and/or utilization

        (1) Gastrointestinal disease

        (2) Endocrine dysfunction

        (3) Infectious disease

        (4) Celiac disease in infants

            (a) Abdominal distension

            (b) Large, pale, foul-smelling stools

            (c) Retardation in growth

            (d) Treatment—dietary control

    d) Increased requirements

        (1) Surgery

        (2) Burns

        (3) Injuries

        (4) Growth

        (5) Pregnancy

        (6) Chronic illness

        (7) Excessive excretion of body fluids

            (a) Burns

            (b) Overusage of diuretic drugs

        (8) Vitamin deficiencies—see Data Summary 5

        (9) Mineral deficiencies

            (a) Iron-deficiency anemia

            (b) Simple goiter—iodine deficiencies

            (c) Rickets—calcium deficiencies

                i) Soft bones

                ii) Beaded ribs (rachitic rosary)

                iii) Deformed thorax (pigeon breast)

                iv) Bowlegs

  2. Treatment

    a) Diet therapy

    b) Nutritional supplements

B. Protein Deficiencies—causes

  1. Acute—rapid, massive loss of plasma and other proteins from the body as in severe hemorrhage, severe burns, etc.

  2. Chronic

    a) Inadequate dietary intake of protein

    b) Impaired intestinal absorption as in chronic diarrhea and steatorrhea

    c) Imperfect metabolism as in liver disease

    d) Excessive loss of protein as in thyrotoxicosis, chronic debilitating illnesses, and draining wounds and fistulae

C. Failure to Thrive

  1. Growth occurs continuously in children but not at the same rate.

  2. Growth rate provides a means of monitoring the child's growth and of recognizing growth and developmental problems.

  3. Causes of deviant growth and development patterns are as follows:

    a) Nutritional factors

DATA SUMMARY 5
Diseases Resulting from Vitamin Deficiencies

Vitamin	Deficiency Manifestations
A	Nightblindness; conjunctival dryness; follicular keratosis
Thiamine (B_1)*	Peripheral neuritis; beriberi
Riboflavin (B_2)	Lip lesions; keratitis; dermatitis
Inositol*	Alopecia
Pyridoxine (B_6)*	Dermatitis
Niacin*	Pellagra
Pantothenic acid*	Gray hair
Folic acid*	Anemia
Choline*	Fatty liver in animals
Biotin*	Dermatitis
B_{12}*	Pernicious anemia; sprue and other macrocytic anemias; nutritional blindness
C	Scurvy (hemorrhages, gingivitis, loose teeth)
D	Rickets; osteomalacia
E	Muscle degeneration; sterility; other lesions; RBC hemolysis
K	Hemorrhagic disease of newborn; prothrombin deficiency in jaundice

*Constituents of vitamin B complex.

---

      b) Disease
      c) Endocrine disturbances
      d) Congenital disturbances
      e) Genetic factors
    4. Treatment includes the following:
      a) Elimination of underlying disease
      b) Correction of nutritional deficiency
      c) Correction of metabolic dysfunction

III. Metabolic Abnormalities
Note: Examples of metabolic abnormalities in different age groups are given below. In a book of this nature it is impossible to discuss each condition. The diseases selected are the more common ones and those the practical nurse would encounter most frequently. The treatments described are limited to those prescribed for metabolic disorders.

  A. Cystic Fibrosis
    1. Etiology—congenital
    2. Symptoms
      a) Delay in regaining birth weight
      b) Large, foul-smelling stools
      c) Respiratory symptoms
    3. Treatments
      a) Adequate pancreatic replacement
      b) Diet of sufficient calories
      c) Adequate protein intake
      d) Reduction of fat intake
      e) Adequate multivitamins

B. Obesity
1. Etiology
a) Excessive fat is stored at various sites in body.
b) Obesity is generally due to excessive intake of calories.
c) Obesity is rarely due to endocrine disorders.
2. Treatment
a) Treatment of any underlying disorders
b) Supervised diet limiting caloric intake

C. Diabetes Mellitus
1. Etiology: disorder of carbohydrate metabolism due to insufficient insulin production
2. Treatment (dietary)
a) Diabetic diet is a normal diet but measured exactly to patient's needs.
b) Regularity of diet is important.
c) Caloric values should be sufficient to maintain approximately ideal weight.

IV. Diet Therapy

A. Role of the Practical Nurse
1. Special knowledge
a) Understand principles of normal diet
b) Understand importance of special diets in treatment of certain diseases
c) Understand how normal diet can be modified for specific therapy
d) Understand psychological reaction of patient
2. Patient feeding
a) Assist patient at mealtime
b) Understand patient's attitudes in regard to food, and interpret them to dietary staff
c) Explain reasons for prescribed diet to patient
d) Record patient's acceptance or rejection of food and relate problems to medical and dietary staff
e) Recognize ethnic food patterns of patient
f) Understand ability of patient to afford diet changes and special foods after leaving hospital

B. Modifications in Normal Diet
1. Consistency
a) Liquid
b) Soft
c) Light
2. Method of preparation
a) Mashing
b) Blending
c) Pureeing
3. Elimination of certain foods
a) Ethnic considerations
b) Allergic reactions
c) Stimulating foods such as meat extractions and highly spiced foods
4. Intervals of feeding—depend on type of disease, e.g., acute peptic ulcer requires more frequent feedings
5. Feeding techniques
a) Tube feeding
b) Intravenous feeding
c) Hypodermoclysis

      6. Amount modification
         a) Amount of nutrients
         b) Roughage increase or decrease
         c) Caloric increase or decrease
      7. Special modifications
         a) Low sodium
         b) Low fat
         c) Low protein
         d) High protein
         e) Low cholesterol

C. Goals of Therapeutic Diets
    1. Improve or continue present nutritive condition
    2. Improve clinical or subclinical nutritive inadequacies
    3. Increase, maintain, or decrease body weight
    4. Relieve or rest specific body organs
    5. Remove allergens from patient's diet
    6. Modify diet according to patient's ability to metabolize specific nutrients

Note: Outline of normal diet modifications that follows is, of necessity, not inclusive of every type of special diet but serves only to illustrate theory in regard to modifications.

V. Therapeutic Diets

A. Diet for Diabetes Mellitus
    1. Indications
        a) Hyperglycemia
        b) Glycosuria
    2. Goals
        a) Correct metabolism of carbohydrates
        b) Maintenance of normal blood sugar
        c) Prevention of glycosuria
        d) Adequate nutrition for patient
        e) Normal life span
    3. Modification of normal diet
        a) Diet must be adequate for excellent nutrition.
        b) Carbohydrate content is restricted and varies from 150 to 250 gm per day.
        c) Protein content is similar to the recommended normal dietary allowances.
        d) Fat content is restricted to prevent ketosis.
        e) Proportions of carbohydrate: protein: fat are adjusted by physician for each patient individually.
    4. Calculation of diabetic diet
        a) Calculation is based on patient's sex, age, height, weight, and activity.
        b) Consideration is given to type of insulin, i.e., slow- or fast-acting.
        c) Consideration is given to severity of diabetic condition.
    5. Dietary treatment
        a) Meals planned using ADA exchange lists
        b) Foods carefully measured according to carbohydrate content and caloric value
        c) Types of foods allowed and to be avoided
            (1) Allowed
               (a) Desserts sweetened with artificial sweeteners
               (b) All other foods except as noted below

        (2) To be avoided
- (a) Sugars and sweetened foods
- (b) Dried fruits and beans
- (c) Soft drinks and alcoholic beverages
- (d) All unknown food mixtures

B. Bland Diet
1. Indications
   a) Peptic ulcer
   b) Gastritis
   c) Hiatus hernia
2. Goals
   a) Dilute gastric juice
   b) Reduce secretion of gastric juice
   c) Reduce peristaltic action of stomach
3. Modification of normal diet
   a) No chemically irritating foods such as coffee, tea, spices, alcohol, acids, meat extracts, or carbonated drinks
   b) No harsh foods such as whole grains or unstrained fruits and vegetables
   c) No hot or cold foods
4. Dietary principles
   a) Multiple small feedings
   b) High fat to delay stomach-emptying time
   c) High protein to combine with gastric juices
   d) Multivitamin supplementation necessary
5. Stages in treatment
   a) Frequent small feedings of milk and cream alternated with alkaline medication
   b) Other soft foods, added gradually, such as eggs, strained cereal, puddings, and junket
   c) Additional foods such as cream cheese, strained fruit, and fruit juices
   d) Ground meat, strained vegetables, pudding

C. Sodium-Restricted Diets
1. Indications
   a) Congestive heart failure
   b) Hypertension
   c) Edema
   d) Ascites
   f) Cirrhosis of liver
   g) Ménière's syndrome
   h) Cortisone therapy
   i) Toxemia of pregnancy
2. Goals
   a) Prevent edema (aid body in eliminating sodium and fluids)
   b) Control sodium intake
   c) Reduce blood pressure
   d) Reduce blood volume
3. Modification of normal diet
   a) Three levels of Na+ restriction possible—mild, moderate, strict
   b) No salt at table
   c) No baking powder and baking soda
   d) No soda water
   e) Low-sodium milk
   f) Restricted use of canned or processed foods, monosodium glutamate
   g) Sodium-free baking powder

D. Low-Cholesterol Diet
  1. Indications
     a) High blood cholesterol
     b) Hypertension
     c) Atherosclerosis
  2. Goal—reduce blood cholesterol
  3. Modification of normal diet
     a) Reduction in foods high in saturated fats without altering caloric intake
        (1) Egg yolk
        (2) Liver
        (3) Kidney, sweetbreads, fish roe
        (4) Whole milk and its products
     b) Reduction in both saturated fat and total calories to control obesity

E. Low-Protein Diet
  1. Indications
     a) Acute nephritis
     b) Chronic nephritis
     c) Acute and chronic glomerulonephritis
     d) Nephrosclerosis
  2. Goals
     a) Reduce work of kidney by reducing waste products
     b) Prevent accumulation of waste products in blood
  3. Modification
     a) Protein in diet reduced to 40-60 gm
     b) Low salt to combat edema

F. High-Protein Diet
  1. Indications
     a) Chronic nephritis, at times
     b) Malnutrition
  2. Goals
     a) Replace albumin lost in urine
     b) Restore protein level in blood
     c) Help to rebuild body tissues
  3. Modification of normal diet
     a) Addition of egg whites to fruit juices
     b) Addition of gelatin to soups
     c) Addition of eggs to milk beverages
     d) Use of concentrated protein beverages

G. Low-Residue Diet
  1. Indications
     a) Diarrhea
     b) Ileitis
     c) Ulcerative colitis
     d) Spastic constipation
     e) Colon surgery
     f) Partial intestinal obstruction
  2. Goals
     a) Decrease peristalsis
     b) Prevent colon distension

3. Modification of normal diet
   a) Omission of bulky and fibrous foods such as the following:
      (1) Whole-grain cereals and breads
      (2) Raw and coarse vegetables
      (3) Raw fruit
      (4) Smoked and tough meat
   b) Omission of rich desserts and fried foods

H. High-Residue Diet
   1. Indication—atonic constipation
   2. Goal—stimulate peristalsis
   3. Modification of normal diet
      a) Increase in fiber content
      b) Addition of foods high in cellulose
         (1) Whole-grain breads and cereals
         (2) Fruits with skins
         (3) Vegetables with fibers and skins

I. High-Protein, High-Carbohydrate, Low-Fat Diet
   1. Indications
      a) Hepatitis
      b) Cirrhosis of liver, early
      c) Gallbladder diseases
   2. Goals
      a) Reduce liver injury and strain
      b) Build up liver tissue
      c) Ease liver function
      d) Reduce gallbladder pain (injured gallbladder is not stimulated)
   3. Modification of normal diet
      a) Low calorie if patient obese
      b) Bland, nonstimulating
      c) Low residue
      d) Easily digested fats but low in amount (reduces gallbladder pain)
      e) High carbohydrate (protein sparing)
      f) High protein
         (1) Regenerates liver tissue
         (2) Increases serum albumin
         (3) Moves fat from liver
      g) Vitamin supplements

J. Low-Calorie Diet
   1. Indications
      a) Slight or moderate excess weight
      b) Obesity
      c) Arthritis
      d) Gout
      e) Diabetes mellitus
      f) Congestive heart failure and cardiac insufficiency
      g) Gallbladder disease with obesity
   2. Goals
      a) Restore and/or maintain good nutrition
      b) Reduce body fat so that gradual loss in body weight results

3. Modification of normal diet
   a) Daily diet about 500 calories lower than actual requirements
      (1) Caloric intake is less than needed.
      (2) Body uses fat reserve for needed calories.
   b) Vitamin supplementation desirable

K. High-Calorie Diet
   1. Indications
      a) Weight less than normal for individual
      b) Fever
      c) Hyperthyroidism
      d) Tuberculosis
      e) Chronic infections
   2. Goals
      a) Accomplish weight gain by storage of body fat
      b) Restore and/or maintain normal nutrition
   3. Modification of normal diet
      a) High protein
      b) 1000-1200 calories above requirement
         (1) Between-meal feedings
         (2) Easily digested foods
         (3) Highly concentrated foods
      c) Vitamin and mineral supplementation (high thiamine)
      d) Foods permitted
         (1) High-calorie foods such as jams and cakes
         (2) Food supplements such as addition of skim-milk powder to milk, cereals, cottage cheese, etc.
         (3) Cream

L. Low-Fat Diet
   1. Indications
      a) Cholecystitis
      b) Cholelithiasis
   2. Goals
      a) Relax the gallbladder
      b) As a result, decrease pain in gallbladder inflammation
   3. Modification of normal diet
      a) Low fat
      b) Bland, nonstimulating foods
      c) Skim milk to replace whole milk
      d) Lean meats
      e) No butter or other dairy products

M. Prenatal Diet
   1. Goals
      a) Adequate nutrition for the mother
      b) Adequate nutrition for the developing fetus
   2. Modification of normal diet
      a) Normal, well-balanced diet
      b) Adequate intake of protein, vitamins, calcium, and iron
      c) Milk or calcium supplementation
      d) If anemic, iron supplementation

N. Miscellaneous Diets
1. Elimination diet for allergies
2. High-iron diet for anemias
3. Diet for urinary calculi
4. Malabsorption-syndrome diet
5. Diet for inborn errors of metabolism
6. Diet for other nutritional deficiencies
7. Postoperative diet

Note: See the following pages for examples of therapeutic diets. For more detailed information, refer to standard textbooks on nutrition and/or nursing.

VI. Sample Therapeutic Diets

NORMAL PREGNANCY

BREAKFAST

Fruit:	Orange juice, grapefruit juice, prune juice, or apple juice.
Cereal:	Strained cereals with milk, such as cream of wheat, farina or oatmeal.
Bread:	Toast with butter or jam.
Eggs:	Two soft-boiled eggs.
Beverage:	Hot or cold milk, cocoa, or Postum.

LUNCH

Soup:	Cream of spinach, asparagus, tomato, consomme or broth.
Meat/Fish:	Roasted or boiled chicken, baked chopped meat, or boiled or baked fish.
Vegetables:	Mashed potatoes, strained carrots, peas, or creamed spinach.
Bread:	White toast or melba toast.
Dessert:	Gelatin, junket, tapioca, chocolate or bread pudding.
Beverage:	Cocoa, light tea, or coffee.

DINNER

Vegetables:	Vegetable dinner consisting of boiled or baked potatoes, squash, strained carrots, and peas. This may be combined with omelet or poached eggs.
Bread:	White toast or melba toast.
Beverage:	Cocoa, milk, light tea, or coffee.
Dessert:	Custard, chocolate or bread pudding, gelatin dessert, or a piece of plain cake.

HYPERTENSION
CHRONIC NEPHRITIS

LOW SODIUM

TOXEMIA OF PREGNANCY

BREAKFAST

Fruit:	Half a grapefruit, sliced orange, peach, apple, or any other fresh or stewed fruit.
Cereal:	Cooked cereal such as farina, cream of wheat, or oatmeal.
Eggs:	Soft boiled, poached, or scrambled eggs.
Beverage:	Milk is the best beverage. Decaffeinated coffee such as Sanka may be used. Tea, coffee, and cocoa should be avoided.

LUNCH

Soup:	Vegetable, spinach, or tomato soup (unseasoned).

Salad:	Mixed vegetable salad or lettuce and tomato salad. NO CONDIMENTS.
Bread:	White or whole wheat or toast.
Beverage:	Milk or decaffeinated coffee.

DINNER

Soup:	Vegetable, spinach, or tomato soup (unseasoned).
Meat:	Small serving of fresh beef, mutton, lamb, chicken, or turkey.
OR	NO SPICED, SALTED OR CANNED MEATS ALLOWED, NO GRAVIES ALLOWED.
Fish:	Fresh fish in small portions. NO CANNED OR SALTED FISH ALLOWED.
OR	
Cheese:	Cottage cheese is best.
Vegetables:	Serving of any of the following vegetables: asparagus, beets, carrots, squash, string beans, eggplant, spinach, lettuce, tomatoes.
Salad:	Lettuce and tomato salad or watercress salad. NO SEASONINGS ALLOWED.
Beverage:	Milk or decaffeinated coffee.
Dessert:	Fruit cup, prune whip, ice cream, junket, or plain cake.

THE FOLLOWING FOODS MUST BE AVOIDED

Canned, salted, or seasoned meats and fish.
Bacon, pork, and veal.
Seasonings, such as salt, pepper, mustard,

chili sauce, and all gravies.
Alcohol, tea, coffee, or cocoa.
Carbonated drinks (vichy, ginger ale).

NO SALT IS ALLOWED TO BE USED AT THE TABLE.

CARDIAC

BREAKFAST

Fruit:	Orange juice with added water; stewed prunes, pears, or apricots.
Cereal:	Cooked cereal, such as farina, cream of wheat, Wheatena.
Egg:	One soft-boiled or coddled egg.
Bread:	Two slices of salt-free bread with UNSALTED butter.
Beverage:	Milk, cocoa, or milk with added chocolate. AVOID tea, coffee.

LUNCH

Soup:	Vegetable soup or clear broth. AVOID creamed soups.
Vegetables:	Choice of one or two of the following: string beans, peas, carrots, cooked spinach, lettuce, tomatoes, boiled potato.
Bread:	Salt-free bread with UNSALTED butter.
Salads:	Grapefruit salad or lettuce and tomato salad (small serving).
Dessert:	Cooked fruit, baked apple, or applesauce. AVOID raw fruit.
Beverage:	Milk, decaffeinated coffee, or Postum.

DINNER

Meat/Fish:	Baked, broiled, or roasted cuts of beef, veal, chicken, liver, turkey, or cooked fresh fish, such as pike, perch, cod, halibut, flounder, or haddock. May be served with the vegetables allowed under LUNCH.
Bread:	Salt-free bread with UNSALTED butter.
Salad:	Vegetable salad or lettuce and tomato salad (small serving).
Dessert:	Cooked fruit or Jell-o, junket or gelatin dessert, tapioca, or bread pudding.
Beverage:	Warm milk, Postum, or decaffeinated coffee.

No salt is to be used in this diet, at table or in cooking. Do not eat too much at one meal, and do not eat unless 4 hours have elapsed since preceding meal. Do not eat in an excited state. Chew food well and eat slowly. Do not drink tea or coffee, vichy or ginger ale, or any alcoholic drinks such as beer, whiskey, or wine. Do not eat too hot or too cold foods or mixtures of both of these at any one meal. REST AFTER EACH MEAL, AND DO NOT EAT JUST BEFORE GOING TO BED.

THE FOLLOWING FOODS MUST BE AVOIDED

Canned, spiced, salted, or preserved meats or fish.
Strong cheese.
Vegetables such as cabbage, cucumbers, corn, onions, peppers, radishes, turnips, baked beans.

Raw fruits.
All HOT BISCUITS, muffins, breads, waffles, cornbreads, cornflakes.

SPASTIC CONSTIPATION

BREAKFAST

Fruit:	Fruit and fruit juices in moderation, diluted orange juice, baked apple, stewed or pureed prunes.
Cereal:	COOKED CEREALS ONLY—farina-type cereals.
Eggs:	Two soft-boiled, coddled, or poached eggs.
Bread:	White bread or toast, buttered.
Beverage:	Weak coffee, weak tea, Postum, or milk.
10:00 A.M.	Baked apple or cooked pears.

LUNCH

Soup:	Clear broth or pureed vegetable soup.
Vegetables:	Cooked vegetables: mashed potato, pureed peas, pureed carrots, pureed beets, pureed turnips. May have macaroni and spaghetti without sauce, tomatoes, or cheese.
Salad:	Shredded lettuce only. May be eaten with cottage or pot cheese.
Bread:	White bread or toast, buttered.
Beverage:	Weak tea, decaffeinated coffee, weak coffee, Postum, or milk.
Dessert:	Rice pudding, tapioca, or chocolate pudding.
4:00 P.M.	Glass of buttermilk and crackers.

DINNER

Soup:	Pureed vegetable soup or clear broth.
Meat/Fish:	Roasted, broiled, or cooked tender cuts of beef, beef steak, roast lamb, scraped beef, chicken, squab, turkey. Baked or boiled fish, such as halibut, pike, perch, bluefish.
Vegetables:	Cooked pureed and mashed vegetables from above list under LUNCH.
Bread:	White bread or toast, buttered.
Beverage:	Weak tea, coffee, coffee, Postum or milk.
Dessert:	Gelatin, junket dessert, or rice pudding.
10:00 P.M.	Glass of buttermilk and crackers.

THE FOLLOWING FOODS MUST BE AVOIDED

All canned, salted, spicy, or smoked meats and fish; also salmon, mackerel, tuna, and herring.
The following vegetables: radishes, corn, cucumbers, cabbage, tomatoes, onions, garlic.

All wholewheat breads and cereals; also hot breads.
Figs, nuts, raisins, preserves, all alcoholic and carbonated drinks.
Candy, pastries, pies, seasoned and thickened soups.

ATONIC CONSTIPATION

On arising, one or two glasses of water. Eat slowly. Chew all foods well.

BREAKFAST

Fruit: A glass of orange juice or half a grapefruit.
Cereal: Shredded wheat, cooked bran, farina-type cereals, cornflakes, oatmeal.
Eggs: Poached or soft-boiled eggs, with two slices of white or whole wheat toast, slightly buttered.
Beverage: Light tea or coffee, buttermilk, or decaffeinated coffee.

10:30 A.M.   Two glasses of water.

LUNCH

Soup: Vegetable soup, clear broth, or clam chowder.
Vegetables: Choice of the following vegetables: string beans, peas, carrots, beets, spinach, celery, tomatoes, lettuce, asparagus, raw cabbage, broccoli, boiled onions, dandelion greens, turnips, corn, rhubarb, or squash.
Bread: Whole wheat or rye, lightly buttered.
Salads: Grapefruit salad, lettuce and tomato salad, or plain lettuce salad.
Dessert: Apples, bananas, blackberries, blueberries, cherries, peaches, pears, plums, or a piece of plain cake.
Beverage: Tea or buttermilk.

3:00 P.M.   Two glasses of water.

DINNER

Appetizer: Fruit cup, tomato juice, or half a grapefruit.
Soup: Clear broth or consomme.
Entree: Baked, broiled, or roasted tender cuts of beef, lamb, chicken, or turkey, or boiled or baked fresh fish. Serve with one potato (boiled or baked) and with at least two green vegetables from the above list under LUNCH.
Bread: Whole wheat or rye, lightly buttered or toasted.
Salads: Vegetable, fruit, or crisp lettuce salad.
Dessert: Applesauce, fresh or stewed fruit, or a small piece of plain cake.
Beverage: Light tea or coffee, buttermilk, or decaffeinated coffee.

Before retiring: Two glasses of water.

THE FOLLOWING FOODS MUST BE AVOIDED

All fried foods, fats, gravies, veal, pork, stews.
All salty, spiced, canned, or preserved meats and fish.

All cream soups and sauces.
All condiments such as catsup, pickles, Worcestershire Sauce, vinegar, spices.
All chocolate, candy, drinks, and pastries.

CHRONIC PEPTIC ULCER

BREAKFAST

Cereal: Cooked cereals only, such as oatmeal, farina-type cereal.
Eggs: Two eggs—poached or soft boiled.
Beverage: Milk, Postum, or decaffeinated coffee.
Bread: White bread (day old) or buttered toast.
Fruit: Strained orange juice well diluted with water at the end of breakfast.

LUNCH

Soups: Vegetable or milk soups. AVOID spicy cream soups, with pepper, etc., and avoid MEAT BROTH.
Vegetables: Carrots, squash, peas, spinach, string beans (pureed or strained only). Boiled or mashed potatoes.
Bread: White bread (day old) or buttered toast.
Salad: Leafy lettuce must not be used. Lettuce must be shredded. Cottage cheese, pot cheese, or farmer cheese may be eaten with the shredded lettuce.
Dessert: Cooked fruits, such as cooked pears, baked apples, applesauce, rice pudding, tapioca pudding, junket, or gelatin desserts.
Beverage: Milk, Postum, decaffeinated coffee, or buttermilk.

DINNER

Soups: Vegetable or milk soups. AVOID spicy cream soups, with pepper, etc., and avoid MEAT BROTH. No canned soups.
Meat/Fish: Broiled, baked, or roasted beef, lamb, liver, chicken, turkey. Baked or cooked fish such as flounder, pike, perch, cod, halibut. Vegetables may be served with this (from above LUNCH list).
Bread: White bread (day old) or buttered toast.
Salad: Shredded lettuce, with cottage or pot cheese.
Dessert: Cooked fruits, cooked pears, baked apple, rice pudding, chocolate pudding, tapioca pudding, blancmange.
Beverage: Milk, postum, or decaffeinated coffee. ONE GLASS OF SWEET MILK BETWEEN MEALS.

THE FOLLOWING FOODS MUST BE AVOIDED

Canned, salted, spiced meats and fish.
Oysters, clams, or lobsters.
Raw fruits and raw vegetables.
The following vegetables: cucumbers, cabbage, peppers, onions, cauliflower, dry beans.

Whole wheat and whole wheat cereals.
All gravies, spices, sauces.
Alcoholic and carbonated drinks.
Pastries, cakes, jams.
Thickened or creamed soups.

EAT SLOWLY—CHEW YOUR FOOD WELL

LOW-FAT, LOW-CHOLESTEROL

BREAKFAST

Fruit: Cooked fruit preferred, or fruit juices well diluted.
Cereal: Farina-type cereal or other COOKED cereal.
Egg: Egg white ALLOWED ONLY.
Beverage: Light tea or coffee, or milk (preferably skimmed).

LUNCH

Soup: Vegetable soup ALLOWED ONLY. Meat soups, chicken soup, or creamed soups not allowed.

Vegetables: Cooked vegetables only, such as carrots, string beans, peas, beets, spinach. Potatoes baked, mashed, or boiled (no butter). The following vegetables MUST NOT BE EATEN either cooked or uncooked: cucumbers, corn, radishes, asparagus, sauerkraut, onions, green peppers, garlic, cabbage.

Bread: White bread (day old) or toast. NO FRESH BREAD ALLOWED.

Beverage: Light tea, coffee, or skimmed milk.

DINNER

Meat: Serving of any lean meat, chicken or turkey. NO FRIED OR FATTY MEATS, including duck or geese, ALLOWED. Meat may be boiled, broiled, or baked. NO STEWS OR GRAVIES PERMITTED.

Fish: Baked fresh fish may be taken only once a week. NO CANNED FISH such as salmon or tuna ALLOWED AT ANY TIME.

Vegetables: Cooked vegetables as above ONLY.

Salad: Lettuce and tomato salad WITHOUT DRESSING. Cottage cheese salad.

Beverage: Light coffee, tea, or milk.

Dessert: Cooked fruits, junket, or gelatin dessert (without cream), angel food cake.

EAT SMALL OR MODERATE-SIZED MEALS

THE FOLLOWING FOODS MUST BE AVOIDED

All fried and fatty foods.

Egg yolks.

Raw vegetables, except lettuce and tomatoes.

Soup except vegetable soup.

Alcoholic drinks, carbonated beverages.

Butter.

Very hot or very cold drinks.

All spicy, salted, or canned meats.

Canned fish of any kind.

Raw fruits, except well-diluted fruit juices.

Gravies.

Condiments or dressings such as mayonnaise or Russian dressing.

The following vegetables: asparagus, corn, cucumbers, green peppers, radishes, cabbage, sauerkraut, onions, garlic.

LOW TRIGLYCERIDE
LOW CHOLESTEROL, LOW FAT

BREAKFAST

Fruit: Any type of fruit juice (at least 4 ounces).

Cereal: Any cooked or uncooked cereal with skimmed milk.

Egg: Egg white ALLOWED ONLY.

Beverage: Skimmed milk, light tea or coffee without cream. Skimmed milk may be added to coffee.

Bread: 1 slice white bread or toast. Use corn oil margarine or safflower oil margarine.

LUNCH

Fruit: Any type of fruit or fruit juices (at least 4 ounces).

Soup: Vegetable soup ALLOWED ONLY (made with skimmed milk). Meat soups or chicken soup NOT ALLOWED.

Meat: Serving of any lean meat, chicken, or turkey. Trim all visible fat from meat and skin of chicken and turkey and leave on plate.

BASIC SCIENCES

Vegetables: Cooked vegetables such as carrots, string beans, peas, corn, onions, beets, spinach, or uncooked vegetables such as lettuce, tomatoes, radishes, sauerkraut, green pepper, or cucumber. Lettuce and tomatoes may be served with corn or cottonseed or safflower oil and vinegar to taste; low-calorie salad dressing allowed.

Bread: 1 slice white bread or toast, without butter. Use corn oil margarine or safflower oil margarine.

Beverage: Skimmed milk, light tea or coffee without cream. Skimmed milk may be added to coffee.

DINNER

Fruit: Any type of fruit or fruit juice (at least 4 ounces).

Meat: NO FRIED OR FATTY MEATS, INCLUDING DUCK OR GOOSE, ALLOWED. NO STEWS OR GRAVIES PERMITTED. Serving of only lean meat, chicken, or turkey. Meat may be boiled, broiled, or baked. Trim all visible fat and discard.

Fish: Baked fresh fish especially good. Fish roe or caviar NOT ALLOWED AT ANY TIME. May have serving of canned salmon or tuna fish, water packed.

Vegetables: Choice of any vegetable as above.

Salad: Lettuce and tomato salad: dressing may be made from corn oil, cottonseed oil or safflower oil and vinegar. Cottage cheese salad. Cottage cheese or farmer cheese may be eaten as often as desired.

Bread: 1 slice white bread or toast, without butter. Use corn oil margarine or safflower oil margarine.

Dessert: Cooked or raw fruits, or gelatin dessert (without cream).

Beverage: Skimmed milk, light tea or coffee without cream. Skimmed milk may be added to coffee.

EAT MODERATE-SIZED MEALS

Limit all fat consumption, including corn oil, cottonseed oil, or safflower oil, to one ounce a day. Limit starches, sugar, and pastries.

THE FOLLOWING FOODS MUST BE AVOIDED

Liver, brains, kidneys, or sweetbreads.
Egg yolks.
Butter or cream.
Whole milk. Olives.
Fried or fatty foods.
Soup except vegetable soup.
Ham, bacon, or other pork products.
Lobster, clams, scallops, shrimps, and oysters.

Dressings such as mayonnaise and Russian dressing.
Gravies.
Cream cheese.
Ice cream.
Spicy, salted, or canned meats, unless fat is trimmed carefully and discarded.
Noodles or spaghetti.

ELIMINATION DIET—ALLERGY

Use the diet listed in the left column below for 2 days. If no symptoms appear, substitute or add ONE of the foods from the right column every 2 days. Keep any diet selected at least 2 days. Add ONE new food in ONE category at ONE time.

BREAKFAST

Juice: Lemon juice
Cereal: Rice (boiled in water without milk)
Baked Goods: Rice muffin
Spread: Grapefruit marmalade

Juice: Grapefruit, pineapple, or pear juice
Cereal: Rice flakes, cornflakes
Baked Goods: Corn or rye bread, rye muffin
Spread: Lemon jelly, pear butter, pineapple jam

LUNCH

Salad: Lettuce
      Cottonseed oil mayonnaise (egg free)
      Pear
Meat or
Other   Lamb or lamb chops
Protein:
Soup: Lamb broth with rice
Vegetables: Cooked spinach
Baked Goods: Rice muffin
Spread: Cottonseed oil
Desserts: Rice pudding without milk
Beverage: Tea

Salad: Carrots, spinach, and beets
      Corn oil mayonnaise (egg free)
      Grapefruit, lemon, pineapple, peach
Meat or Roasted chicken, veal, bacon,
Other   oysters, soybeans, lima beans,
Protein: and peas
Vegetables: Carrots, beets, squash and
      potatoes
Spread: Carefully washed butter
Desserts: Tapioca or corn starch pudding
      or gelatin pudding

SUPPER

Repeat lunch meal.

Ethical and Legal Aspects of Nursing

VOCABULARY

assault   threat or attempt to do harm to a person that is neither consented to nor privileged

attorney   a lawyer; a person who legally has power to act for another

battery   performing treatment on a patient without his or her consent

contract   binding agreement between two or more parties, enforceable by law

crime   any act, or failure to act, that violates a law; the nature of the act is against the whole of society

false imprisonment   unlawful physical restraint of a patient by hospital personnel; the unwarranted detention of a patient in a hospital for any reason

invasion of privacy   intrusion upon a person's right or desire to remain secluded from the scrutiny of others; unauthorized disclosures about a patient

legal   lawful; recognized by law rather than equity

malpractice   negligent performance of professional duties

negligence   failure to carry out ordinary precautions expected of a responsible person, thereby causing harm to another person

tort   wrongful act committed by one person against another person

will   written, legal declaration for disposition of a person's possessions after death

I. **Ethical Responsibilities of the Nurse**

  A. Code of Ethics for Medical Doctors: Medical doctors follow the Hippocratic Oath.

  B. Code of Ethics for Professional Registered Nurses: Registered nurses follow a code of ethics prepared by the American Nurses Association.

  C. Code of Ethics for Licensed Practical Nurses
    1. A code of ethics has been adopted by the National Federation of Licensed Practical Nurses.
    2. As a licensed practical nurse, you should adhere to the following rules of conduct:
      a) Respect and obey nursing rules, hospital regulations, those in authority, and the state nurse practice act.
      b) Adjust to the rules and work methods of the institution in which you are employed.
      c) Recognize that those who work with you and for whom you work form their opinions based on your work habits and behavior both on and off the job.
      d) Be punctual in reporting on and off duty and carrying out patient assignments.

    e) Exercise your rights and privileges as a citizen and accept responsibility for the health and welfare of others in your community.

    f) Participate in nursing organizations.

II. Legal Aspects of Nursing Practice

A. Negligence

1. The practical nurse may be sued if any harm comes to a patient under her/his care because of negligence. For example:
   a) A patient receives a burn from a hot-water bottle.
   b) The nurse administers the incorrect medicine.
   c) An unconscious patient falls from an unprotected crib or bed.
2. The nurse may be sued for libel or slander for making damaging and/or untrue statements about another person.
3. The nurse may be sued for damages in the following cases:
   a) She/he fails to meet hospital standards for safe patient care.
   b) A patient, visitor, or fellow employee receives an injury as the result of neglect on the nurse's part.
4. The nurse rendering aid at the scene of an emergency is liable for any injuries resulting from negligent acts.

B. Patient's Rights

1. The nurse can be held legally responsible for damages due to an invasion of the patient's personal rights.
2. The nurse may be charged with assault and battery for performing or threatening to perform a treatment on a patient without his/her consent or the consent of a parent, legal guardian, or nearest relative.
3. It is the nurse's responsibility to protect the patient from harm or injury; however, false imprisonment is unlawful.
4. The nurse must obtain written permission from the doctor to use restraints.

C. Consulting an Attorney

1. The nurse should seek advice from an attorney if she is involved in any legal action.
2. The nurse should encourage a patient to consult a lawyer if the patient wishes to obtain legal advice or to draw up a will; the fact that a will was made should be recorded on the patient's chart.
3. The nurse should avoid being a witness to wills.

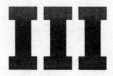

III

Basic Nursing Procedures

UNIT 1: BASIC PATIENT CARE

VOCABULARY

alopecia	natural or abnormal deficiency of hair
axilla	armpit
decubitus	bedsore
dentifrice	powder or other substance for cleaning teeth
dentures	set of teeth, either artificial or natural
deodorant	agent that destroys or neutralizes foul odor
deodorize	to remove foul odor
enema	injection of water, often containing drugs, into rectum and colon to empty lower intestines or for therapeutic treatment
epistaxis	nosebleed
excoriate	to scrape away an outer layer of tissue by chemical or physical means
flatus	gas in the digestive system
incontinence	inability to retain urine or feces
parotitis	inflammation of the parotid gland
pediculosis	infestation with lice
pneumonia	inflammation of the lungs caused by microbes, chemical irritants, vegetable dusts, or allergy
sordes	foul matter; excretions; dregs about the mouth
specimen	a portion of something that reflects the quality of the whole

I. **The Nurse's Role**

   A. General Principles
     1. Promote and maintain health
     2. Be able to identify
       a) Patient's needs
       b) Factors affecting patient's perception of his/her illness
       c) Factors affecting patient's response to his/her illness

   B. Features
     1. Maintenance of good hygiene and physical comfort
     2. Promotion of optional activity—exercise
     3. Provision of rest and sleep
     4. Promotion of safety through prevention of accident, injury, or other trauma and through the prevention of the spread of infection
     5. Maintenance of good body mechanics and prevention and correction of deformities

BASIC NURSING PROCEDURES

II The Health Team

A. The Physician
1. Diagnoses patient's illness by
   a) Taking a complete history
   b) Performing a thorough physical examination
   c) Ordering necessary diagnostic tests
   d) Requesting necessary consultations
2. Establishes a medical care plan for patient that includes
   a) Orders for medications
   b) Orders for specific therapeutic diets
   c) Orders for physiotherapy when necessary
   d) Orders for patient's degree of activity
3. Records daily progress notes describing patient's reaction to therapeutic regimen
4. Records statement of medical goals for patient

B. The Registered Nurse (R.N.)
1. Diagnoses and treats human responses to actual or potential health problems through
   a) Case finding
   b) Health teaching
   c) Health counseling
   d) Providing care supportive to or restorative of life and well-being
2. Executes medical regimens prescribed by licensed physician or dentist
3. Assesses total patient care needs
4. Develops nursing care plan based upon patient's diagnosis and psychological, emotional, and physical needs
5. Implements nursing interventions based upon medical regimen and nursing care plan
6. Evaluates patient care plan
7. Revises and modifies nursing care plan to meet patient's changing needs
8. Supervises and evaluates members of nursing team who assist in implementing nursing care plan
9. Collaborates with other members of health care team
10. Audits and maintains nursing records.

C. The Licensed Practical Nurse (L.P.N./L.V.N.)
1. Functions under direction of the registered nurse, licensed physician, or dentist in
   a) Case finding
   b) Health teaching
   c) Health counseling
   d) Providing supportive or restorative care
   e) Administering medication and therapeutic treatments
2. Makes pertinent observations, reports, and records
3. Assists in meeting patient's physical, emotional, and psychological needs
4. May, under direction of R.N., supervise nurse's aides and/or orderlies
5. Is familiar with laws that govern nursing (nurse practice act) in state where he/she practices; duties will vary with policies of different agencies and with conditions of employment

D. The Medical Social Worker
1. Aids patient in dealing with social service agencies and community facilities that can be of assistance
2. Helps patient with third-party financial aid (application for Medicaid, etc.)

    3. Aids patient in making plans for future care

    4. Studies patient's home situation and counsels patient and family on adjustment to patient's illness

E. The Nutritionist
1. Supervises preparation of patient's therapeutic diet
2. Consults with patient in regard to diet

F. The Physiotherapist
1. Follows the prescription of the physician (physiatrist) to aid patient in the rehabilitation and restoration of normal bodily function after illness or injury
2. Uses physical agents, massage, manipulation, therapeutic exercises, hydrotherapy, and forms of electrotherapy in the treatment methods

G. The Occupational Therapist
1. Aids in socialization of the patient
2. Uses group therapy techniques in working with handicapped patients
3. Aids patients who have limited motion in hand and fingers
4. Assists patients in achieving the activities of daily living

H. The Recreational Therapist
1. Has supportive role in preparation of patients for hospitalization
2. Provides a nonthreatening environment for children
3. Provides continuing education programs
4. Serves as advocate for children
5. Aids in socialization of nursing home patients

I. The Nurse's Aide (Nursing Assistant)
1. Gives direct nursing care to patients under supervision of the R.N. and L.P.N.
2. Helps to maintain the proper patient environment

J. The Orderly (Nursing Assistant)
1. Helps other members of the nursing staff in giving direct patient care
2. Helps to maintain the proper patient environment

K. The Spiritual Advisor
1. Helps patient to identify any emotional and psychological problems
2. Helps patient to resolve these problems
3. Gives spiritual comfort to patient

III. **The Patient's Unit and Environment**

A. Definition of **Unit**: Patient's room, furniture, and equipment

B. Requirements
1. Room should be at a comfortable temperature (68°–74°F); humidity should be maintained at 30–60%; adequate ventilation is necessary, but the room must be free from drafts.
2. Room should have adequate lighting, provided by reading lights, overhead lights, nightlights, and/or television lights; call light should function properly.
3. Room must be kept noise free; this necessarily precludes loud talking, banging of equipment, and high volume levels on radios and television sets.
4. Room and furniture must be cleaned and tidied daily.
5. Room and furniture must be kept SAFE; all equipment must be in good working order,

floors must be clean, dry, and object free.
6. All procedures in the unit should be performed with efficiency and minimal inconvenience to patient.

IV. Patient Admission and Discharge

A. Admission
1. Treat new patient like guest.
2. Orient new patient to hospital; explain hospital routine.
3. Give admission bath if necessary and if hospital policy.
4. Check clothing and valuables according to hospital policy.
5. Report any unusual reaction of patient.
6. Report to charge nurse any medication brought in by patient.
7. Observe patient carefully while assisting him/her, and note general condition, discomfort, etc.
8. Assist patient into bed.
9. Follow routine procedure of admission.
10. Chart time of admission, observations, temperature, pulse and respiration, blood pressure, weight, and other pertinent information.

B. Discharge
1. Check doctor's orders for discharge.
2. Provide safe conveyance.
3. Prepare patient for departure from hospital.
4. Return patient's personal belongings and valuables.
5. Assist patient in dressing.
6. Be sure patient has proper instructions before leaving hospital.
7. Assist patient to wheelchair.
8. Follow detailed procedure of discharge.
9. Chart time of discharge, method, observations, and condition of patient; close chart.

V. Personal Hygiene Procedures

A. Purposes of Personal Hygiene
1. To cleanse, soothe, and refresh patient
2. To stimulate circulation and movement
3. To prevent skin breakdown
4. To contribute to self-esteem

B. Baths
1. Bed bath is given to patients who are confined to bed or are unable to bathe themselves.
2. Showers or tub baths are given to patients who are up and have no dressings.
3. Room temperature should be 75°–80° F, and room should be free from drafts.
4. Bath water should be 110° F.
5. Privacy is essential and should be ensured.

C. Oral Hygiene
1. Purpose is to help keep patient's mouth and teeth clean, healthy, and odor free.
2. It is very important that mouth be cleansed thoroughly to help prevent sordes, surgical parotitis, and pneumonia.
3. Routine or special mouth care should be given daily.

D. Care of Removable Dentures
1. Use only cold water, brush, and dentifrice to clean dentures.
2. If patient is irrational or unconscious, or is going to surgery, remove dentures from his/her mouth.
3. If dentures are occluding the patient's airway, remove them.

E. Care of the Hair
1. Comb hair daily and groom as needed.
2. Shampoo as needed.
3. Give pediculosis treatment when needed.

F. Care of Nails, Hands, and Feet
1. Care of nails, hands, and feet may be done as part of bed bath.
2. Good nail care helps to prevent transmission of infection into torn cuticles or by scratching into skin.
3. Nail care includes cleaning beneath nails, pushing back the cuticle, and removing hangnails.

G. Care of Decubitus
1. Care includes dressings and special cleansing as ordered by doctor or hospital protocol.
2. Prevention is best treatment; measures that may prevent decubitis are turning patient frequently, keeping patient dry and clean, keeping bed linen dry, clean, and free from crumbs and wrinkles, giving special back care frequently, avoiding pressure, and maintaining adequate nutrition.

H. Care of the Incontinent Patient
1. Incontinence refers to inability of sphincter muscles of bladder or rectum to function properly.
2. Patient may be incontinent of feces or urine or both.
3. Condition may be temporary, as in an acute illness, or permanent, as in senility or paralysis.
4. Usually this condition causes much embarrassment to patient; practical nurse can help relieve this embarrassment by teaching patient to care for self as soon as possible and by remaining calm.
5. Bathing buttocks, genitals, and back with mild soap and water is essential; skin is then dried by patting gently, and the back is rubbed to refresh patient and stimulate circulation.

I. Meticulous Skin Care
1. This is most important to prevent decubitus ulcers from developing.
2. Back rub is essential.

J. Shaving
1. Daily shaving is important for cleanliness and morale.
2. Care should be taken to avoid cuts.
3. Care should be taken to avoid folliculitis (shaving bumps).
a) Use brush to dislodge hairs.
b) Use depilatory cream if necessary.

VI. Morning and Evening Care

A. A.M. or Morning Care
1. Give bath, including face and hands.

2. Comb hair.
3. Brush teeth.
4. Care for nails.
5. Make bed with clean linen, and adjust bed.
6. Change patient's position.

B. P.M. Care
   1. Repeat procedures of A.M. care.
   2. Give back rub.

VII. Bedmaking

A. Types of Beds
   1. Occupied—provides safety and comfort for patient who remains in bed
   2. Open—is clean, safe, and comfortable bed in use by patient who may be out of bed
   3. Closed—is clean, safe, and comfortable bed ready to receive new patient
   4. Surgical—is prepared for patient who is recovering from anesthesia
   5. Cradle—is made with a cradle to prevent bedclothes from touching part or all of patient's body

B. Equipment: For all types, includes linen pack containing daily change of linen

C. Precautions
   1. Use proper body mechanics.
   2. Lock bed wheels.
   3. If bed is occupied, avoid motions that might cause patient to fall out of bed.
   4. Prepare safe working space.
   5. Have adequate working space.
   6. Keep soiled linen away from uniform.
   7. Check side rails carefully.
   8. Wash hands before and after performing procedures.
   9. Work quickly and quietly.
   10. Prevent exposure of patient while making bed.

D. Review
   1. Review procedures with which you are most comfortable for detailed information on making a specific bed.
   2. Remember modifications necessary in bedmaking to provide comfort and safety to patient.

VIII. Assisting the Patient from Bed to Chair

A. Introduction
   1. In assisting patient safely from bed to chair or chair to bed, it is necessary to move or support patient without injury to patient or nurse.
   2. All principles of good body mechanics must be applied by nurse.

B. Purposes of Moving Patients
   1. To assist patient in regaining physical strength
   2. To stimulate interest and avoid unnecessary invalidism
   3. To prevent respiratory, circulatory, and muscular complications
   4. To provide activity for patient
   5. To provide rest after activity
   6. To transport patient from one location to another

C. Precautions
1. Use proper body mechanics.
2. Check doctor's orders.
3. Lock bed.
4. Prepare chair or bed before moving patient.
5. Prevent drafts.
6. Attach signal cord within easy reach of patient.
7. Check patient frequently.
8. Check patency of tubes, e.g., catheters.
9. Limit patient's activity as appropriate.
10. Ensure patient safety.

D. Items to Chart
1. The procedure—bed to chair or chair to bed
2. Patient's tolerance
3. Observations noted by nurse

IX. Elimination

A. Procedure for Bedpan/Urinal
1. Offer bedpan or urinal to patient before meals, before visiting hours, at bedtime, and whenever else patient requests.
2. Reassure patient about using bedpan so that he/she will not be embarrassed or self-conscious.
3. Cover bedpan both before and after use; patient should have privacy when using bedpan.
4. If patient needs assistance, place hand under small of back to help lift him/her; if patient is helpless, turn him/her on side, put bedpan against buttocks, and turn gently back on bedpan.
5. Place patient in Fowler's position, unless contraindicated.
6. Give helpless patient appropriate personal hygiene care; provide patient with materials for hand washing.
7. Record frequency of use and contents of bedpan; measure urine if output is being monitored; save, label, and properly store specimen if indicated.

B. Procedure for Incontinent Patient
1. Offer bedpan or urinal frequently.
2. Provide good skin care.
3. Use absorbent pads under patient to facilitate frequent changing.
4. Keep patient clean and dry to prevent skin breakdown.
5. Provide reassurance and encouragement.

X. Body Mechanics

A. Definition of **Body Mechanics:** Coordinating movements of the body

B. General Principles
1. Good body mechanics allows the body to work smoothly with the least amount of strain.
2. Use of good body mechanics is necessary for the following purposes:
   a) Prevent strain or injury to patient and nurse
   b) Prevent fatigue to patient and nurse
   c) Maintain good body alignment for patient and nurse

3. When nurse or patient walks, sits, stands, or lies down, the body should be in the correct position required for the type of movement to be executed.
4. Head and trunk must be kept erect.

IX. Body Positions

A. General Principles
1. Special positions are necessary for patients who are receiving treatments involving certain parts of the body.
2. The body must be moved correctly to prevent injury or pain.

B. Basic Positions
1. Standing—necessary to observe neurologic and orthopedic conditions
2. Supine (horizontal recumbent)—usually used for physical examination
3. Prone—used for examination of spine or back
4. Dorsal recumbent—preferred for rectal and vaginal examination
5. Sims's—used for rectal examinations and treatments of colon
6. Dorsal lithotomy—preferred for rectal, vaginal, and bladder examinations
7. Trendelenburg—used when patient is in shock
8. Fowler's—used following an operation when drainage from the upper part of the body is expected; this is one of the most comfortable positions

XII. Feeding Orthopneic Patients

A. Definition of **Orthopnea:** Condition in which the person can breathe comfortably only when sitting erect or standing

B. Serving Foods and Fluids
1. Fluids and foods are served by the dietary department personnel; however, nurse may be required to serve and feed some patients.
2. Patient should be made as comfortable and relaxed as possible for his/her meal.
3. Nurse washes her/his hands before feeding patients.
4. Patient's hands should be washed before eating.
5. Patient should be encouraged to eat.
6. Patient should be allowed to feed self, with assistance as necessary.
7. Fluids should be offered at intervals, and charted if tolerated.
8. Patient's dislikes and complaints in regard to food served should be reported to charge nurse and dietician.
9. Amounts of food eaten and fluid taken, time, and any unusual observations associated with the meal should be recorded.

XIII. Nursing Care of the Surgical Patient

A. Preoperative Process
1. Preoperative assessment
2. Nursing plans
3. Patient education
   a) Assess patient needs.
   b) Educate regarding postoperative activities.
      (1) Breathing (diaphragmatic)
      (2) Coughing
      (3) Turning
      (4) Leg exercises

BASIC NURSING PROCEDURES

4. Operative permit (informed consent)
   a) Procedures for which it is required
      (1) Any surgical procedure
      (2) Entrance into a body cavity
      (3) Anesthesia (general, local, regional)
   b) Possible forms
      (1) Written document with witness
      (2) Signature of emancipated minor
      (3) Telephone or telegram
      (4) Permission through courts

B. Ambulatory Surgery
   1. Frequently performed procedures
      a) Dilatation and curettage
      b) Tubal ligation
      c) Excision of skin lesions
      d) Excision of superficial lipomas
      e) Myringotomy
      f) Cystoscopy
      g) Oral surgery (tonsillectomy and adenoidectomy, gingevectomy, etc.)
      h) Diagnostic laproscopy
      i) Vasectomy
      j) Cataract excision
      k) Carpal tunnel surgery
      l) Repair of simple hernia
   2. Nursing management of ambulatory surgery patients
      a) Preoperative information
         (1) In all centers, a prepared package which nurse explains is given to patient; it contains the following:
            (a) A consent form
            (b) Instructions to patient
         (2) Psychological status of patient is considered.
      b) Preoperative preparation
         (1) Check vital signs.
         (2) Give preanesthetic medication.
      c) Postoperative care
         (1) Check vital signs until stable.
         (2) Change patient's position as necessary.
         (3) Ascertain patient's recovery before discharge.

C. Nonambulatory Surgery
   1. Preoperative preparation
      a) Skin preparation of particular operative areas
         (1) Shaving as necessary
         (2) After-shave cleansing
      b) Psychological attention to patient
         (1) Provide emotional support.
         (2) Explain procedures.
         (3) Observe patient's emotional condition.
         (4) Warn patient of unpleasant sensations.
         (5) Touch patient during procedure.
         (6) Inform other members of health team about patient's emotional condition.
      c) Preanesthetic medication

        (1)   Administer at exact time ordered.

        (2)   Give on-call medications as ordered.

    d) Transporting patient to operating room

        (1)   Check patient's identity.

        (2)   Identify O.R. attendants to patient.

        (3)   Complete chart, and add all information that may be needed in operating room.

    e) Attention to patient's family

        (1)   Acquaint family with the surroundings, procedures, and expectations of outcome of surgery.

        (2)   Interview family as to what patient wants to know about his/her condition.

2. Nursing process in immediate postoperative period

    a) Immediate nursing assessment

        (1)   Observe patient's airway and note skin color.

        (2)   Verify patient's identity, procedure performed, and surgeon.

        (3)   Request briefing on surgery and any problems encountered or expected.

        (4)   Check vital signs.

        (5)   Inspect operative site for drainage.

        (6)   Make safety checks.

    b) Nursing plans

        (1)   Ensure function of airway and respiratory function.

        (2)   Assess status of circulatory system.

        (3)   Promote comfort and maintain safety.

        (4)   Continue constant observation of patient until he/she has completely reacted.

        (5)   Recognize stress factors, and be aware that hearing is first sense to return.

        (6)   Transfer patient to his/her unit, giving complete report to unit nurse.

3. Postoperative discomforts

    a) Nausea and vomiting

    b) Thirst

    c) Pain

    d) Constipation

4. Postoperative complications

    a) Shock

    b) Hemorrhage

    c) Phlebitis

    d) Hiccups

    e) Pulmonary complications

    f) Pulmonary embolism

    g) Urinary difficulties

    h) Intestinal obstruction

    i) Wound complications

D. Nursing Care of Patient Undergoing Intracranial Surgery

  1. Preoperative management

    a) Assist patient undergoing neurologic examinations and diagnostic tests.

    b) Record patient's symptoms and signs so to have a postoperative evaluation basis.

    c) Explain postoperative care, indicating devices and equipment that may be used on patient.

    d) Assist patient with neurologic defects.

    e) Safeguard the confused patient.

    f) Prepare patient for surgery.

    (1) Shampoo and clip hair, saving clippings.
    (2) Give treatments and medications as ordered.
    (3) Attach an indwelling catheter to patient's thigh.
  2. Postoperative management
    a) Assess patient's airway to see that proper respiratory exchange can occur.
    b) Note patient's level of responsiveness.
    c) Assess patient for signs and symptoms of increasing intracranial pressure.
      (1) Vital sign changes
      (2) Restlessness
      (3) Decreased response to stimuli
      (4) Headache
      (5) Vision changes
      (6) Weakness and paralysis of extremities
    d) Record urinary specific gravity periodically.
    e) Note electrolyte status.
    f) Monitor blood pressure.
    g) Elevate head of bed to reduce intracranial pressure.

UNIT 2: BASIC DIAGNOSTIC PROCEDURES

VOCABULARY

apnea	temporary absence of respiration
asepsis	condition free from germs, infection, or pathogenic bacteria
	medical asepsis—refers to all procedures used to protect the patient and others from disease-producing organisms
	surgical asepsis—refers to all procedures used to render objects or areas free of all microorganisms
bradycardia	pulse rate lower than normal
clammy	cold and moist
diagnosis	science and art of differentiating one disease from another
dyspnea	shortness of breath
hypertension	condition in which blood pressure is higher than normal
hypotension	condition in which blood pressure is lower than normal
jaundice	condition characterized by yellow coloration of skin, mucous membranes, and eyes due to bile pigment in blood
metabolism	sum total of all the chemical and physical processes by which organized substance is produced and maintained
mottling	condition indicated by spotted areas of the body
myositis	inflammatory condition of a muscle
orthopnea	difficulty in breathing that is relieved by sitting in an upright position or by standing
pulse	beat of heart as felt through walls of arteries
respiration	act of breathing
rhythm	pattern or spacing of heart beats
seizure	attack of uncontrolled contraction and relaxation of muscles
symptom	perceptible change in the body or its function which may indicate deviation from normal
	objective symptom—observed by nurse (sometimes called sign)
	subjective symptom—evident only to patient; of internal origin
tachycardia	unusually high pulse rate
tachypnea	rapid breathing

BASIC NURSING PROCEDURES

temperature   measurement of body heat; clinical thermometers measure body temperature; reading represents balance between heat produced and heat lost by the body

vital signs   temperature, pulse, respiration, and blood pressure

I. Patient's History

General Principles
1. Usually taken by the physician or registered nurse; the practical nurse can contribute in the collection of data
2. Important in helping with diagnosis and in planning total patient care

II. Physical Examination

A. Purposes
1. To obtain a determination of patient's physical status
2. To diagnose illness
3. To help maintain and preserve health through early detection of disease

B. Methods
1. Inspection—looking at the body; good light is essential
2. Percussion—tapping the body to detect changes in sound in chest and abdomen
3. Palpation—feeling parts of the body with the hands to discover evidence of abnormalities in various organs
4. Auscultation—using stethoscope to listen to sounds within the body

C. Responsibilities of the Practical Nurse
1. Assist patient onto examination table or bed and drape him/her to avoid unnecessary exposure
2. Prepare patient both physically and mentally for each step of examination; help patient to relax by reassuring him/her
3. Ensure privacy
4. Maintain adequate lighting and ventilation
5. Properly position patient
6. Arrange necessary equipment for examination—tongue blades, percussion hammer, flashlight, ophthalmoscope (for eye examination), otoscope (for ear examination), stethoscope, rubber gloves, lubricants, vaginal speculum
7. Assist doctor during examination

D. Body Positions Used (see figure on next page)
1. Dorsal recumbent
2. Sims's or lateral
3. Trendelenburg
4. Dorsal lithotomy
5. Knee-chest
6. Jackknife

III. Collecting Specimens

A. General Principles
1. All specimens must be collected at correct time.
2. All specimens must be labeled correctly and sent to laboratory promptly with correct laboratory slip.
3. Inside of container must not become contaminated.

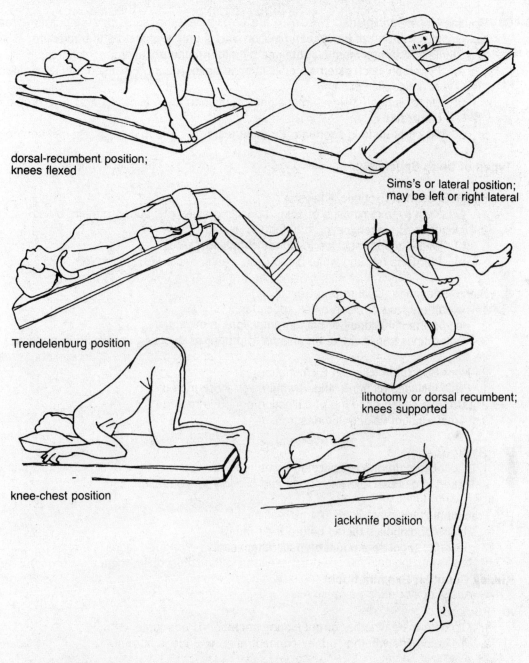

dorsal-recumbent position;
knees flexed

Sims's or lateral position;
may be left or right lateral

Trendelenburg position

lithotomy or dorsal recumbent;
knees supported

knee-chest position

jackknife position

4. Correct amount of specimen must be collected.
5. Medical and/or surgical asepsis techniques must be utilized when indicated.
6. Universal precautions must be observed.

B. Routine Sputum Specimens
1. Collect sputum early in the morning.
2. Instruct patient to cough deeply and to expectorate material brought up from lungs and bronchi.
3. Use proper container for collection.
4. Do not contaminate outside of container with sputum.
5. Label correctly.
6. Use proper asepsis precautions.

BASIC NURSING PROCEDURES

C. Routine Urine Specimens
   1. Urinalysis is part of health examination and is part of admissions procedure.
   2. Sterile specimens must be obtained by either catheterization or "clean catch."
      a) For clean catch external genitalia must be thoroughly cleansed with soap and water or antiseptic solution.
      b) Urine is then voided into sterile container after allowing first few drops to be discarded.
   3. 50-100 cc of urine is adequate for most tests.

IV. Types of Urine Specimens

A. Single Specimen (Routine Analysis)
   1. Qualitative—examination of color, specific gravity, pH, sugar, protein, blood
   2. Microscopic—examination of urinary sediment
      a) Gives important clues to kidney condition
      b) Identifies red and white blood cells, casts, bacteria

B. Sterile Specimen (Culture and Sensitivity)
   1. Is catheterized or clean-catch specimen
   2. Is important in kidney or bladder infections
   3. Determines sensitivity of organisms to proper antibiotics or chemotherapeutics

C. 24-Hour Specimen (Special Examination)
   1. This includes all urine voided within a 24-hour period.
   2. Urine is saved and time of collection period is recorded.
   3. Total amount voided is measured.

D. Timed Specimens
   1. Collection of urine at specified times
   2. Used in glucose tolerance tests and dilution-concentration tests

E. Fractional Urine
   1. Urine of diabetics tested before their meals
   2. Used to regulate amount of insulin necessary

V. Kidney Function Examinations

A. Purposes
   1. To determine whether or not kidney secretion is adequate
   2. To determine whether kidney concentration of urine is normal

VI. Stool Specimens

A. General Principle—important in disorders of GI tract

B. Types of Examination
   1. Laboratory examination for occult blood
      a) Patient should not eat either meat or fish for 3 days before the examination (may give a false positive for blood).
      b) Test is important in inflammations and ulcerations causing bleeding in tract.
   2. Microscopic examination for ova and parasites
      a) Stool must be kept warm until examined.
      b) Specimen must be delivered immediately to laboratory.

BASIC NURSING PROCEDURES

     c) Nurse must be careful to avoid contamination of hands.
     d) Tongue blade is used to transfer specimen from bedpan to container.
     e) Container must be labeled correctly.

VII. Blood Examinations

  A. General Principles
    1. Specimens are usually collected by physician, R.N., or laboratory technician.
    2. Small amount of blood is taken from finger or earlobe for hemoglobin, coagulation time, bleeding time, and cell counts.
    3. Venipuncture is done for serology, blood chemistry, and sedimentation rate.
    4. Blood chemistry, Wasserman test, and sedimentation rate tests use blood drawn from the vein (venipuncture).

VIII. Vomitus

  A. General Principles
    1. Observe and report symptoms associated with vomiting, and note type of vomiting, e.g., projectile vomiting.
    2. Save specimen of vomitus if it contains any unusual matter such as fecal material, pus, blood, or mucous.
    3. Save specimen if it is suspected that patient has been poisoned.

IX. Spinal Fluid

  A. General Principles
    1. Specimen is obtained by lumbar puncture (spinal tap).
    2. Pressure, cell count, and presence of blood or protein are important.
    3. It is nurse's responsibility to assemble necessary equipment.
    4. Fluid is to be taken immediately to laboratory for examination.
    5. Patient is kept in supine position after procedure unless contraindicated.
    6. Dressing at puncture site must be monitored.

X. Vital Signs

  A. Temperature
    1. Average body temperature is 98.6° F; there may be a slight variation of one degree in the temperature of a normally healthy person.
    2. Body heat is produced by the burning of food, which is generated in the muscles and secreting glands, and is distributed to other parts of the body by the blood and blood vessels.
    3. Body heat is eliminated through lungs by the breath, through skin by perspiration, and through urine, feces, and saliva by evaporation.
    4. Body temperature is taken with a clinical thermometer (see Figure 8).

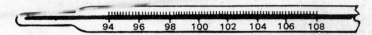

Figure 8

    5. Sudden fall in temperature may indicate shock, collapse, hemorrhage, or approach of death.
    6. Sudden rise in temperature may indicate indigestion, constipation, onset of disease, fatigue, worry, fear, or undue excitement.

BASIC NURSING PROCEDURES

7. Usual methods of taking body temperature depend on patient's state of health and understanding.
   a) Mouth (oral)—normal temperature is 98.6° F; thermometer is placed under tongue with lips closed for 3 minutes
   b) Axilla (axillary)—normal temperature is 97.6° F; axillary temperature should not be taken when the patient is so thin that there is a hollow under the arm or when patient is perspiring so profusely that axilla cannot be kept dry for allotted time; thermometer is placed in the armpit and left in place for 10 minutes
   c) Rectum (rectal)—normal temperature is 99.6° F; thermometer is inserted into rectum approximately 1 inch and left in place for 2 minutes; usually used for infants and children (although routine in some hospitals) and always for unconscious patients
8. Certain precautions must be observed in taking oral temperatures.
   a) Patient should not have had anything hot or cold in the mouth for 10 minutes before thermometer is placed in mouth.
   b) Thermometer should be held with lips closed and not teeth.
   c) If patient is unconscious, delirious, or disoriented, or has oral lesions, oral method should not be used.
9. Certain precautions must be observed in using rectal method.
   a) Rectal temperature is most accurate of all methods used.
   b) Rectal thermometer should be held in place in children or in very ill patients.
   c) The thermometer should be well lubricated.
   d) Thermometer should not be inserted too far.
   e) Rectal method should not be used if patient has any disease of the rectum, has had an operation of the rectum, or has hemorrhoids.
   f) Rectal thermometer should be cleansed and disinfected according to hospital routine.

B. Pulse
1. Taking the pulse
   a) The pulse is a shock wave that travels along the fibers of the arteries with each contraction of the heart.
   b) The pulse is taken by pressing an artery against a bone with the fingers and counting the pulsations for 1 minute.
   c) Arteries most commonly used for taking the pulse are the radial, temporal, carotid, and femoral arteries.
   d) Only equipment needed is a watch with a second hand, a pencil, and a pad.
   e) Pulse is taken whenever the temperature is taken.
2. Pulse rate
   a) Normal pulse rate varies according to sex, age, size, position of patient, and many other factors.
   b) Average pulse rates are as follows:
      (1) Women—70–80 beats per minute
      (2) Men—60–70 beats per minute
      (3) Children (over 7 years)—80–90 beats per minute
      (4) Children (1 to 7 years)—80–120 beats per minute
      (5) Infants—110–130 beats per minute
   c) Increase in pulse rate may be caused by excitement, emotional disturbances, use of certain drugs, elevated temperature, shock, some forms of heart disease, and exercise.
   d) Decrease in pulse rate may be caused by certain drugs, poisons, chronic disease, mental depression, and accidents; the pulse is slower during sleep.
3. Rhythm—may be regular or intermittent; the spacing of beats is referred to as *rhythm;* any irregularity must be reported to the charge nurse at once

    4. Volume—refers to force of the pulse; varies with strength of the heart contraction and elasticity of blood vessels

C. Respiration
1. Definition of **Respiration:** The inhaling of oxygen and the exhaling of carbon dioxide
2. Techniques of taking
    a) Normally, respiration is counted immediately following taking of pulse, while the hand is still placed on the artery.
    b) The respiratory rate is counted by watching the chest or abdomen rise and fall.
    c) The respirations are described by rate, by adjectives such as *deep, shallow,* and *wheezing,* and by regularity.
3. Respiratory rate
    a) Normal respiration rates are as follows:
        (1) Women—18–20 respirations per minute
        (2) Men—14–18 respirations per minute
        (3) Children—20–26 respirations per minute
        (4) Infants—30–38 respirations per minute
    b) Some causes of variations of normal respiration are nervousness, excitement, exercise, sleep, injuries, disease, certain drugs, shock, pain, gas poisoning, elevated body temperature, obstruction of the air passages, and high altitudes.

D. Blood Pressure
1. Definition of **blood pressure:** Pressure exerted by the blood against the walls of the arteries
2. Types
    a) Systolic pressure is the arterial pressure at the time of the contraction of the ventricles.
    b) Diastolic pressure is the arterial pressure during dilation of the ventricles when the heart relaxes between contractions.
3. Range
    a) Average range for healthy adults is 120/80–140/90; pressure may change from hour to hour and day to day.
    b) Blood pressure varies with age, sex, and muscular development.
        (1) It should be taken when the patient is quiet and relaxed.
        (2) It is usually lower in women than in men.
    c) Sphygmomanometer is used to measure pressure, and stethoscope to listen to the sounds.
4. Important points to remember
    a) Take blood pressure when patient is quiet and relaxed.
    b) Have patient in a comfortable position (sitting or reclining); this ensures a more accurate reading.
    c) Check sphygmomanometer and stethoscope before using them; place sphygmomanometer on firm, flat surface.
    d) Avoid applying excessive pressure on patient's arm.
    e) Chart blood pressure on nurse's notes or graphic chart immediately after taking pressure.
    f) Notify charge nurse of any change in patient's pressure.

XI. The Patient's Chart

A. General information
1. Recording of symptoms of patient's condition is called *charting.*
2. Practical nurse must consult with nurse in charge to find out what the practical nurse's responsibilities are and how charting is done in the hospital.

3. Patient's chart is kept in a safe central place on each ward.
4. Patient's chart is a legal document.
5. Included on chart are the following:
    a) Identifying information
    b) Doctor's orders and progress notes
    c) Doctor's notes—patient's history; present and past illnesses, including complaints and reasons for admission; diagnosis; physical examination, including special examinations and laboratory reports
    d) Graphic sheet—temperature, pulse, respiration, blood pressure, intake, output
    e) Nurse's notes—pertinent observations that describe all changes related to patient, including therapeutic responses to medication and treatment
    f) Other special forms—e.g., laboratory sheets, diabetic sheet, or social history

B. Charting Procedures
    1. Be aware that charting procedures vary in different hospitals, e.g., problem-oriented chart is used in some hospitals.
    2. Consult charge nurse if in doubt.
    3. Know the basic rules that apply in most situations.
    4. Print notes in small letters and figures, with capital letters to begin sentences.
    5. Sign each entry.
    6. Erase nothing; mistakes are to be crossed out and initialed, and a correct entry made.
    7. Use a minimum amount of abbreviations and only those approved by the hospital.
    8. Never use ditto marks.
    9. Fill out page headings completely.
    10. Record all treatments and pertinent information at exact time given.

C. Important Points to Remember
    1. Everything relating to patient's condition and progress must be charted when it occurs.
    2. The exact time must be recorded with all statements on chart.
    3. A marked or sudden change in patient's condition must be recorded.
    4. All symptoms observed by nurse must be recorded accurately.
    5. Nursing care given must be recorded, and doctor's orders must be carried out and recorded.

UNIT 3: THERAPEUTIC AND SUPPORTIVE MEASURES

VOCABULARY

congestion	presence of excessive amount of blood in tissues or an organ
constitution	physical makeup and functional habits of the body
contagious	transmitted readily from one person to another
contract	to reduce in size
contusion	bruise or black-and-blue spot due to injury, causing rupture of small blood vessel
cyanosis	discoloration of skin; may be bluish, dark purple, or grayish
debridement	removal of infected or necrotic tissue from a wound
ecchymosis	spot or blemish on skin appearing in large, irregularly formed hemorrhagic areas
erythema	redness of skin resulting from a number of causes
exudate	pus containing dead phagocytes, bacteria, cells, and tissue fluid
penetrate	to enter into the interior of

BASIC NURSING PROCEDURES

sterile   free of microorganisms
suppurative   agent producing pus formation
swelling   enlargement appearing on surface of body
therapeutics   special branch of medicine dealing with treatment of disease
vasoconstrictor   that which narrows the caliber of blood vessels

I. **Cold Applications**

   A. Types
     1. Dry cold
       a) Ice caps
       b) Ice collars
       c) Ice bags
     2. Moist cold (more penetrating than dry cold)
       a) Cold packs
       b) Compresses

   B. Effects
     1. Aid in prevention of swelling
     2. Help to control hemorrhage
     3. Prevent discoloration
     4. Prevent suppuration
     5. Check process of inflammation
     6. Constrict blood vessels and reduce circulation of blood to particular area
     7. Help to relieve pain
     8. May be very harmful when used on very weak or aged patients

   C. Safety Factors
     1. Observe condition of part of body where ice has been used.
     2. Remove cold application at frequent intervals.
     3. Use cold applications on doctor's order only.
     4. Observe infants, young children, or aged patients every 15–20 minutes when cold applications are applied.

   D. Methods of Application
     1. Ice bags, ice caps, ice collars
       a) Fill ice bag, collar, or cap no less, but no more, than two-thirds in order to avoid putting too much weight on part.
       b) Test for leakage before filling.
       c) Expel as much air as possible from bag.
       d) Screw on top, dry outer surface, cover bag, and apply to area.
       e) Remove cold application at regular intervals to prevent tissue damage.
       f) Refill or replace ice bag every 1 to 2 hours.
       g) Observe condition of skin each time application is removed.
     2. Cold compresses—may be applied to eyes, head, or other parts of body; usually ordered for eyes or head
       a) Wash hands and assemble following equipment: tray with basin; cracked ice; covered basin with solution ordered; gauze flats; cotton balls; four towels; bath towel; and paper bag.
       b) Explain procedure to patient.
       c) Change compresses every 15–20 seconds for the prescribed time, usually 15–20 minutes.
       d) Upon completion make patient comfortable; then remove, clean, and replace equipment.

II. Hot applications

A. Effects
1. Help localize infection
2. Produce muscular relaxation
3. Promote suppuration
4. Relieve congestion (by dilating the blood vessels, thereby increasing the flow of blood locally)
5. Increase metabolic rate
6. Relieve pain

B. Important Points to Remember
1. Elderly persons and infants do not tolerate heat as well as others.
2. Moist heat is more penetrating than dry heat.

C. Methods of Application
1. Hot water bottle
   a) Have water at a temperature of 120°–130° F.
   b) Apply only when ordered by doctor.
   c) Fill bag halfway; expel air.
   d) Cover bag to prevent burning.
   e) Refill bottle as necessary.
   f) Check to prevent burning.
2. Electric heating pads
   a) Apply only when ordered by doctor.
   b) Check to see if pad is in good order.
   c) Set thermostat on low.
   d) Cover pad.
   e) Check skin for redness.
3. Hot compresses
   a) Assemble necessary equipment before starting procedure.
   b) Apply to eye or other areas of body only when ordered by doctor.
   c) Be aware that temperature of solution should be higher than desired because compresses will cool considerably when wrung out and applied.
   d) Use compresses that are as hot as patient can bear without burning or causing discomfort.
   e) Observe patient during procedures.
   f) Record results.

III. Enemas

A. Types
1. Cleansing—given to relieve distension and to remove feces from the lower bowel and rectum
2. Oil retention—given to soften feces, to aid in expulsion of gas, and to relieve distension
3. Emollient—given to soothe irritated mucous membranes
4. Anthelmintic—given to destroy intestinal parasites (used only when patient cannot tolerate medication by mouth)
5. Carminative—given to stimulate peristalsis and to aid in expelling gas
6. Commercially prepared sets are available for enemas of many kinds; directions for use are given with each set and should be read carefully.

BASIC NURSING PROCEDURES

B. Precautions
1. Explain procedure to patient.
2. Check doctor's order.
3. Use correct solution, amount, and temperature.
4. Expel air from tubing.
5. Administer solution from proper height—approximately 18 inches above patient's buttocks.
6. Stop solution when patient complains of discomfort.
7. Discontinue treatment in case of pain.
8. Check patient frequently after giving enema.

C. Items to Chart
1. Time enema was given
2. Amount of solution
3. Kind of solution
4. Temperature of solution
5. Observations—color of stool returned, consistency, amount, flatus expelled, any unusual material expelled, reaction of patient

IV. Irrigations

A. General Principles
1. Procedure must be ordered by doctor.
2. Solutions, strength, and temperature must be accurate.
3. Gentle, steady stream is necessary to cleanse area being irrigated.
4. Pressure used should be sufficient to reach desired area but not enough to force fluid beyond this area.
5. Irrigating tip should not touch area to be irrigated.

B. Types
1. Eye irrigation
   a) Conditions for which doctor may order irrigation
      (1) Superficial irritation of the eye
      (2) Discharge of the eye
      (3) Infection of the eye
      (4) Inflammation of the eye
   b) Procedure
      (1) Temperature of prescribed solution should be 95°–100°F.
      (2) Patient's head should be turned toward eye that is to be irrigated.
      (3) Solution should flow from inner canthus to outer canthus.
      (4) Irrigation may be given to patient while in bed or sitting in a chair.
      (5) Patient assists with procedure by holding basin used to collect irrigating return flow and retracting lower eyelid.
   c) Items to chart
      (1) Time of procedure
      (2) Temperature
      (3) Reaction of patient to treatment
      (4) Observations made of patient
      (5) Nature of return
2. Mouth and throat irrigation
   a) Purposes for which doctor may order mouth and throat irrigation
      (1) To cleanse oral wound
      (2) To remove secretions

        (3)   To relieve inflammation of throat

        (4)   To relieve pain and congestion in throat

   b) Procedure

        (1)   Temperature of the prescribed solution shoud be 100°–120° F.

        (2)   Patient should be protected from getting wet.

        (3)   Patient's head should be held forward and tilted from one side to the other during procedure.

        (4)   Solution should be directed toward area being treated.

        (5)   Irrigation is usually given to patient in sitting position; if patient is unable to sit in chair, head of bed is elevated and patient placed in sitting position.

        (6)   Patient may assist by holding irrigating tube and directing flow of solution.

   c) Items to chart

        (1)   Time of procedure

        (2)   Reaction of patient to treatment

        (3)   Observations of patient

        (4)   Nature of return

3.   Ear irrigation

   a) Purpose for which doctor may order ear irrigation—to cleanse external auditory canal

   b) Procedure

        (1)   Temperature of prescribed solution should be 105°–108° F.

        (2)   Normal saline, boric acid, water, or bicarbonate of soda are usual solutions used for ear irrigations.

        (3)   Patient's head should be tilted in direction of ear to be irrigated.

        (4)   Flow of solution should be directed toward side of external ear canal (do not direct flow toward eardrum).

        (5)   Patient may assist by holding basin for return flow.

        (6)   Irrigation may be given while patient is in sitting position or lying in bed.

   c) Items to chart

        (1)   Time of procedure

        (2)   Reaction of patient to treatment

        (3)   Observations made of patient

        (4)   Nature of return

4.   Vaginal irrigation

   a) Purposes for which doctor may order vaginal irrigation

        (1)   To treat inflammation and congestion

        (2)   To cleanse and deodorize in cases of discharge

        (3)   To neutralize secretions in vaginal canal

        (4)   To change pH of vagina from alkaline to acid

   b) Procedure

        (1)   Bed protector should be placed under patient's hips.

        (2)   Patient's privacy should be ensured.

        (3)   Patient should be encouraged to empty bladder before irrigation.

        (4)   Patient may assist by inserting douche nozzle.

        (5)   Temperature of prescribed solution should be 105°F.

        (6)   Solution should be placed 12–18 inches above vulva.

        (7)   Solution should flow slowly, while douche nozzle is rotated, until prescribed amount of solution is given.

   c) Items to chart

        (1)   Time of procedure

        (2)   Reaction of patient to treatment

        (3)   Observations made of patient

        (4)   Results obtained

5. Wound irrigations
    a) Purpose for which doctor may order—to remove excessive discharge or secretions from body cavities or surfaces and apply moist heat
    b) Items needed
        (1) Protection for patient and bedding
        (2) Irrigator
        (3) Basin to hold solution
        (4) Basin for return flow
        (5) Thermometer to measure temperature of solution
        (6) Other items that may be needed for certain types of irrigation
6. Colostomy irrigations (method of cleansing colon through artificial opening in intestines)
    a) Purposes
        (1) To remove feces from colon
        (2) To help establish regularity of bowel movements
    b) Important points to remember
        (1) Procedure should be done at the same time each day to help patient establish bowel regularity.
        (2) Patient is taught how to manage colostomy before being discharged from hospital.

V. Inhalations

A. Purposes
    1. To relieve spasms and cough
    2. To loosen secretions in bronchial tubes
    3. To soothe irritated membranes
    4. To relieve inflammatory conditions of respiratory tract

B. Procedure
    1. Patient must be protected from direct flow of steam.
    2. Patient should be kept comfortable during procedure.
    3. Steam nozzle should be 18–24 inches from patient.
    4. Medication may be ordered in steam inhalator (menthol or tincture of benzoin); otherwise plain steam is used.
    5. Treatment must be given for entire length of time ordered.

C. Items to Chart
    1. Time of procedure
    2. Type of inhalation given
    3. Whether relief was obtained by patient

VI. Catheterization

A. Purposes
    1. To relieve urinary retention
    2. To keep perineum dry after surgery
    3. To empty bladder before surgery or decompress bladder during surgery
    4. To obtain sterile urine specimens
    5. To obtain urine specimen during the female menstrual period
    6. To determine presence of urine in the bladder
    7. To keep the incontinent patient dry (by use of an indwelling or Foley catheter)

B. Procedure
   1. Small catheter is introduced into urinary bladder.
   2. The procedure must be done under sterile conditions.

VII. Bandages

A. Purposes
   1. To immobilize a limb
   2. To apply pressure
   3. To hold dressing
   4. To give support

B. Types
   1. Cotton
   2. Strips of gauze
   3. Flannel or elastic material
   4. Montgomery straps
   5. Different widths are used, depending on part of body to be bandaged and purpose of bandage.

C. Basic Forms
   1. Figure-of-eight
   2. Circular
   3. Spiral
   4. Spiral reverse
   5. Recurrent

VIII. Binders

A. Purposes
   1. To hold dressings in place
   2. To apply pressure
   3. To provide support

B. Types
   1. Tailed—Scultetus' bandage, T-binder, or four-tailed
   2. Straight—chest or abdomen

C. Precautions
   1. Purpose of binder specifies how it should be applied.
   2. Binders must be smooth; irritation due to wrinkles may cause decubiti.
   3. If too tight, binders will interfere with normal circulation.

UNIT 4: ASEPTIC TECHNIQUES

VOCABULARY

antiseptic	substance that retards or inhibits growth of pathogenic organisms
asepsis	freedom from bacteria or microorganisms; prevention of infection
astringent	substance that contracts or hardens tissue
contamination	soiling with infected material or with anything else that may cause infection
counterirritant	substance that produces irritation to relieve inflammation
disinfect	to make something free from infection

BASIC NURSING PROCEDURES

infection   invasion of the body or part of the body by microorganisms or parasites, resulting in a disease condition

irrigation   washing of body cavity with a medicated solution or with water

isolate   to limit contact of patient suffering from a communicable disease with other people and equipment to prevent spread of disease

pustulant   agent that causes the formation of pustules

pustule   small elevation of skin filled with pus or lymph

sterilize   to make something free from microoganisms

vesicant   agent that causes blisters

I. Introduction

A. Definition of **Aseptic Techniques:** Techniques used to prevent infection and spread of disease-producing organisms; nurse must assume responsibility for preventing spread of disease

B. Standard Precautions
   1. Wash hands before and after every contact with a patient; hand washing is the most important precaution to prevent the spread of disease.
   2. Wash hands before handling food.
   3. Wash hands after using the toilet.
   4. Avoid off-duty contact with persons who have communicable diseases.
   5. Use special procedures to prevent contact with infectious organisms; e.g., use gloves.
   6. Hold soiled linen away from uniform.
   7. Wrap soiled dressings so they can be handled safely.
   8. Do not shake bed linen; use special laundry bags provided; use a dampened dust cloth to avoid spreading dust particles.
   9. Wash patient's hands after patient uses bedpan or urinal.
   10. Give special attention to all equipment that comes in contact with patients with communicable diseases.
   11. Follow hospital procedures.

C. General Principles
   1. The term *surgical aseptic technique* is accepted as including all steps performed in sterilization of articles, as well as measures used to prevent contamination of sterile material.
   2. An article is either sterile or unsterile.
   3. If in doubt as to whether an article is sterile or unsterile, the article should be considered unsterile.
   4. Contact with an unsterile surface contaminates a sterile object.
   5. Air currents are capable of carrying contaminants.
   6. Nurse must assist with, set up, and perform sterile procedures in as clean an environment as possible; must practice good personal hygiene; and must observe established procedures in all hospital housekeeping duties, especially in discarding waste and in maintaining a dust-free work area.
   7. Nurse must wash hands thoroughly before beginning any sterile procedure (in order to make hands as clean as possible and free of surface bacteria).
   8. Any object that becomes contaminated must be discarded.

II. Disinfection, Sterilization, and Isolation

A. Medical Aseptic Techniques
   1. Carrying out of procedures to control and prevent contact with disease organisms

  2. Destruction of organisms after they leave the body

  3. Example—isolation

 B. Surgical Aseptic Techniques

  1. Carrying out of procedures to make and keep articles and areas sterile (free from all microorganisms)

  2. Examples—sterilization, disinfection

 C. Disinfectants

  1. May not kill all organisms but will check their growth

  2. Examples—sunlight, fresh air, soap and water

 D. Hospital Procedure—All equipment for nursing treatments generally is sterilized in a central supply room.

 E. Organisms

  1. Enter body through

   a) Breaks in mucous membrane and skin

   b) Respiratory system

   c) Urinary and reproductive systems

   d) Gastrointestinal system

  2. Leave body through

   a) Vomitus and feces

   b) Sneezing, coughing, and sputum

   c) Mucous discharge and urine

   d) Exudates from surface wounds

Note: See Chapter 1, Unit 2, on microbiology for description of pathogenic organisms and methods of sterilization.

III. Medical Asepsis

 General Principles

  1. Terms used to describe objects in patient's unit are *clean* and *contaminated*.

  2. Terminal disinfection is carried out in relation to routine nursing care.

  3. When working in an isolation unit, the nurse must follow hospital procedure regarding use of mask, gown, and hand-washing techniques.

  4. All dishes, linen, and other equipment used for patient in isolation should be disinfected (follow instruction given in hospital).

IV. Surgical Asepsis

 General Principles

  1. Surgical asepsis means "sterilization of all items coming into contact with operative field."

  2. Terms used are *sterile* and *unsterile*.

  3. All items are sterilized in a central supply unit.

V. Sterile Pick-up Forceps (used to handle and lift sterile articles)

 General Principles

  1. While placing articles on tray, do not touch sterile equipment or tray with anything but sterile forceps.

2. Hold tip end of forceps pointed downward and keep above waist level.
3. Replace forceps so they do not touch inside of holder.
4. Do not breathe directly onto sterile field or bend over sterile field.
5. Do not turn back on sterile field.

VI. Dressings

A. General Principles
   1. Dressings may be defined as any material applied to a wound or incision to protect it, promote healing, or absorb drainage.
   2. Dressings are always sterile to prevent introducing organisms into wounds.

B. Types of Materials
   1. Gauze
   2. Cotton
   3. Silk
   4. Paper
   5. All of the above are held in place by bandage or adhesive.

C. Types of Dressings
   1. Dry sterile
   2. Clean
   3. Grease gauze
   4. Colostomy

D. Nurse's Role
   1. May be required to change dressing and assist doctor or registered nurse
   2. Must know when to apply sterile dressing

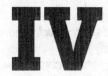

IV

Nursing Care of the Adult Patient

UNIT 1: THE INTEGUMENTARY SYSTEM: Skin and Accessory Organs

VOCABULARY

absorb	to suck up
derma-	refers to the skin
dermis	true skin
duct	tubular vessel conveying blood or other secretions of the body
epidermis	outer layer of the skin
excretory	pertaining to elimination
fissure	cracklike lesion
follicle	small excretory duct or sac
intertrigo	chafing
kerato-	refers to a callus
-oma	refers to a tumor
pruritis	itching
scale	thin, dry flake shed from upper layers of skin
sclero-	refers to condition of hardening
sebaceous glands	oil-secreting glands
sudoriferous glands	sweat-producing glands
urticaria	inflammatory condition, characterized by eruption of pale wheals associated with severe itching

I. **Functions and Structure**

    A. Definition of **Skin:** The outer covering of the body; the skin is both a system and an organ

    B. Functions
        1. Covers the body
        2. Protects deeper tissues from injury and infections if unbroken
        3. Contains endings of many sensory nerves
        4. Plays important part in regulation of body temperature
        5. Has limited excretory functions through sebaceous and sudoriferous glands
        6. Has limited absorption functions
        7. Contains bacteria normally

    C. Structure
        1. Epidermis
           a) Has four layers

b) Contains skin pigments
c) Has as its main purpose to protect the dermis
2. Dermis (also called *corium*)
a) Consists of several layers of connective tissue
b) Contains a network of nerves and blood vessels
c) Contains hair follicles, sudoriferous glands, and sebaceous glands
d) Has pronounced projections causing ridging (fingerprints)

D. Accessory Organs
1. Hair
a) Appears on all parts of body except palms and soles
b) Exists in greater amount on scalp
c) Has color due to pigment in hair shaft
2. Nails
3. Sebaceous glands
4. Sudoriferous glands

II. Assessment of Skin

A. Common Symptoms and Signs
1. Abnormal color: pallor, jaundice, flushing, cyanosis, ashen
2. Erythema
3. Change in temperature
4. Pruritis
5. Weeping
6. Rash (see Data Summaries 6 and 7)
7. Fissuring
8. Changes in pigment
9. Scaling
10. Loss of hair
11. Ulcers
12. Change in texture
13. Change in sensation

B. Causes of Skin Abnormalities
1. Allergic reactions
a) Definition: Skin reaction to foreign substance
b) Signs and symptoms
(1) Itching
(2) Erythema
(3) Lesions
c) Causes
(1) Clothing and household products
(2) Toxic plants
(3) Foods, e.g., shellfish
(4) Medications, e.g., penicillin, codeine
(5) Environmental factors, e.g., dust, chlorine in water, hair sprays, nail polish
d) Treatment
(1) Cleansing of skin
(2) Local applications
(3) Systemic drugs (steroids, adrenaline)
2. Pathogens
a) Causes

        (1)   Bacterial
        (2)   Viral
        (3)   Fungal
        (4)   Mycotic
        (5)   Parasitic
   b) Assessment
        (1)   Itching
        (2)   Lesions
        (3)   Erythema
        (4)   Pain
   c) Treatment
        (1)   Maintain cleanliness.
        (2)   Keep lesions dry.
        (3)   Apply antibiotics locally.
        (4)   Isolate patient's clothing, towels, etc.

3. Nutritional defects
   a) Avitaminosis
   b) Protein deficiency
4. Extremes of temperature
   a) Burns
   b) Extreme cold
5. Chemicals
   a) Burns
   b) Ulcerations
6. Drug reactions
7. Disease in other systems
8. Neoplasms
9. Normal aging process
10. Unknown factors

C. Diagnosis
   1. History, taken by physician
   2. Diagnostic tests and procedures
      a) Visual examination of skin lesions under daylight or strong white light
      b) Complete physical examination of patient
      c) Skin cultures (especially in suspected fungus infections)
      d) Patch tests (used for allergy detection)
      e) Intradermal tests
      f) Biopsy (stained sections of the skin)
      g) Urinalysis
      h) Complete blood count
      i) Basal metabolic rate
      j) Blood serology (important in syphilis)
      k) Blood chemistry
      l) Stool examination for ova and parasites

III. Common Skin Disorders

Note: Because dermatology can be bewildering to the novice, some common disorders of the skin are listed below in a particular classification that may help the practical nurse become familiar with the terminology. No attempt is made to give the complete etiology, diagnosis, or treatment. General nursing procedures referrable to disorders of the skin will follow this section. The one exception is burns, which are more fully described.

A. Seborrheic Dermatoses
   1. Acne
   2. Seborrheic dermatitis

B. Eczematous Dermatoses (Eczema)
   1. Contact dermatitis
   2. Atopic eczema

C. Erythematous Rashes
   1. Urticaria
   2. Erythema multiforme
   3. Erythema nodosum

D. Drug Eruptions

E. Pyogenic Infections
   1. Erysipelas
   2. Impetigo contagiosa
   3. Folliculitis
   4. Furunculosis

F. Viral Infections
   1. Herpes simplex
   2. Herpes zoster

G. Diseases Caused by Animal Parasites
   1. Scabies
   2. Pediculosis

H. Fungus Infections
   1. Tinea capitis
   2. Tinea corporis
   3. Dermatophytosis
   4. Tinea cruris
   5. Moniliasis

I. Common Dermatoses of Unknown Etiology
   1. Psoriasis
   2. Lichen planus
   3. Pityriasis rosea
   4. Alopecia areata
   5. Vitiligo
   6. Sarcoidosis
   7. Lupus erythematosus
   8. Scleroderma

J. Lymphoblastomas

K. Tuberculosis of the Skin

L. Syphilis

M. Benign tumors

    1. Warts
    2. Nevi
    3. Moles
    4. Keloids
    5. Keratoses

N. Malignant Tumors
    1. Basal cell epithelioma
    2. Melanoma
    3. Paget's disease
    4. Squamous cell carcinoma

IV. Fundamentals of Nursing Care

A. Goals
    1. Make patient more comfortable, physically and emotionally
    2. Relieve itching
    3. Encourage patient
    4. Assist in administering prescribed treatment
    5. Help provide for personal hygiene of patient

B. Drug Therapies
    1. Types
        a) External
            (1) Ointments—antibiotic, analgesic, antipruritic, hormonal, etc.
            (2) Lotions—antibiotic, analgesic, antipruritic, hormonal, etc.
            (3) Solutions—antibiotic, analgesic, antipruritic, hormonal, etc.
            (4) Creams—antibiotic, analgesic, antipruritic, hormonal, etc.
            (5) Medicated Baths
                (a) Starch
                (b) Oatmeal or bran
                (c) Potassium permanganate
            (6) Powders
        b) Internal
            (1) Analgesics
            (2) Sedatives
            (3) Antibiotics
            (4) Antipruritics
            (5) Vitamins
            (6) Hormones
                (a) Adrenaline
                (b) Cortisone
                (c) ACTH

    2. Purposes
        a) To relieve itching
        b) To dry moist and weeping lesions
        c) To soothe inflamed areas of skin and reduce inflammation
        d) To remove hard lesions and crusts
        e) To supply a protective coating
        f) To kill bacteria, parasites, and fungi by direct application of medication

C. Diet Therapy
    1. Purpose—generally to relieve allergic condition
    2. Generally preceded by an elimination diet

DATA SUMMARY 6 Classification of Primary Skin Lesions		
Lesion	*Description*	
Macule	A discolored spot on the skin; not elevated; depressed; cannot be felt.	MACULE (flat)
Papule	A solid elevation of the skin; not larger than a split pea.	PAPULE (solid)
Vesicle	A small sac; not larger than a split pea; containing serous fluid.	VESICLE (clear fluid)
Pustule	A small elevation of the skin; filled with pus.	PUSTULE (pus-filled)
Bulla	A sac; larger than a split pea; containing fluid.	
Nodule	A solid formation of the skin; larger than a split pea.	
Tumor	A solid formation of the skin; larger than a hazelnut.	
Wheal	A temporary elevation of the skin.	WHEAL (smooth, slightly elevated)
Scale	A mass of exfoliating skin.	
Cyst	A closed sac or pouch containing fluid.	CYST (fluid- or solid-filled sac)
Polyp	A protruding growth from mucous membrane.	POLYP (growth)

DATA SUMMARY 7
Description of Primary Skin Lesions

Lesion	Description
Crust	A mass formed upon the surface of the skin from the accumulation of dried exudate.
Excoriation	A superficial scraping of the skin.
Fissure	A crack in the skin. FISSURE (slit, groove)
Ulcer	An open erosion or sore of the skin or mucous membrane. ULCER (open sore)
Scar	A mark left in the skin by the healing of a wound through the growth of connective tissue in the wound.

D. General Nursing Procedures
1. Colloidal baths—relieve skin irritation and pruritus (itching); contain the following:
   a) Oatmeal
   b) Bran
   c) Starch
   d) Combination
2. Moist dressings
   a) May be warm or cold, open or closed
   b) Are made with various solutions, depending on lesion
      (1) Normal saline
      (2) Epsom salts
      (3) Burrow's solution
      (4) Boric acid (highly poisonous—no longer recommended for antiseptic use in powder form)
3. Soaks
   a) Loosen dead tissue
   b) Bring abscesses to a head
4. Unna paste boot—gelatin-impregnated bandage
   a) Used—to treat leg ulcers
      (1) Gives support to veins, relieving venostasis
      (2) Relieves edema of area
   b) Method of application
      (1) Sterile dressing laid over ulcer
      (2) Unna paste painted on from metatarsals to knee
      (3) Layer of 3-inch bandage applied
      (4) Paste and bandage repeated for 2-3 thicknesses
      (5) After bandage dries, toes checked for edema and color
      (6) Boot changed every 14-21 days

E. Summary of Principles and Goals of Nursing Care
    1. Relieve itching and pain
        a) Observe area and record signs in detail.
        b) Promote rest of area to reduce stimuli.
        c) Omit stimulating foods from diet, e.g., coffee, tea, condiments, alcohol.
        d) Use tub baths.
        e) Apply local anesthetic, analgesic, or antipruritic medications.
        f) Administer sedatives or tranquilizers orally or parenterally to control severe discomfort.
    2. Reduce inflammation
        a) Apply wet dressings continuously or intermittently as ordered.
        b) Remove scaling and crusting before application of topical medications.
            (1) Adequate applications of medications into skin to increase penetration
            (2) Periodic observation of lesion to note response to therapy
            (3) Recording of observations
    3. Curb weeping, oozing, and prevent formation of crusts
        a) Apply wet dressings.
        b) Gently remove old medications with mineral oil.
        c) Use astringent, drying solutions, and lotions to decrease oozing.
        d) Use antibiotics orally, topically, or parenterally.
        e) Give high-protein diet to offset severe serum loss.
    4. Prevent further skin damage
        a) Avoid excessively hot wet dressings.
        b) Avoid excessive friction by blotting skin in drying.
        c) Shield healthy skin to prevent maceration during application of wet dressings.
    5. Help educate patient
        a) Explain why treatments are necessary and how they are to be performed.
        b) Encourage patient's cooperation in assisting with own care if not contraindicated.

V. Burns

A. Etiology
    1. Caused by injury to skin
        a) Heat
        b) Electricity
        c) Irradiation
        d) Chemicals
    2. Classified according to depth of skin involvement
        a) Erythema—*first degree*
        b) Erythema plus blisters—*second degree*
        c) Destruction of skin and of underlying tissues—*third degree*
    3. Estimated in extent by the rule of 9's (see Figure 9)
        a) Adults

(1) Entire head and neck		9%
(2) Entire right arm		9%
(3) Entire left arm		9%
(4) Anterior surface of upper trunk		9%
(5) Posterior surface of upper trunk		9%
(6) Anterior surface of lower trunk		9%
(7) Posterior surface of lower trunk		9%
(8) Right leg		9%
(9) Left leg		9%
(10) Genitals		1%

NURSING CARE OF THE ADULT PATIENT

b) Infants and children—percentages vary
c) Lesser parts of body surfaces—percentages vary

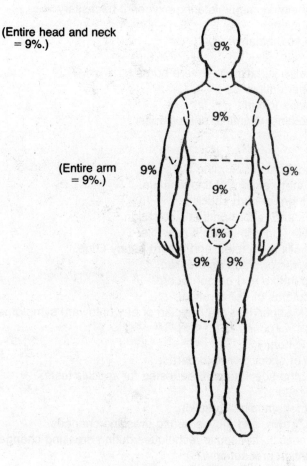

(Entire head and neck = 9%.)

9%

9%

(Entire arm = 9%.) 9% 9%

9%

(1%)

9% 9%

ADULT
("Rule of Nines")

Figure 9

B. Bodily Changes Caused by Severe Burns
    1. Electrolyte imbalance
    2. Fluid loss
    3. Inhalation injuries
        a) Lung burns
        b) Obstruction of air passages
        c) Pulmonary edema
    4. Kidney involvement
        a) Decreased urinary output
        b) Urinary tract infection
    5. Gastrointestinal involvement
        a) Short-term results: gastric dilatation, paralytic ileus
        b) Long-term result: ulcer of gastric mucosa (Curling's ulcer)

C. Immediate Treatment
    1. Removal of cause

2. Applying cold water to small first- and second-degree burns
3. Noting and recording extent of burn
4. Checking vital signs
5. Maintaining adequate airway; administering oxygen if necessary
6. Control of shock, if present
7. Careful monitoring of fluid balance
8. Relieving pain
9. Maintaining strict reverse isolation in severe burns
10. Administration of proper antibiotics
11. Administration of tetanus toxoid
12. Giving diet high in proteins, vitamins, and calories

   D. Summary of Principles and Goals of Nursing Care
Note: Nursing care is most important treatment of this disease.
   1. Prevention and treatment of burn shock
      a) Carefully observe and record patient's condition.
         (1) Weigh patient on admission if possible.
         (2) Insert indwelling catheter, and record hourly urine.
      b) Administer fluids and/or blood as ordered.
      c) Maintain detailed intake and output record.
      d) Observe for symptoms of dehydration.
      e) Immediately notify supervisor or physician of any untoward symptoms.
   2. Evaluation of patient's response to therapy
      a) Record vital signs hourly.
      b) Notify laboratory of specific tests ordered.
      c) Obtain 24-hour urine specimens if requested for specific tests.
   3. Prevention of complications
      a) Use careful regimens against infection.
         (1) Use mask, gown, and gloves during dressing changes.
         (2) Observe meticulous aseptic techniques during dressing changes.
      b) Use reverse isolation precautions.
      c) Obtain wound cultures as ordered.
      d) Maintain meticulous personal hygiene of patient.
         (1) Frequent oral hygiene.
         (2) Meticulous attention to patient's eyes, ears, nose, and hair.
         (3) Attention to meatus around catheter.
      e) Observe for respiratory difficulties.
      f) Maintain good body alignment of patient to prevent contractures and deformities.
      g) Observe for temperature elevations.
   4. Promotion of wound healing
      a) Maintain good nutritional status.
         (1) Encourage high-protein diet.
         (2) Give supplementary protein feedings.
         (3) Keep accurate record of amount eaten.
      b) Assist with local wound care—*very important.*
      c) Prepare patient for surgical or grafting procedures.
   5. Promotion of restoration of patient's health
      a) Maintain patient in correct position.
         (1) Use bed cradle.
         (2) Use footboard
         (3) Use splints or hand rolls as necessary.
         (4) Elevate extremities and immobilize in functional position.

b) Employ passive exercise and range-of-motion movements as ordered by physician.
c) Encourage and assist patient in adjusting to physical limitations.
d) Educate patient in regimen and methods of self-help.
6. Relief of pain—medicate if warranted and ordered.

UNIT 2: THE MUSCULOSKELETAL SYSTEM

VOCABULARY

aligned	arranged in line; in correct anatomical position
arthritis	inflammation of a joint
articular surface	site of connection of bones
congenital	occurring during fetal life
contraction	shortening of a muscle or muscle group
decalcification	loss of calcium
immobilize	to make immovable
joints	point of juncture between two bones
orthopedics	branch of medical science that deals with treatment of disorders involving locomotor structures of the body; e.g., skeleton, joints, muscles
osteomalacia	metabolic bone disease; decreased absorption of calcium by bones
osteoporosis	softening of bone due to impaired mineralization
prosthesis	artificial substitute for a missing part
spica	reverse spiral bandage; body cast usually applied to anatomical areas of different dimensions
torticollis	stiff neck caused by spasmodic contraction of neck muscles

I. **Components of Musculoskeletal System**
  A. Bones
    1. Types
      a) Long bones as in extremities
      b) Short bones as in hands and feet
      c) Flat bones as in skull and thorax
      d) Irregularly shaped bones such as vertebrae
    2. Functions
      a) Provide hardest connective tissue of body
      b) Form framework of body
      c) Support body
      d) Serve as storage place for minerals
      e) Help in formation of blood cells (red marrow)
      f) Surround and protect vital organs
      g) Give points of attachment for muscles
  B. Joints
    1. Functions
      a) Provide union of two or more bones
      b) Make motion possible
    2. Types (see Figure 10)
      a) Immovable—between bones of skull
      b) Slightly movable—between vertebrae
      c) Freely movable
        (1) Ball and socket—shoulder and hip joint have rotating movement which includes all movements
        (2) Hinge joints—elbow and knee have flexion and extension movements

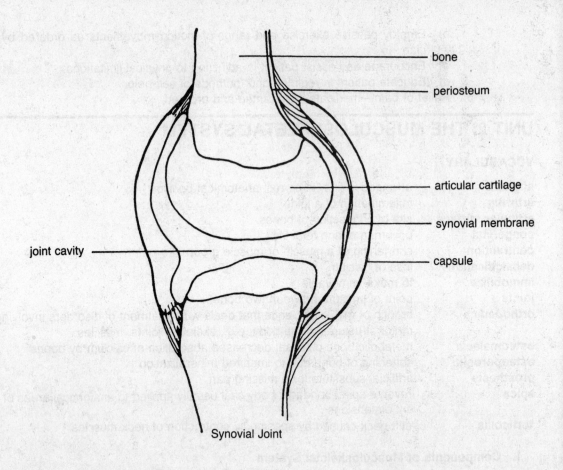

Synovial Joint

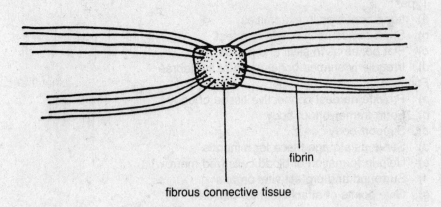

Figure 10

C. Cartilage
   1. Elastic tissue without blood supply or nerves
   2. Functions
      a) Lines bones and joints
      b) Lies between vertebrae
      c) Helps movements of the spine

D. Ligaments
   1. Flexible, fibrous connective tissue
   2. Functions
      a) Connect articular ends (joints) of bones
      b) Support muscles

E. Skeletal Muscles
   1. Spindle-shaped
   2. Attached to bones by tendons
   3. Fixed point of attachment is origin; movable point of attachment is insertion
   4. Function—contraction, which causes movement of joint

F. Tendons
   1. Fibrous connective tissue
   2. Function—to attach muscles to bones

E. Bursa
   1. Pouch or sac found in connective tissue
   2. Function—to reduce friction around tendons and bony prominences

F. Synovial Membrane
   1. Lines joint capsule
   2. Function—secretes fluid that lubricates joint

II. Classification of Musculoskeletal Disorders

A. Congenital Disorders
   1. Club foot (talipes)
      a) Bilateral or unilateral
      b) Mild or severe
   2. Dislocation of hip
      a) Bilateral or unilateral
      b) Mild or severe
   3. Spina bifida and spina bifida occulta: defects in walls of spinal canal that can result in neurologic symptoms
   4. Torticollis (congenital wryneck)
      a) Is generally believed to be due to birth injury
      b) Affects sternocleidomastoid muscle
      c) Is unilateral
   5. Craniofacial abnormalities
      a) Cleft lip and cleft palate
      b) Small-mandible defects
   6. Congenital scoliosis

B. Traumatic Disorders
   1. Fractures of bones
      a) Greenstick—only part of thickness of bone is involved
      b) Simple—bone is completely broken, but ends do not puncture skin
      c) Compound—broken ends of bone puncture skin
      d) Cumminuted—bone is fragmented in area of break
      e) Impacted fracture—one end of bone is wedged into interior of other end
   2. Dislocations of joints
      a) Ends of bones forming joint are in abnormal position within joint capsule

b) Bones are not displaced.
3. Strains of muscles or tendons—due to excessive overuse, pulling, or twisting of muscles or tendons

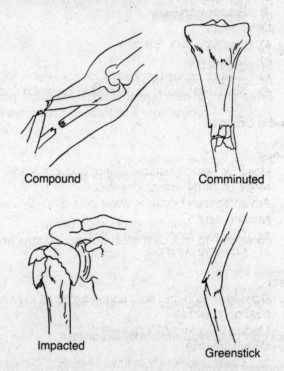

Compound   Comminuted

Impacted   Greenstick

C. Arthritis
  1. Definition of **arthritis:** Joint affections characterized by inflammation and other changes depending upon type
  2. Types
     a) Metabolic (gout)
     b) Traumatic
     c) Neurotropic (Charcot joint)
     d) Allergic
     e) Suppurative
     f) Hemorrhagic disease (hemophilia)
     g) Toxic
     h) Chronic rheumatoid
     i) Chronic osteoarthritis

III. Diagnostic Tests

A. X-ray Study and Bone Scan
  1. X-rays are used to determine bone changes in the following:
     a) Size
     b) Contour
     c) Density
  2. Bone scan, using radioactive isotopes, is useful in detecting tumors, usually of metastatic origin.

B. Laboratory Tests
  1. Blood tests
     a) Complete blood count

      b) Sedimentation rate
      c) Serology
      d) C-reactive protein
      e) Uric acid
      f) Serum enzymes
  2. Other tests
      a) Synovial fluid analysis
      b) Urinalysis
      c) Culture, to determine the responsible organisms in bone infection
      d) Sensitivity tests, to determine the most useful antibiotic in bone infection

IV. Orthopedic Devices

A. Splints
  1. Used for immobilization, union, and protection
  2. Made of metal, wood, or plaster
  3. Advantageous because allow care of injuries requiring observation and dressings
  4. Nursing care
      a) Observe for pressure points.
      b) Observe position.

B. Casts
  1. Used to immobilize, hold bone fragments in reduction, protect, and permit early weight-bearing activities
  2. Made of plaster of Paris
  3. Disadvantages
      a) Casts, especially spicas, impede patient's movements.
      b) Immobilization sometimes causes emotional and physical problems.
  4. Nursing care
      a) Preparation of bed depends on type of cast.
      b) Careful movement of patient is necessary to prevent damage to cast.
      c) Careful observation is necessary.
         (1) Cast must not cut into patient's flesh or exert pressure over a bony prominence (pain is a warning signal).
         (2) Circulation of extremity must be checked at intervals as long as cast remains (observe for swelling, blanching, pain, tingling, numbness, loss of movement in fingers or toes, edema, change in color).
         (3) Abdominal distension must be watched for in patients in body spicas (rectal tubes inserted for short periods to provide relief).
         (4) Any unusual odor should be reported.
      d) Perineal care is important.
      e) Routine turning of patient is important.
      f) Well-balanced diet, low in calories, is necessary for patients in body spica.
      g) Active exercise of uninvolved joints is necessary
  5. Care of cast
      a) Allow cast to dry properly.
      b) Pad cast edges and keep clean.
      c) Give special attention to bowel and bladder hygiene.
      d) Observe cast for soft spots and discoloration.
      e) Support cast.
  6. Cast removal
      a) Cast is generally bivalved for removal.
      b) Care is needed in moving patient or part after cast is removed.

   (1) Decalcification of bone may result in fracture.
   (2) Loss of muscle tone and some disuse atrophy are present.
   (3) Skin may need gentle cleansing to remove exudate.
  c) Support, such as elastic bandage, is generally necessary.
  d) Physical therapy is indicated to help muscles regain tone.
  e) Immediate weight bearing is generally not indicated.

C. Traction
 1. Definition of **traction**: force applied in two directions
 2. Purposes
  a) To relieve muscle spasm
  b) To regain normal length and alignment
  c) To reduce and immobilize fracture
 3. Types
  a) Skin—adhesive material applied directly to skin
   (1) Russell traction in fractures of femur or hip
   (2) Buck's extension when partial or temporary immobilization is desired
   (3) Bryant's traction for fractures of femur in children
  b) Skeletal—pins or wire placed through bone (Kirchner wire)
  c) Crutchfield tongs—attached to skull for cervical traction
 4. Nursing care
  a) Observe:
   (1) Skin for abrasion and/or irritation
   (2) Wire or pin wounds for infection
   (3) Circulation of extremities
   (4) Pressure points for irritations
   (5) Traction apparatus for alterations
  b) Inspect sacral area when patient is lifted for care.
  c) Use special bedpans and urinals for these patients.
  d) Give meticulous oral care.
  e) Give diet high in iron, protein, calcium, roughage, and vitamins.
  f) Urge patient to breathe deeply, cough, and actively exercise unaffected joints.

D. Frames
 1. Types used for patients in traction
  a) Balkan—placed on bed before traction is set up
  b) Bradford—similar to Balkan
  c) Stryker—allows for changing patient's position without interfering with his/her body alignment
  d) Foster—similar to Stryker
 2. Nursing care
  a) Balkan and Bradford frames
   (1) Sheets must be tightened several times daily.
   (2) Patients must be protected from falling.
  b) Stryker and Foster frames
   (1) Care is easier because frames pivot and position of patients can easily be changed.
   (2) Patients can more easily help themselves.
   (3) Caution is needed in turning patient.

E. Additional Orthopedic Devices
 1. Collars, corsets and back braces, crutches, braces
 2. Purposes—to immobilize and/or aid in locomotion

V. General Nursing Care of Orthopedic Patients

A. Nursing Procedures
   1. Certain bed equipment necessary
      a) Bed boards
      b) Firm mattress
      c) Overhead trapeze
   2. Protection and observation of orthopedic devices for malfunction
   3. Excellent personal hygiene
   4. Constant observation of skin for pressure
   5. Constant observation of extremities for circulation
   6. Adequate fluid intake
   7. Observation for problems of elimination
   8. Active exercise of unaffected joints to maintain muscle tone and function
   9. Protection of all open wounds from infection

B. Body Mechanics and Positioning
   1. Positioning is important to prevent contractures and development of deformities.
   2. Active and passive exercise, including range-of-motion movements of joints, is needed.
   3. Patients must be turned periodically.
      a) Purposes
         (1) To prevent pulmonary complications
         (2) To stimulate circulation
         (3) To prevent decubiti
      b) Use of tilt table helpful
         (1) In relieving postural hypotension, if present
         (2) In retarding osteoporosis
         (3) In preventing pooling of urine in bladder and thus cystitis
   4. Practical nurse should educate patient in proper use of body when sitting, standing, walking, and stooping.

VI. Treatment of Traumatic Disorders

A. Fracture
   1. Reduction
      a) Closed—bones manipulated without breaking skin
      b) Open—operative procedure
   2. Immobilization
      a) Splint
      b) Plaster cast
      c) Traction
      d) Internal fixation (nails, wires, plates)
   3. Immediate nursing care
      (1) Fracture to be immobilized without causing further injury
      (2) Wound of compound fracture to be covered with clean cloth
      (3) Patient to be observed for shock and vital signs recorded
      (4) Patient to be covered and kept warm
      (5) Clothing to be removed without disturbing injured part
   4. Types of casts
      a) Short-leg or long-leg casts cover part or all of lower extremity.
      b) Casts for upper extremities may be of several types, depending upon type of fracture.

      c) Walking casts have extra material and an appliance added to the sole for weight bearing.

      d) Body spica covers trunk and possibly extremities.

  5. Preparation of patient for cast application

      a) Skin is thoroughly washed and rinsed.

      b) Shaving may be required if surgery is to be done.

  6. Care of fresh cast

      a) Patient is positioned gently in bed.

      b) Rough handling of cast is avoided.

      c) Wet cast must always be handled by palm of hand, not by fingertips.

      d) Supports are placed beneath curves of cast to prevent distortion.

      e) Patient is turned frequently to help cast dry evenly.

      f) Cast drier helps circulate air around cast.

      g) Cast must be completely dry before covering.

  7. Care of patient in cast

      a) Observation of patient's fingers or toes for proper circulation

      b) Proper alignment of patient and part

      c) Meticulous skin care

  8. Care of patient in traction

      a) Monitor position.

      b) Maintain weight prescribed by physician.

      c) Keep rope on pulley

      d) Observe for signs of irritation over coccyx and around pin

      e) Adjust bedclothes so that pull of traction is maintained and patient is kept warm

      f) Give proper skin care.

      g) Observe for circulatory changes.

      h) Check for edema.

      i) Prevent footdrop.

         (1) Foot plate

         (2) Dorsiflexion exercises

  9. Care of patient on crutches

      a) Strengthening of muscles through exercise should precede crutch walking.

      b) Proper gait with crutches and use of crutches should be demonstrated.

      c) Crutches should be proper length.

B. Sprains

  1. Intermittent cold compresses

  2. Temporary elastic compression bandage

  3. Immobilization of joint

  4. Elevation of joint

  5. X-ray study to rule out fracture

C. Strains

  1. Cold compresses

  2. Immobilization

  3. Operative repair if necessary

VII. Treatment of Inflammatory Disorders

A. Arthritis

  1. Removal of foci of infection (if associated with a specific disease)

  2. Complete rest during inflammatory phase; frequent periods of rest thereafter to take weight off joints

    3. Proper positioning
    4. Medication as ordered—analgesics, steroids, Colchicine (gout)
    5. Frequent change in position
    6. Observation of bony prominences
    7. Cradle to avoid pressure from bedclothes
    8. Heat, if ordered
    9. Maintenance of joint mobility and muscle power
   10. Proper elimination
   11. Range-of-motion exercises, if ordered
   12. Special diets, if necessary, e.g., low purine for gout
   13. Rehabilitation

  B Bursitis
    1. Heat
    2. Procaine hydrochloride injected into joint
    3. Restful position

  C. Tendonitis
    1. Infiltration of Novocain
    2. Heat
    3. Rest

VIII. Treatment of Infectious Disorders

  A. Osteomyelitis
    1. Definition of **osteomyelitis:** Inflammation of bone caused by a pyogenic organism; it may remain localized or may spread through the bone to involve the marrow, cortex, cancellous tissue, and periosteum
    2. Type: may be acute or chronic
    3. Treatment
      a) Medical
        (1) Large doses of penicillin or other antibiotics as ordered
        (2) Part put at rest with splints
      b) Surgical
        (1) Incision and drainage if necessary
        (2) Exploration for removal of sequestra
      c) Nursing care
        (1) That for surgical procedure, pre- and postoperative
        (2) Psychological support

  B. Tuberculosis of Bone
    1. Definition of **tuberculosis:** Chronic infection with bacterium *Mycobacterium tuberculosis,* characterized by the formation of tubercles and casseous necrosis
    2. Types
      a) Occuring in spine
        1. Bone softening may result in deformity.
        2. Treatment is by immobilization of spine and antituberculosis drugs.
        3. Surgery may be required.
        4. Nursing care includes medical asepsis.
      b) Occurring in hip
        1. Treatment is by immobilization.
        2. Surgery is usually required

IX. Treatment of Neoplasms

A. Benign Osteomas (Bone Tumors)
   1. Treatment may be surgical (biopsy after removal of tumor to rule out malignancy)
   2. Nursing care: psychological support.

B. Malignant Tumors
   1. They may be primary and metastasize to other parts of body.
   2. They may be secondary and the results of metastasis.
   3. Treatment is dependent upon extent of involvement and type.
   4. Amputation of extremity may be necessary.

X. Surgery of the Musculoskeletal System

A. Hip Fracture
   1. Occurrence—most frequent in elderly women
   2. Preoperative nursing care
      a) Give skin care.
      b) Maintain proper position.
      c) Assist patient in eating, bathing, etc.
   3. Operative procedures
      a) Surgical fixation with nails, plates, or screws
      b) Possibly replacement
   4. Postoperative nursing care
      a) Follow surgeon's orders in regard to turning.
      b) Carry out routine postoperative orders.

B. Hip Replacement
   1. Procedure: Femoral head is replaced by steel ball and stem, and acetabulum is replaced by plastic or metal cup.
   2. Nursing care
      a) Follow surgeon's orders.
      b) Encourage patient to follow orders of physiotherapist.

C. Total Knee Replacement
   1. Follow postoperative orders.
   2. Encourage patient to follow exercises suggested by physiotherapist.

D. Amputation
   1. Procedure: Surgical removal of a diseased limb or part due to
      a) Severe trauma
      b) Malignancy
      c) Gangrene
   2. Preoperative care
      a) Special orthopedic skin preparation
      b) Psychological preparation
      c) Other routine preoperative care
      d) Plans for fitting an artificial limb
   3. Postoperative care
      a) Use fracture bed.
      b) Observe and record vital signs.
      c) Elevate stump.
      d) Keep patient prone for part of time.

e) Elevate stump for 24 hours.
f) Encourage deep breathing and coughing to aerate lungs.
g) Observe carefully for hemorrhage.
h) Record intake and output.
i) Apply pressure on stump for relief of phantom pain.
j) Give medication as ordered for pain.
k) Prepare plans for referral to physiotherapy for exercises, balancing, crutch walking, and gait training after prosthesis is fitted.
l) Continue psychological support.

UNIT 3: THE NERVOUS SYSTEM

VOCABULARY

asthenia	loss of strength
ataxia	lack of muscle coordination
coma	state of unconsciousness from which patient cannot be aroused
encephalitis	inflammation of brain
esthesia	feeling, sensation
flaccid	flabby or relaxed; lacking muscle tone
hemiplegia	paralysis of half of the body
meningitis	inflammation of brain meninges (three connective tissue membranes that enclose and protect the brain)
neuralgia	pain along course of nerves
neuro-	pertaining to nerves
neurology	study of the nervous system and its diseases
nystagmus	constant involuntary movement of the eyeball
papilledema	edema and inflammation of optic nerve at its point of entrance into eyeball
paralysis	impairment or loss of muscle function
paraplegia	paralysis of lower portion of body and of both legs
quadriplegia	paralysis of all four limbs
seizure	convulsion
spasm	involuntary contraction of muscles
spastic	pertaining to spasm or uncontrolled skeletal muscle contraction
syncope	temporary loss of consciousness
syndrome	all the symptoms of a disease considered as a whole
tonic spasm	continued involuntary contraction of muscles

I. Introduction

    A. Functions and Structure
       1. Functions
          a) Helps to regulate body functions
          b) Receives and responds to stimuli
       2. Structure
          a) Includes
             (1) Brain
             (2) Cranial nerves
             (3) Spinal cord
             (4) Spinal nerves
             (5) Autonomic ganglia
             (6) Ganglionated trunks
             (7) Peripheral nerves

   b) Is connected to sense organs
      (1) Eye
      (2) Ear
      (3) Organs of taste
      (4) Organs of smell
      (5) Skin
   c) Is divided into three parts:
      (1) Central nervous system: the brain and spinal cord
      (2) Autonomic nervous system
      (3) Peripheral nervous system: the cranial and spinal nerves
   d) Is protected by
      (1) Cranial bones, which surround brain
      (2) Vertebrae, which surround spinal cord
      (3) Meninges—tough membrane, which covers brain and spinal cord and is com-
          posed of three layers:
          (a) Dura mater
          (b) Arachnoid
          (c) Pia mater
      (4) Cerebrospinal fluid, which circulates
          (a) Inside ventricles of brain
          (b) Inside spinal canal
          (c) Through ventricles and into subarachnoid space, whence it bathes brain
              and spinal cord
   e) Has as its basic unit the nerve cell (see Figure 11), or neuron, which consists of
      (1) Cell body
      (2) Processes of the cell body, which are of two types
          (a) Dendrite—carries impulses toward cell body
          (b) Axon—carries impulses away from cell body

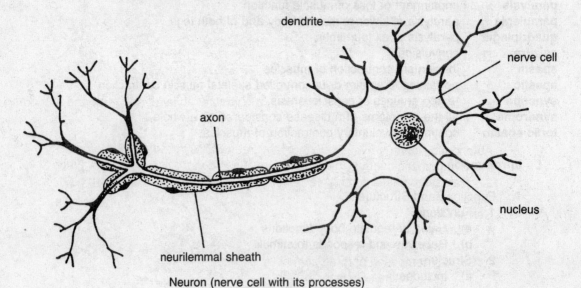

Neuron (nerve cell with its processes)

Figure 11

B. Nerve Cell
   1. Each nerve cell has a single axon and several dendrites.

2. Synapse is the functional junction between the axon of one neuron and the dendrite of another neuron.
3. Impulse travels from the end of the axon of one neuron to the dendrites of another neuron.
4. There are three kinds of nerve cells:
   a) Sensory neurons—transmit impulses to spinal cord and brain
   b) Motor neurons—transmit impulses away from spinal cord and brain out to muscles and glands
   c) Central neurons—transmit impulses from sensory neurons to motor neurons

C. The Brain—three parts
   1. Cerebrum
      a) Is largest part of brain
      b) Has cerebral cortex
      c) Has gray matter and white matter
      d) Controls all mental processes
      e) Controls voluntary movements
   2. Cerebellum
      a) Is second largest part of brain
      b) Coordinates and makes muscular movements precise
   3. Medulla oblongata
      a) Is lowest part of brain
      b) Contains vital centers—relays impulses to heart, blood vessels, and respiratory muscles

D. The Spinal Cord
   1. Lies inside spinal column
   2. Provides communication between brain and other parts of body
   3. Serves as a center for many reflexes
   4. Extends from occipital foramen down to the bottom of first lumbar vertebra

E. The Cranial Nerves
   1. Exist in 12 pairs (see Data Summary 8)
   2. Attach to undersurface of brain
   3. Conduct impulses between brain and structures in head and neck and in thoracic and abdominal cavities

F. Autonomic Nervous System (Sympathetic and Parasympathetic Systems)
   1. Sympathetic controls involuntary functions in opposition to parasympathetic
   2. Parasympathetic controls involuntary functions in opposition to sympathetic

G. Sense Organs
   1. The eye
      a) Is organ of vision
      b) Is composed of three coats:
         (1) Retina—sensory for light
         (2) Uvea (choroid, ciliary body, iris)
         (3) Sclera and cornea—protective
      c) Has accessory attachments
         (1) Conjunctiva—thin membranous lining covering front of eyeball and eyelids
         (2) Lacrimal gland—located in upper outer part of each eye socket; produces tears to keep eyeball lubricated and to act as cleansing agent
      d) Functions by refracting (bending) light rays so that they focus on the retina
      e) Has four refracting media:

DATA SUMMARY 8
The Twelve Pairs of Cranial Nerves

Number	Name	Function	Origin	Distribution
I	Olfactory	Sensory	Nasal lining	Cerebrum
II	Optic	Sensory	Retina	Cerebrum
III	Oculomotor	Motor	Midbrain	Muscles of eyeball
IV	Trochlear	Motor	Midbrain	Muscles of eyeball
V	Trigeminal	Mixed	Pons	1st branch: Ophthalmic—around the eye 2nd branch: Maxillary—upper part of face 3rd branch: Mandibular—temple, ear, lower lip, teeth, gums of mandible, muscles of mastication
VI	Abducens	Motor	Pons	Muscles of eyeball
VII	Facial	Mixed	Pons	Muscles of face, taste buds, middle ear
VIII	Auditory	Sensory	Pons	1st branch: Cochlear—cochlea of inner ear 2nd branch: Vestibular—semicircular canals
IX	Glossopharyngeal	Mixed	Medulla	Tongue and pharynx
X	Vagus	Mixed	Medulla	Heart and abdominal viscera
XI	Spinal accessory	Motor	Medulla	Muscles of neck
XII	Hypoglossal	Motor	Medulla	Tongue and muscles of hyoid

    (1) Aqueous humor—watery liquid between cornea and lens

    (2) Lens—situated just behind pupil; functions to focus rays so they form a perfect image on retina

    (3) Vitreous body—transparent jellylike mass that fills cavity of eyeball between lens and retina

    (4) Cornea—transparent portion of coat of eyeball

2. The ear

    a) Is organ of hearing

    b) Is composed of three parts:

        (1) External ear

            (a) Pinna (auricle)

            (b) Auditory canal

        (2) Middle ear

            (a) Auditory bones—malleus, incus, and stapes

            (b) Mucous membrane lining—continuous with lining of throat and eustachian tube

            (c) Opening to eustachian tube which connects throat with middle ear

            (d) Opening to mastoid sinuses of temporal bone

        (3) Internal ear

            (a) Vestibule

            (b) Semicircular canals

            (c) Cochlea

            (d) Organ of Corti (sense organ of hearing), which lies in cochlea

NURSING CARE OF THE ADULT PATIENT

        (e) Sense organ of equilibrium, which is in vestibule and semicircular canals
- 3. Taste organs
  - a) Are found in tongue
  - b) Consist of taste buds
- 4. Olfactory organs
  - a) Are end organs of olfactory nerve
  - b) Are located on surface of upper part of nasal septum and on turbinates
- 5. Skin—serves as sense organ through its many appendages. See Unit 1.

II. Neurologic Assessment

A. Symptoms
  1. Headache
  2. Visual disturbances
  3. Dizziness
  4. Weakness
  5. Speech disturbances
  6. Nausea and vomiting
  7. Memory and thinking disturbances
  8. Motor disturbances

B. Signs
  1. Levels of consciousness, including confusion, delirium, stupor, coma
  2. Pupillary signs
     a) Reaction to light
     b) Size and bilateral status
  3. Sensory function—reaction to pain, touch, pressure
  4. Motor function
     a) Reflexes—Babinski, biceps, triceps, scrotal
     b) Voluntary movement
     c) Paralyses—hemiplegia, paraplegia, quadriplegia
     d) Involuntary movement—tremors, spasms, convulsions
  5. Vital signs
     a) Temperature
     b) Respiration: rate and type
     c) Blood pressure and pulse

III. Common Disorders of the Nervous System

A. Trauma
  1. Cerebral concussion
  2. Cerebral contusion and laceration
  3. Skull fracture
     a) Linear
     b) Depressed
  4. Spine fracture and compression of spinal cord
  5. Ruptured intervertebral disc

B. Infections
  1. Meningitis
  2. Encephalitis
  3. Poliomyelitis

    4. Brain abscess
    5. Herpes zoster

  C. Degenerative Diseases
    1. Multiple sclerosis
    2. Parkinsonism (Parkinson's disease, paralysis agitans)
    3. Myasthenia gravis
    4. Alzheimer's disease

  D. Cerebrovascular Accident

  E. Convulsive Disorder (epilepsy)

  F. Tumors (Neoplasms)
    1. Benign
    2. Malignant

  G. Neuritis and Neuralgia

III. **Nursing Care of Patients with Neurologic Injuries of Various Types and According to State of Consciousness**

  A. Signs of Complicating Factors
    1. Neurologic
      a) Abnormal and unequal pupillary reflexes
      b) Abnormal response to pain, touch, and pressure
    2. Respiratory
      a) Skin color: pallor, cyanosis
      b) Abnormal rate, rhythm, depth of respiration
      c) Breath sounds: stertorous
      d) Accumulation of secretions in mouth
    3. Cardiovascular
      a) Falling blood pressure
      b) Thready pulse
      c) Edema
      d) Arrhythmias
      e) Shocklike state
    4. Musculoskeletal
      a) Paralysis
      b) Poor muscle tone
      c) Deformities/contractures
    5. Skin
      a) Color: pallor, excoriation
      b) Pressure-point abnormalities
    6. Gastrointestinal
      a) Constipation
      b) Impaction
      c) Diarrhea
      d) Paralytic ileus
    7. Bladder
      a) Incontinence
      b) Urinary stasis (bladder distension)
      c) Inadequate output

       8. Nutritional
          a) Dehydration
          b) Acid-base imbalance

B. General Nursing Care
    1. Positioning
        a. Ensure good body alignment with support of head and limbs in functional anatomic position.
        b. Avoid complete immobility if possible.
    2. Skin—observe for
        a) Changes in color
        b) Ulcerations due to pressure
        c) Sensation losses
    3. Eyes
        a) Observe for corneal and conjunctival irritation.
        b) Irrigate prn.
    4. Nose
        a) Observe for trauma or infection.
        b) Secure nasogastric tube after physician has changed it.
        c) Lubricate nares
    5. Mouth
        a) Provide excellent oral hygiene.
        b) Lubricate mucous membranes if patient is breathing.
    6. Ears
        a) Observe for drainage of cerebrospinal fluid in cases of cerebral injury.
        b) Apply dry, sterile dressing over ear.
    7. Nutrition and fluid and electrolyte balance
        a) Tube feedings
           (1) Check position of tube.
           (2) Measure gastric contents and subtract from proposed feeding—DO NOT OVERLOAD STOMACH.
           (3) Prevent air from entering stomach.
           (4) Place patient in semi-Fowler's position, right side.
           (5) Monitor and record intake and output.
        b) Oral feedings
           (1) Give semiliquid purees or soft diet high in protein, vitamins, and calories.
           (2) Place patient in semi-Fowler's position.
           (3) Have suction apparatus available.
    8. Elimination
        a) Give catheter care if Foley has been inserted.
        b) Prevent constipation—laxative/enema, fluid intake, regular routine.
    9. Psychological support
        a) Encourage and reassure patient.
        b) Explain procedures to family, and reassure them.
        c) Encourage physical therapy and optimal physical activity.

III. Specific Diagnostic Tests

A. Neurologic Examination (done by a neurologist)

B. X-ray Studies
    1. Skull
    2. Spine

C. Spinal Tap (Lumbar Puncture)
1. Spinal needle is inserted between vertebrae into spinal canal below level of cord.
2. Pressure of fluid is noted.
3. Specimen of fluid is taken for laboratory examination.

D. Electroencephalogram (EEG; Tracing of Electrical Waves of Brain)

E. Pneumoencephalogram
1. Air is injected into spinal canal.
2. Ventricles in brain become visible on X ray as air rises.
3. X-ray study is made.

F. Arteriogram
1. Dye is injected into carotid artery.
2. Arteries become visible on X ray.

G. Myelogram
1. Dye is injected into spinal canal.
2. Lesions or defects within vertebral column can then be visualized on X ray.

H. Ventriculogram (operating room procedure)
1. Air is injected into ventricles of brain through burr holes (openings in skull).
2. Ventricles are then visible on X ray.

I. Brain Scan
1. Radioactive drugs are given.
2. Brain is scanned to pinpoint areas of concentration of drug.

J. Magnetic Resonance Imagery (MRI; new technique)
1. It avoids invasive techniques.
2. Lesions of brain and spinal cord are projected (supplanting myelogram).
3. Test cannot be used on patient with pacemaker.

K. CAT (Computerized axial tomography) Scan

IV. **Cerebral Injury**

A. Assessment
1. Loss of consciousness—may or may not occur
2. Pain (headache)
3. Local bleeding
4. Signs of increased intracranial pressure
   a) Bleeding from ears, nose, mouth
   b) Clear liquid draining from ears and nose—cerebrospinal fluid
   c) Visual disturbances
      (1) Double vision
      (2) Blurring of vision
   d) Inequality of pupils; dilation of pupil on injured side
   e) Papilledema—edema and inflammation of the optic nerve at its point of entrance into the eyeball
5. Secondary cerebral infection

B. Cerebral Concussion
1. Is caused by blow to head
2. May result in slight bruising of brain to severe injury
3. Assessment
    a) Unconsciousness
    b) Nausea and vomiting
    c) Headache
    d) Weak pulse
    e) Nystagmus

C. Cerebral Contusion
1. Injury causes rupture of small blood vessels, which leads to formation of a hematoma.
2. There are two types of hematoma.
    a) Extradural hematoma
        (1) Clot is formed above dura mater.
        (2) Symptoms are produced early, within 24–48 hours.
        (3) Surgery may be needed to remove clot.
    b) Subdural hematoma
        (1) Clot is formed below dura mater.
        (2) Symptoms may occur late.
        (3) Surgery may be needed to remove clot.

D. Skull Fracture
1. Linear fracture—X ray shows a fracture resembling a line
    a) There are no specific symptoms except pain.
    b) No surgery is needed.
2. Depressed fracture—fragments of skull are pushed into brain
    a) Signs and symptoms of increase in intracranial pressure
        (1) Bleeding from ears, nose, or throat
        (2) Clear liquid draining from nose and ears
        (3) Papilledema
        (4) Dilated pupil on injured side
        (5) Visual disturbances
        (6) Convulsions
        (7) Weakness or paralysis
    b) Residual symptoms
        (1) Headache
        (2) Secondary infection
    c) Nursing care
        (1) Maintain strict bedrest for patient.
        (2) Observe and record vital signs frequently.
        (3) Observe for symptoms of increase in intracranial pressure.
            (a) Change in vital signs: elevated blood pressure, decrease in pulse rate, labored breathing, increase in body temperature
            (b) Change in level of consciousness: knowledge of orientation, change in awareness, decreasing response to stimulation
            (c) Change in pupillary size: unilateral dilatation (may be sign of cerebral hemorrhage), bilateral dilatation
            (d) Increased restlessness
            (e) Muscle weakness or paralysis
        (4) Check for bleeding or drainage from nose, ears, or mouth.
        (5) Observe pupillary reaction.
        (6) Record intake and output accurately.

(7) Check for urinary retention and fecal impaction.
(8) Turn patient frequently.
(9) Carry out range-of-motion exercises frequently.
(10) Provide frequent mouth care.
(11) Attach side rails if patient is restless.
(12) Give strict attention to physician's orders.

V. Spinal Injury

A. Assessment
   1. Pain
   2. Paralysis
      a) Paralysis of body below level of injury—may be temporary
      b) Loss of sensation of body below level of injury—may be temporary or permanent

B. Spinal Fracture
   1. May cause injury to spinal cord
      a) Partially destroyed
      b) Completely severed
   2. Requires specific treatment and close observation for progression of symptoms
      a) Vertebrae must be kept motionless.
      b) Traction or hyperextension is used.
      c) Body cast may be applied.
      d) Skin care is needed to prevent bed sores (decubiti).
      e) Alternating pressure mattresses are used.
      f) Intake and output must be recorded correctly.
      g) Urinary retention and constipation must be observed; catheterize and give enemas as necessary.
      h) Correct position is required to prevent contractures and footdrop.
      i) Deep breathing is to be encouraged.
      j) Patient requires help in rehabilitation.
         (1) Activities of daily living
         (2) Transfer from bed to wheelchair
         (3) Bowel and bladder training
         (4) Gaining independence

C. Ruptured Intervertebral Disc
   1. Cause—nucleus pulposus slips outward when covering separating vertebrae are injured
   2. Symptoms
      a) Low back pain
      b) Intensification of pain when lifting, bending, coughing, or sneezing
      c) Loss of sensation and/or weakness in area supplied by spinal nerves coming from affected area
   3. Treatment
      a) Bedrest
      b) Reconditioning exercises
      c) Heat and massage
      d) Traction
      e) Braces
      f) Surgery if no relief is obtained from other measures
   4. Nursing care
      a) Preoperative

        (1)   Teach deep breathing exercises.
        (2)   Reassure patient; allow verbalization of fears/concerns.
        (3)   Teach patient how to turn self (log-rolling).
        (4)   Follow physician's orders for preoperative preparation.

   b) Postoperative
        (1)   Check vital signs frequently.
        (2)   Inspect wound for evidence of hemorrhage.
        (3)   Turn patient frequently to relieve pressure.
        (4)   Evaluate motor movements.
        (5)   Check for sensation in toes.
        (6)   Check for voiding.
        (7)   Record intake and output.
        (8)   Medicate as ordered.
        (9)   Give diet as tolerated.
     (10)   Reassure patient.
     (11)   Maintain safe environment.
        (a)   Call bell in place
        (b)   Side rails up
     (12)   Body cast may be applied and worn 6–8 weeks.
     (13)   Brace may be worn for an additional 3–6 months.

VI. Infectious Diseases

  A.   Meningitis
     1.   Definition of **meningitis:** Inflammation of meninges
     2.   Causes
        a) Bacteria
        b) Virus
     3.   Diagnosis—by lumbar puncture
        a) Pressure of fluid is measured.
        b) Fluid is tested for blood and sugar.
        c) Culture and sensitivity test are done.
     4.   Assessment
        a) Severe headache and stiff neck
        b) General malaise and fever
        c) Sensory disturbances
        d) Central nervous system disturbances such as convulsions, irritability, loss of consciousness
     5.   Nursing care
        a) Follow specific orders of physician.
        b) Give antibiotics specific for organism as ordered.
        c) Record intake and output accurately.
        d) Monitor vital signs as ordered, and do neurologic check.
        e) Observe strict isolation techniques.
        f) Provide general nursing care for unconscious patient with infection.

  B.   Encephalitis
     1.   Definition of **encephalitis:** Inflammation of brain
     2.   Causes
        a) Viral infection
        b) Chemicals
        c) Protozoa
     3.   Assessment

        a) Headache
        b) Fever
        c) Drowsiness
        d) Increasing intracranial pressure
        e) Generalized signs of cerebral dysfunction
    4. Treatment—symptomatic
    5. Nursing care—as above

C. Poliomyelitis
    1. Definition of **poliomyelitis:** Infectious viral disease that affects the central nervous system
    2. Two forms
        a) Bulbar polio—affects medulla oblongata
        b) Acute anterior polio—affects anterior portion of gray matter of spinal cord
    3. Assessment
        a) General malaise
        b) Headache
        c) Fever
        d) Sore throat
        e) Stiff neck
        f) Pain, weakness, and spastic paralysis of muscles affected
        g) Gradual atrophy of affected muscles
        h) Disappearance of acute symptoms after about 6 weeks
    4. Nursing care
        a) Complete bedrest
        b) Isolation techniques
        c) Proper positioning to prevent deformities
        d) Application of warm, moist packs to affected muscles
        e) Early physical therapy
        f) Continued physiotherapy and braces for deformities if needed

D. Brain Abscess
    1. Cause—any infection entering skull or body and invading brain
    2. Assessment
        a) Headache
        b) Inflammation (elevated temperature, pain)
        c) Increased intracranial pressure
    3. Treatment
        a) Medical—antibiotics
        b) Surgical—craniotomy
    4. Pre- and postoperative care similar to that for other neurologic surgery

E. Herpes Zoster
    1. Definition of **herpes zoster:** Viral infection causing inflammation and vesicles distributed along nerve trunks
    2. Assessment
        a) Intercostal neuralgia
        b) Vesicles
        c) Pain
        d) Possible loss of vision if ophthalmic nerve involved
    3. Treatment
        a) Analgesics
        b) Warm packs

NURSING CARE OF THE ADULT PATIENT

F. Brain Tumor
   1. Definition of **brain tumor:** Abnormal growth of cells within brain
   2. Forms
      a) Benign or malignant
      b) Primary or secondary
   3. Assessment
      a) Severe, persistent headache
      b) General malaise
      c) Disturbances of vision
      d) Dilation or inequality of pupils
      e) Projectile vomiting
      f) Convulsive seizures
      g) Occasional muscular weakness and/or paralysis
      h) Choked disk seen on fundoscopic examination
   5. Treatment
      a) Treatment is surgical, if possible.
         (1) Relief of intracranial pressure by removal of part of skull
         (2) Removal of tumor (or as much of it as possible)
      b) Pre- and postoperative care is meticulous for postneurological surgery.
   6. Nursing care (under supervision of R.N.)
      a) Maintain airway.
      b) Position patient with slight hyperextension of head when lying on back or side.
      c) Slightly elevate head of bed (lessens pressure on diaphragm).
      d) Encourage coughing and deep breathing unless contraindicated (coughing is con-
         traindicated in patients with increased intracranial pressure).
      e) Suction as necessary (care must be taken not to traumatize tissues).
      f) Report and record food intake accurately.
      g) Provide good oral hygiene care.
      h) Give small, frequent feedings.
      i) Change patient's position frequently to prevent contractures and/or pneumonia.
      j) Provide footboard to prevent footdrop.
      k) Provide good skin care to prevent decubiti.
      l) Report and record all changes in vital signs and/or levels of consciousness.
      m) Observe and report signs of neck rigidity.
      n) Record intake and output.
      o) Report episodes of diarrhea immediately.
      p) Keep accurate record of bowel movements.
      q) If patient is unconscious, make sure side rails are in place.
      r) Protect patient from drafts.
      s) Reassure family.

H. Tumor of the Spinal Cord
   1. Definition of **spinal cord tumor:** Abnormal growth of cells within or on the spinal
      cord
   2. Forms
      a) May be benign or malignant
      b) May be primary or secondary
   3. Symptoms
      a) There is persistent pain in area of tumor and in area supplied by nerve supply from
         tumor area.
      b) There is increasing numbness in affected area.
      c) Paralysis—partial or complete—of body areas below level of tumor develops grad-
         ually.

        d) Brown-Sequard syndrome may be present.
           (1) Loss of sensation on one side of body below lesion
           (2) Increased sensation on other side of body below lesion
    4. Treatment
        a) Surgery—removal of tumor, if possible, after laminectomy
        b) Routine neurological pre- and post-operative care

VII. Degenerative Diseases

  A. Multiple Sclerosis
    1. Definition of **multiple sclerosis:** Progressive disease of nerve fibers
    2. Characteristics
        a) Degeneration of myelin sheaths of nerves
        b) Foci of sclerosis scattered through nervous system
    3. Assessment
        a) Tremors
        b) Slurred speech
        c) Involuntary eyeball movement
        d) Emotional instability
        e) Spasticity
        f) Increased deep reflexes
        g) Contractures and deformities
    4. Treatment
        a) Symptomatic treatment
        b) Steroids in acute phase
        c) Routine nursing care
        d) Supportive and emotional care of patient and family

  b. Parkinsonism (Parkinson's Disease)
    1. Definition of **Parkinsonism:** Chronic, degenerative disease of nervous system
    2. Assessment
        a) Rigidity
        b) Fine tremor
        c) Pill-rolling movement of hand and fingers
        d) Masklike face
        e) Dragging gait
        f) Typical stooping position of body
        g) Drooling
        h) Paralysis
        i) Slurred speech
        j) Tendency to perspire
        k) Fatigue
    3. Treatment
        a) Symptomatic treatment
        b) Drugs
           (1) Antispasmodic
           (2) Muscle relaxants
           (3) L-Dopa
           (4) Cerebral stimulants
        c) Surgical treatment for selected cases
        d) Modification of diet for swallowing difficulties
        e) Physiotherapy
           (1) Prevention of deformities

    (2) Strengthening of muscular function
   f) Training in activities of daily living
   g) Control of constipation
 C. Myasthenia Gravis
  1. Definition of **myasthenia gravis:** Chronic disease of adult life, of unknown etiology, that affects muscles
  2. Characteristics
   a) Muscular fatigue
   b) Ptosis
   c) Difficulty in swallowing and speaking
   d) Double vision
   e) Exhaustion
  3. Treatment—prostigmin
  4. Nursing care
   a) Symptomatic treatment
   b) Measures to aid patient in conserving energy and to prevent pulmonary infections

 D. Cerebrovascular Accident (CVA)
  1. Definition of **CVA:** abnormal condition in which hemorrhage or blockage of blood vessels in brain leads to oxygen lack
  2. Causes
   a) Compression of blood vessel due to tumor
   b) Occlusion of blood vessel due to clot formation (thrombus)
   c) Hemorrhage into brain tissue due to rupture of blood vessel
   d) Closure of blood vessel due to spasm
  3. Remote cause—atherosclerosis
  4. Assessment
   a) Dizziness
   b) Anxiety
   c) Speech disturbances
   d) Coma
   e) Dilated, inactive pupils
   f) Loss of deep and superficial reflexes
   g) Incontinence
   h) Stertorous breathing
   i) Eyes may deviate to affected side
   j) Spastic hemiplegia
   k) Aphasia
  5. Diagnosis—by cerebral angiography
  6. Treatment and nursing care
   a) Give symptomatic care during acute attack.
   b) Administer anticoagulants, antihypertensives, analgesics, laxatives as ordered.
   c) Turn patient's head to side, and keep airway cleared of secretions, elevate head of bed.
   d) Check vital signs frequently.
   e) Record blood pressure hourly for first 24 hours.
   f) Reassure patient.
   g) Position patient properly.
   h) Provide proper support of paralyzed side.
   i) Provide daily speech training in aphasia; establish means of communicating.
   j) Meet dietary needs.
   k) Provide bladder and bowel care; record input and output.

        l) Provide physiotherapy: passive and then later active exercises
            (1) Range of motion exercises
            (2) Exercises to prevent footdrop and contractures
       m) Observe for seizures.
       n) Observe for change in condition.
       o) Help with activities of daily living.

VIII. Convulsive Disorders

A. Epilepsy: a syndrome characterized by recurrent episodes of convulsive seizures and impaired consciousness
  1. Causes
     a) Symptomatic epilepsy—caused by brain injury
     b) Essential or idiopathic epilepsy—no definite cause known
  2. Three types
     a) Grand mal
        (1) Preceded by a premonition (aura)
        (2) Loss of consciousness
        (3) Fall to ground
        (4) Tonic convulsions (muscular rigidity)
        (5) Clonic convulsions
     b) Status epilepticus: several convulsions in succession
     c) Petit mal
        (1) Loss of consciousness for very short time
        (2) No fall to ground
        (3) May or may not have a few jerking convulsions

B. Jacksonian Epilepsy
        (1) There is jerking in one part of body for a very short time.
        (2) This can precede grand mal.

C. Treatment and Nursing Care
  1. Correct diagnosis by physician is important.
  2. Anticonvulsant drugs (phenobarbital, Dilantin) may be used as ordered.
  3. Surgery may be indicated if brain tumor is present.
  4. Dentures and removable bridges should be removed at night.
  5. Adequate rest and stress-free existence should be maintained.
  6. Symptoms and reactions to medication should be observed and recorded.
  7. Seizure precautions must be taken.

D. Nursing Care During Seizure
  1. Maintain airway.
  2. Protect patient from injury.
  3. Loosen clothing.
  4. Avoid restraining limbs.
  5. Avoid forcing object into mouth.
  6. Record seizure activity.
     a) Aura
     b) Time seizure begins
     c) Duration of seizure
     d) Incontinence
  7. Give anticonvulsant medication as directed.
  8. Assist with diagnostic evaluation as to cause.

IX. **Other Disorders of the Nervous System**

    A. Neuritis
        1. Definition of **neuritis:** Inflammation of a nerve or nerves
        2. Causes
            a) Infections
            b) Injury
            c) Vitamin deficiencies
            d) Imbalances of metabolism, such as diabetes mellitus
            e) Bacterial toxins and chemical poisons
            f) Pressure from enlarging tumor
        3. Symptoms
            a) Pain
            b) Weakness in area supplied by affected nerve
        4. Types
            a) Polyneuritis—several nerves are inflamed
            b) Mononeuritis—one nerve is affected
        5. Treatment
            a) Analgesics as ordered
            b) Correction of underlying cause if possible
            c) Observation and recording of symptoms

    B. Trigeminal Neuralgia
        1. Definition of **trigeminal neuralgia:** Syndrome characterized by severe pain along course of fifth cranial nerve (trigeminal nerve)
        2. Cause—sometimes, infected teeth
        3. Assessment
            a) Face appears relaxed.
            b) There is severe pain.
            c) Malnourishment may be present because chewing may start pain.
            d) Pain can be triggered by various stimuli.
        4. Treatment
            a) Analgesics and other drugs are given as ordered.
            b) Surgery may be necessary in some cases.
               (1) Severing of branch of nerve
               (2) Stripping of dura mater from section of nerve
               (3) Routine postoperative care
               (4) Special eye care

    C. Sciatica
        1. Definition of **sciatica:** Syndrome characterized by pain and numbness or tingling along course of sciatic nerve
        2. Causes
            a) Injury to nerve
            b) Lumbosacral sprain
            c) Inflammation of nerve
        3. Treatment
            a) Removal of cause if possible
            b) Observation and recording of symptoms

X. **Disorders of the Sense Organs**

    A. Eye Abnormalities
        1. Assessment

   a) Persistent headache
   b) Lacrimation
   c) Itching
   d) Redness
   e) Blurred vision
   f) Distortion of vision
   g) Intolerance of light
   h) Night blindness
2. Visual defects
   a) Myopia (nearsightedness)
   b) Hyperopia (farsightedness)
   c) Astigmatism (images do not properly focus on retina)
   d) Presbyopia (inability to accommodate due to age)
3. Diagnostic tests
   a) Visual acuity
      (1) Snellen chart used for distance testing; normal—20/20
      (2) Jaeger's tests used for testing of near vision
   b) Measurement of intraocular pressure (tonometry)
      (1) Pressure is measured by tonometer.
      (2) Increased pressure is indication of glaucoma.
   c) Field test for temporal and peripheral vision—most important test in following course of glaucoma
4. Abnormalities
   a) Stye
      (1) Definition of **stye:** Inflammation of a sebaceous gland near edge of eyelid, ending in suppuration
      (2) Assessment—redness, burning, and itching of lid
      (3) Treatment—warm, moist compresses to localize pustule
      (4) Surgical incision and drainage if necessary
   b) Conjunctivitis
      (1) Definition of **conjunctivitis:** Inflammation of lining of eye
      (2) Cause—may be bacterial infection
      (3) Assessment
         (a) Redness
         (b) Swelling
         (c) Itching
         (d) Tearing
      (4) Treatment
         (a) Moist compresses
         (b) Antibiotics
         (c) Steroids
   c) Cataract
      (1) Definition of **cataract:** Opacity of lens, which may be due to aging but occasionally is congenital
      (2) Symptom—decreased vision
      (3) Treatment
         (a) Frequent refractions
         (b) Chronic pupillary dilation
         (c) Lens extraction
      (4) Preoperative care
         (a) Relieve anxiety.
         (b) Obtain conjunctival culture if requested.
         (c) Administer local antibiotics as prescribed.

         (d)   Instill mydriatic if ordered.

         (e)   Give tranquilizers and antiemetics as ordered.

     (5) Postoperative care

         (a)   Patient rests for 2 hours.

         (b)   Nurse monitors signs and symptoms before discharge.

         (c)   Patient is discharged if no complaints.

         (d)   Patient returns to ophthalmologist the following day.

     (6) Postoperative follow-up

         (a)   Cataract spectacles

         (b)   Contact lenses

         (c)   Intraoperative implantation of prosthetic lens

  5. Glaucoma

     a) Definition of **glaucoma:** Increased pressure within eyeball which leads to blindness if untreated

     b) Cause—improper drainage of aqueous humor via Schlemm's canal

     c) Early symptoms—mild

     d) Late symptoms—blurred vision, rainbow-colored rings around lights, difficulty in adjusting sight to darkened rooms, decrease in side vision

     e) Treatment

        (1) Use of drugs to constrict pupils (miotics)

        (2) Surgery in some forms of glaucoma

          (a)   Laser trabeculopexy

          (b)   Filtering surgery

  6. Color blindness—characterized by inability to identify one or more of the primary colors

B. Hearing Abnormalities

  1. Types

     a) Nerve deafness—pathology of eighth cranial nerve

     b) Conduction deafness—blocked transmission of sound waves from outside auditory nerve

  2. Causes

     a) Injury or disease of part of brain controlling hearing center

     b) Hysteria

     c) Injury from loud noises

     d) Disease of labyrinth (internal ear)

  3. Diagnostic tests conducted by use of

     a) Tuning fork—determines whether patient has nerve deafness or conduction deafness

     b) Audiometer—measures the ability to hear

  4. Common ear disorders

     a) Otosclerosis

        (1) Definition of **otosclerosis:** formation of spongy bone in the capsule of the labyrinth of the ear; growth of bone around the oval window of the ear blocks transmission of sound waves from stapes to inner ear, causing conduction deafness

        (2) Treatment

          (a)   Hearing aid

          (b)   Surgery

     b) Otitis media

        (1) Definition of **otitis media:** Infection of middle ear, secondary to upper respiratory infection

        (2) Assessment

           (a)   Pain
           (b)   Red and/or bulging eardrum
           (c)   Fever
           (d)   Purulent discharge from ear
           (e)   Temporary loss of hearing
       (3)   Treatment
           (a)   Systemic antibiotics
           (b)   Irrigation of canal
           (c)   Instillation of specific solution in ear canal
   c)   Mastoiditis
       (1)   Definition of **mastoiditis:** Inflammation and infection of mastoid sinus process
       (2)   Cause—extension of infection from middle ear
       (3)   Assessment
           (a)   Pain
           (b)   Headache
           (c)   Tenderness of mastoid
       (4)   Treatment and nursing care
           (a)   Antibiotic therapy
           (b)   Bedrest
           (c)   Surgery if required

UNIT 4: THE CARDIOVASCULAR SYSTEM

VOCABULARY

agglutination	clumping of either microorganisms or blood cells
cardiac decompensation	cardiac failure
cholesterol	substance found in fats and oils
CPK	creatine phosphokinase; blood enzyme
dextrocardia	condition in which the heart is located on the right side of the body
diuretic	drug that increases production of urine
ductus arteriosus	communicating channel between aorta and pulmonary artery in fetus; normally closes at birth
fluoroscopy	use of fluoroscope for diagnosis
hypertrophy	increase in size of an organ or part due to enlargement of individual cells
LDH	lactic dehydrogenase; blood enzyme
pallor	lack of color; paleness
petechiae	tiny, hemorrhagic spots on skin
productive cough	cough with production of phlegm
phlebotomy	opening of a vein
protoplasm	essential, living material in all organisms
recurrent	returning at intervals
SGOT	serum glutamic-oxalacetic transaminase; blood enzyme
thromboplastin	substance found in tissues that acts with calcium and prothrombin to help in blood clotting
valve	structure for temporarily closing an opening

NURSING CARE OF THE ADULT PATIENT

I. **Components of Cardiovascular System**

    A. Heart

    B. Blood vessels
        1. Arteries
        2. Veins
        3. Capillaries

    C. Blood

II. **The Heart**

    A. Definition of **Heart:** Hollow, muscular organ, situated a little to the left of midline of chest, that pumps blood throughout the body

    B. Structure
        1. Is covered by thin membrane—pericardium
        2. Has inner lining—endocardium
        3. Has thick muscular walls—myocardium
        4. Has four chambers:
            a) Right and left ventricles—lower chambers
            b) Right and left auricles (atria)—upper chambers
        5. Has four valves:
            a) Aortic—between left ventricle and aorta
            b) Pulmonary—between right ventricle and pulmonary artery
            c) Tricuspid—between right atrium and right ventricle
            d) Bicuspid (mitral)—between left atrium and left ventricle

III. **The Blood Vessels**

    A. Functions and Structure
        1. Arteries
            a) Carry blood away from heart
            b) Carry oxygenated blood (except pulmonary artery; see Figure 12)
            c) End in tiny arteries called *arterioles*
        2. Veins
            a) Carry blood from body back to heart
            b) Carry nonoxygenated blood (except pulmonary veins; see Figure 12)
            c) Have valves to direct flow of blood
            d) End in tiny veins called *venules*
        3. Capillaries—connect arterioles and venules

IV. **The Blood**

    A. Definition of **blood:** Fluid tissue that is pumped by heart through blood vessels; total volume is between 4 and 6 quarts in adult

    B. Functions
        1. Carries oxygen and carbon dioxide
        2. Carries products of digestion throughout body
        3. Carries products of endocrine glands (hormones) throughout body
        4. Carries waste products from tissues to kidneys and intestines for excretion
        5. Regulates body temperature
        6. Maintains bodily water balance
        7. Carries immune bodies throughout body

B. Parts
   1. Red blood cells (erythrocytes)
      a) Range normally from 4.5 to 5.5 million per cubic millimeter
      b) Are produced in red bone marrow
      c) Do not contain nuclei and therefore cannot reproduce themselves
      d) Have life span of 3-4 months
      e) Are removed by spleen and liver
      f) Contain hemoglobin, which
         (1) Is composed of protein and iron
         (2) Gives red color to blood
         (3) Transports oxygen by forming chemical compound with it
         (4) Aids in transport of carbon dioxide
         (5) Is part of buffer system of blood
   2. White blood cells (leukocytes)
      a) Range normally from 5 to 10 thousand per cubic millimeter
      b) Are produced in bone marrow and some (lymphocytes and monocytes) in lymph tissue
      c) Defend body against pathogens and other harmful substances
      d) Three types:
         (1) Granulocytes
            (a) Neutrophils
            (b) Eosinophils
            (c) Basophils
         (2) Lymphocytes
         (3) Monocytes
   3. Platelets (thrombocytes)
      a) Range normally from 500 to 800 thousand per cubic millimeter
      b) Are fragments of protoplasm without nuclei
      c) Form thromboplastin upon disintegrating
      d) Are important in clotting mechanism of blood (thrombin combines with fibrinogen to form clot)
   4. Plasma
      a) Is straw-colored fluid part of blood
      b) Is composed of
         (1) Plasma proteins
            (a) Albumin
            (b) Globulin
            (c) Fibrinogen
            (d) Prothrombin
         (2) Inorganic salts
         (3) Organic products of excretion (urea, uric acid, amino acids, glucose, lipids, enzymes, hormones)
      c) Is changed to serum when fibers are removed

C. Blood Classification
   1. Types
      a) A
      b) B
      c) AB (universal recipient)
      d) O (universal donor)
   2. Rh factor
      a) Is protein factor found in blood of 85% of humans
      b) Is inherited factor and dominant

c) Can be acted upon by anti-Rh factor, causing clumping and destruction of red blood cells

V. Way in Which the Heart Works

A. Heart as Pump
1. Heart has four separate compartments—two above and two below.
2. Heart acts as pump divided by a septum, down the center from top to bottom, into two separate sides—left and right—with no communication between the two.

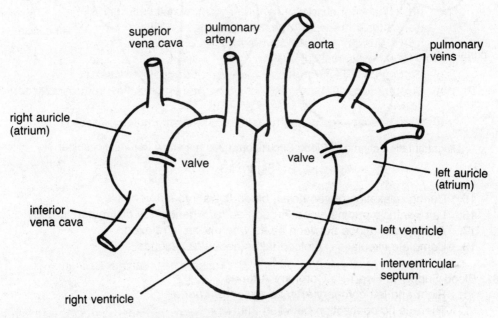

The Heart (diagrammatic scheme only)

Figure 12

3. Two upper compartments (atria) are receiving compartments only and are thin-walled.
4. Two lower compartments (ventricles) are dispensing compartments only and are thick-walled.
5. Right side contains only blue (deoxygenated) blood.
6. Left side contains only red (oxygenated) blood.
7. A large tube extends from each lower compartment; these are the two large arteries leading from heart.
8. Right tube (pulmonary artery) carries blood to lungs.
9. Left artery (aorta) carries blood to rest of body.
10. Right atrium is separated from right ventricle by tricuspid valve.
11. Left atrium is separated from left ventricle by mitral valve.
12. Blood coming from body via inferior and superior venae cavae with its waste products flows into right atrium and down into right ventricle.
13. Blood is then pumped by right ventricle through pulmonary artery to lungs, where it is oxygenated.
14. From lungs blood returns to left atrium through pulmonary veins.

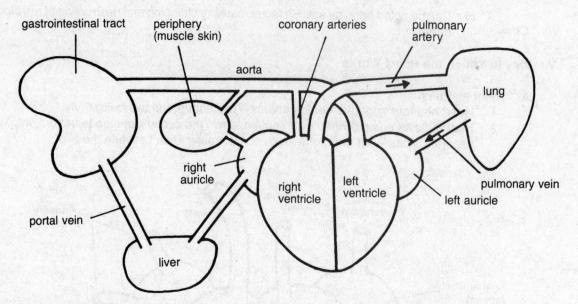

gastrointestinal tract · periphery (muscle skin) · coronary arteries · pulmonary artery · aorta · lung · right auricle · right ventricle · left ventricle · pulmonary vein · left auricle · portal vein · liver

Diagrammatic Scheme of Blood Circulation (does not show true relationships)

Figure 13

15. During relaxation of ventricles, blood flows into left ventricle.
16. Left ventricle pumps blood through aorta, whence it is distributed to body.
17. Atria fill with blood between beats when heart is relaxed.
18. Complete circulation of blood takes about 22 seconds.

B. Blood Supply to Heart via Coronary Arteries
   1. Right and left coronary arteries arise from aorta.
   2. There is no connection between the two.
   3. Drainage is via coronary veins.

VI. Blood Pressure

A. Process
   1. As heart forces blood into circulation, pressure is exerted on wall of arteries
   2. Amount of pressure exerted by heart depends on
      a) Rate of heart beat
      b) Amount of blood in circulation
      c) Elasticity of arteries
      d) Strength of heart beat

B. Types of Blood Pressure
   1. Pressure exerted by heart at beginning of its contraction (systole) is *systolic pressure.*
   2. Pressure exerted at point of greatest cardiac relaxation (diastole) is *diastolic pressure* (represents resistance of arteries to force of heart).
   3. Blood pressure is written as a fraction with systolic pressure on top and diastolic on bottom: $\frac{\text{systolic}}{\text{diastolic}}$, e.g., 120/80, 160/90, 110/70.
   4. Pulse pressure is the difference between the systolic pressure and the diastolic pressure; e.g., 120-80=40.

NURSING CARE OF THE ADULT PATIENT

VII. Circulation

   A. Process
1. Arteries carry blood *away from* heart.
2. Veins carry blood *to* heart.
3. All arteries, *except pulmonary artery,* have bright red blood (oxygenated).
4. All veins, *except pulmonary veins,* have blue blood (deoxygenated).
5. Auricles receive blood.
6. Ventricles pump out blood.
7. Left side of heart has bright red blood.
8. Right side of heart has blue blood.

VIII. Fundamentals of Nursing Care for Cardiac Patients

   A. Goals
1. Recognize signs of cardiovascular dysfunction.
    a) Skin color—cyanosis, flushing, pallor, petechiae
    b) Temperature—elevated, depressed
    c) Heart rate
    d) Heart rhythm—regular, irregular
    e) Respiration—rate, depth, character, patient position
    f) Blood pressure
    g) Pain—location, radiation, duration, intensity
    h) Cough—productive, nonproductive, sputum color, blood
    i) Patient response to treatment
2. Assist in administering prescribed treatment.
3. Make patient more comfortable.
4. Help calm patient's fears and anxieties.
5. Assist patient to return to as healthful a state as possible.

   B. Types of Cardiovascular Disease
1. Those related to heart itself
2. Those related to coronary arteries
3. Those related to blood vessels
4. Those related to lymphatic system
5. Those related to blood

   C. Specific Nursing Care depends upon diagnosis
1. Maintain bedrest if necessary.
    a) Activity is prescribed by physician.
    b) Activity depends upon state of circulation.
2. Administer sedative drugs as ordered by physician.
    a) Relaxed mind during waking hours aids in repair.
    b) Adequate sleep is necessary.
3. Administer digitalis preparations as ordered.
    a) Dosage is adjusted according to condition of the heart.
    b) Check pulse rate before administering medication; hold medication if pulse is less than 60 or over 120 and notify R.N.
    c) Observe and record effects of medication.
4. Administer diuretics as ordered.
    a) Retention of fluid is common in cardiac failure.
    b) Diuretics may be given orally or by injection.
      (1) Purpose is to relieve edema.

(2) Amount of urine is increased by preventing reabsorption of water from tubules of kidneys.
  c) Patient must be observed for signs of dehydration.
5. Administer antibiotics, if necessary and if ordered.
  a) Observe for any reaction.
  b) Record patient's response.
6. Monitor and record intake and output of fluids.
7. Weigh patient daily.
  a) Serves as additional check of fluid balance
  b) Gives indication of fluids lost by perspiration and involuntary urination
8. Monitor low-sodium diet if prescribed.
9. Observe for symptoms of need for oxygen therapy.
  a) Dyspnea and cyanosis indicate need for oxygen.
  b) Oxygen may be given by tent, nasal catheter, or mask.
10. Record intestinal elimination.
11. Add understanding, sympathy, and empathy to all nursing relationships with patient.

IX. **Diagnostic Tests and Procedures**

A. Physical Examination
  1. Inspection, percussion, and auscultation
  2. Pulse
    a) Rate
    b) Volume—strong, bounding, steady or weak, irregular
    c) Rhythm—regular, irregular, intermittent
  3. Blood pressure
  4. Pulse pressure

B. Laboratory Examination
  1. Complete blood count
  2. Sedimentation rate
  3. Blood culture and sensitivity
  4. Cholesterol
  5. Triglycerides
  6. Lipoproteins
  7. Enzymes—elevation indicates damage to heart muscle
    a) CPK—most sensitive but returns to normal quickly
    b) SGOT—reaches its peak in 48 hours and returns to normal in 96 hours
    c) LDK—starts to rise a few days after damage and takes up to 3 weeks to return to normal
  8. Sternal and iliac crest punctures for bone marrow studies

C. Radiology Techniques
  1. Chest X ray and fluoroscopy
    a) Reveal changes in the shape of the heart; distortions of blood vessels
    b) Reveal relationship of heart to areas around it
  2. Angiography
    a) Is X-ray study of heart after special dye has been injected
    b) Outlines chambers of heart and large blood vessels

D. Electrocardiogram
  1. Gives information concerning rhythm of heart
  2. Gives information concerning state of cardiac muscle

E. Stress Cardiogram
   1. Procedure determines level at which heart can work without symptoms or change in EKG.
   2. Treadmill, Master's Two-Step Test, and bicycle ergometer are devices used together with EKG.

F. Vectorcardiogram
   1. Measures activity of heart in more than two dimensions
   2. Is more sensitive than EKG in recording thickening of heart muscle
   3. Records photographically

G. Echocardiogram: gives information concerning valves, muscle, pericardium, and chambers by analysis of the echo (similar to sonar)

H. Phonocardiogram
   1. Heart sounds beyond range of human ear are picked up and recorded.
   2. Permanent recording on paper is made.

I. Dynamic Electrocardiogram
   1. Records all changes in heart rate and rhythm over a specific length of time, usually 24 hours
   2. Used for conditions (abnormal rhythms, etc.) reported by patient but not noticed in normal EKG

J. Catheterization
   1. Catheter is passed into heart to get precise information about structure of heart and valves.
   2. Procedure is combined with cardioangiography.

K. Thermography
   1. Is helpful in evaluating peripheral vascular disorders such as thrombophlebitis.
   2. Records heat variations.

L. Circulation Time
   1. Blood-flow speed is computed.
   2. Arm-tongue time is 12–15 seconds.

M. Central Venous Pressure
   1. Measures pressure of blood in veins
   2. Is monitored in acute states such as shock

X. **Specific Drug Therapy for Cardiac Disorders and Congestive Heart Failure**

   A. Digitalis, Digitalis Derivatives, and Purified Glycosides
      1. Treat cardiac arrhythmias
      2. Stimulate heart muscle
      3. Improve circulation by slowing and strengthening heart beat

   B. Diuretics
      1. Increase output of urine
      2. Improve general circulation
      3. Increase excretion of sodium, thus reducing edema and blood volume

    4. May increase excretion of potassium
    5. Help to lower blood pressure (certain diuretics)

C. Sedatives—calm patients and allay fears; e.g., phenobarbital in prescribed doses

D. Analgesics—relieve pain; e.g., aspirin, codeine, morphine

E. Cathartics—promote evacuations and thus prevent straining; e.g., cascara sagrada, Milk of Magnesia, stool softeners

F. Nitroglycerine
    1. Increases diameter of coronary arteries
    2. May produce tachycardia (side action)
    3. May produce orthostatic hypotension (side action)

XI. Diseases of the Cardiovascular System

A. Diagnostic Tests Performed
    1. Complete blood count
        a) Determination of number of red blood cells and white blood cells per cubic millimeter
        b) Microscopic examination of smear to determine size, shape, color of cells
        c) Hemoglobin determination
    2. Platelet count
    3. Bleeding time determination
    4. Clotting time determination
    5. Prothrombin time
    6. Reticulocyte count
    7. Capillary resistance

B. Hemophilia
    1. Definition of **hemophilia**: Hereditary disease of males transmitted by females
    2. Characteristics
        a) Tendency to hemorrhage from slight wounds
        b) Increase in blood coagulation time
        c) Normal capillary resistance
        d) Normal prothrombin, calcium, and fibrinogen
    3. Treatment
        a) Prevention of injury
        b) Transfusions
        c) High-iron, high-protein diet

C. Anemia
    1. Definition of **anemia**: Deficiency of red blood cells, hemoglobin, or both in circulating blood
    2. Types (see Data Summary 9)
        a) Acute
        b) Chronic
        c) Aplastic
        d) Sickle-cell
        e) Pernicious
    3. Possible causes
        a) Loss of blood

NURSING CARE OF THE ADULT PATIENT

      b) Increased destruction of blood
      c) Defective formation of blood
   4. Assessment
      a) Fatigue
      b) Dizziness
      c) Paleness of skin
      d) Headache

DATA SUMMARY 9
Classification of Anemias

Type	Cause	Treatment
Acute anemia	Sudden hemorrhage trauma to blood vessels peptic ulcer ruptured ectopic pregnancy placenta previa pulmonary tuberculosis poisoning overwhelming infection postoperative	Stopping hemorrhage Transfusions of blood Removal of cause
Chronic anemia	Continued bleeding hemorrhoids uterine lesions hepatic cirrhosis	Removal of cause Transfusions when indicated
Aplastic anemia	Destruction of red bone marrow poisoning severe sepsis nephritis at times	Removal of cause
Sickle-cell anemia	Hereditary condition in persons of African descent	Symptomatic; no known treatment
Pernicious anemia	Primary anemia absence of "intrinsic factor"	Liver therapy Vitamin B

---

      e) Shortness of breath
      f) Quickened pulse and pounding heart on slightest exertion
   5. Treatment and nursing care
      a) Drug therapy
         (1) Iron may be given by mouth or by intramuscular injection in cases of iron deficiency anemia.
         (2) Vitamin B_{12} and liver extract are given, with dramatic results, for pernicious anemia.
      b) Blood transfusions
         (1) Transfusions are given in both acute and chronic anemia.
         (2) Bloods of donor and recipient must be compatible.
         (3) Patient must be carefully watched for adverse reaction to the transfused blood, such as itching, edema, chills, fever, shortness of breath

D. Leukemia
   1. Definition of **leukemia:** Malignant disease of white blood cells, characterized by rapid and abnormal growth of leukocytes
   2. Classification—according to type of leukocyte predominating
      a) Acute
      b) Chronic
   3. Assessment (symptoms depend on type)
      a) Acute—usually in children and generally fatal, with fever, pallor, enlarged tender lymph nodes present
      b) Chronic—usually in older persons, with enlarged lymph nodes, anemia, fatigue
   4. Treatment
      a) Symptomatic treatment
      b) Radiation therapy in some cases
      c) Steroids in some cases
      d) Chemotherapy in some cases

E. Lymphoma
   1. Definition of **lymphoma:** Progressive, painless enlargement of lymphatic tissue, usually malignant
   2. Diagnosis by biopsy
   3. Treatment symptomatic by chemotherapy

F. Purpura
   1. Characteristics
      a) There are spontaneous hemorrhages into skin and venous membranes.
      b) Purpura is a symptom of many diseases.
   2. Treatment—symptomatic

G. Acute Infectious Mononucleosis
   1. Definition of **acute infectious mononucleosis:** Infectious disease caused by the Epstein-Barr herpes virus
   2. Characteristics
      a) Fever
      b) Enlarged lymph nodes
      d) Increase in mononuclear leukocytes
   3. Diagnosis—by positive heterophile antibody agglutination test (Paul-Bunnell)
   4. Treatment—symptomatic

H. Hodgkin's Disease
   1. Characteristics
      a) Painless, progressive enlargement of lymph nodes
      b) Fever
      c) Wasting
      d) Anemia
      e) Enlarged spleen
   2. Diagnosis—by biopsy
   3. Treatment
      a) Radiation
      b) Chemotherapy

XII. **Diseases Related to the Heart**

A. Congenital Heart Disease (results from abnormality in heart chambers or valves of one or more of the great vessels present at birth)

    1. Cause—improper development of heart, possibly due to
       a) Maternal rubella during first trimester of pregnancy
       b) Other maternal viral diseases
    2. Characteristics
       a) Cyanosis in most cases
       b) Dyspnea upon exertion
       c) Failure to thrive
       d) Clubbing of fingers and toes
       e) Loud murmurs
    3. Frequent manifestations
       a) Coarctation of aorta
       b) Patent foramen ovale
       c) Tetralogy of Fallot
       d) Patent ductus arteriosus
       e) Dextrocardia
    4. Diagnosis
       a) Physical examination
       b) X-ray study
       c) Cardiac catheterization
       d) Angiocardiography
    5. Treatment
       a) Supportive measures
          (1) Prevention of infection
          (2) Maintenance of sufficient oxygen level
       b) Surgery where possible

B. Arteriosclerotic Heart Disease
    1. Causes—atherosclerosis
       a) Formation of fatty deposits under lining of blood vessels
       b) Narrowing of lumen of arteries
    2. Characteristics
       a) Hypertension
       b) Hypertrophy of left ventricle
       c) Premature systoles
       d) Auricular fibrillation
       e) Cardiac decompensation
    3. Diagnosis
       a) Physical examination
       b) X-ray study
       c) EKG
    4. Treatment
       a) Treatment of symptoms
       b) Moderation in daily living
       c) Diet modification—diet may be low sodium and low cholesterol

C. Hypertension
    1. Definition of **hypertension:** Disorder, often with no symptoms, in which the blood pressure is persistently above 140/90 mm Hg
    2. Causes
       a) Adrenal and kidney disorders
       b) Thyroid disorders
       c) Toxemia of pregnancy
       d) Emotional stress
       e) Unknown factors

3. Two types
   a) Essential hypertension
      (1) Constriction of arterioles throughout the body
      (2) Necessity for heart to beat more forcefully to counteract resistance of arterioles
      (3) No known cause
   b) Malignant hypertension
      (1) Occurs in youth
      (2) Affects kidneys adversely
      (3) Rapidly results in uremia and death

D. Hypertensive Heart Disease (results in left ventricular failure)
   1. Cause—long-standing, untreated hypertension
   2. Characteristics
      a) Fatigue
      b) Dyspnea
      c) Edema of extremities
      d) Cyanosis
      e) May lead to
         (1) Left ventricular failure
         (2) Cerebral hemorrhage
         (3) Chronic nephritis
   3. Treatment
      a) Attempt to reduce blood pressure
      b) Weight reduction if necessary
      c) Moderation in daily living
      d) Avoidance of stimulants
      e) Symptomatic treatment

E. Angina Pectoris
   1. Cause—spasm of one of coronary arteries due to
      a) Atherosclerosis of coronary vessels
      b) Syphilitic heart disease
      c) Severe anemia
   2. Assessment
      a) Sudden severe pain in substernal area radiating to left shoulder and inner left arm
      b) Ashen color
      c) Cold, clammy perspiration
      d) Normal pulse rate with little or no change in blood pressure
   3. Precipitating factors
      a) Effort
      b) Walking against wind
      c) Exposure to cold
      d) Emotional upset
      e) Heavy meal
   4. Treatment
      a) Rest
      b) Relaxation
      c) Protection from cold
      d) Avoidance of precipitating factors
      e) Nitroglycerin sublingually
      f) Treatment of hypertension, if present

F. Myocardial Infarction
  1. Cause—occlusion of one of coronary arteries
  2. Assessment
     a) Crushing substernal pain
     b) Shock
     c) Fever
     d) Nausea and vomiting
  3. Diagnosis
     a) EKG—may be normal or abnormal
     b) Increased leukocyte count after 24 hours
     c) Increased sedimentation rate
     d) Sometimes, low-grade fever
     e) Change in enzymes
  4. Treatment
     a) Relief of pain immediately by administration of morphine or Demerol
     b) Administration of oxygen
     c) Frequent check of vital signs
     d) Anticoagulant therapy
     e) Strict bedrest
     f) Digitalis if ordered by physician
     g) Later, passive exercise of patient's extremities
     h) Supportive, emotional care

G. Rheumatic Fever
  1. Definition of **rheumatic fever:** Acute infectious disease of children and young adults that affects the heart and also involves joints, tendons, the nervous system, subcutaneous tissues, and larger arteries.
  2. Cause—toxins from streptococcus after strep throat
  3. Assessment
     a) Migratory joint pains
     b) High fever
     c) Sore throat
     d) Leukocytosis; high sedimentation rate
     e) Usually more than one attack
  4. Treatment
     a) Salicylates, steroids
     b) Antibiotics
     c) Bedrest
     d) Support of painful joints
     e) Footboards
     f) Heat
     g) Warm baths
     h) Bed cradle
  5. Complications
     a) Damage to heart valves
     b) Possible damage to heart muscle

H. Rheumatic Heart Disease
  1. Cause—damage to heart valves, resulting from rheumatic fever
  2. Type of damage
     a) Scar tissue may cause valve to leak—insufficiency
     b) Scar tissue may cause stenosis of valve

I. Congestive Heart Failure
    1. Causes
        a) Heart unable to do its work
        b) Underlying cardiovascular disease
            (1) Rheumatic heart disease
            (2) Arteriosclerotic heart disease
            (3) Endocarditis
            (4) Myocarditis
            (5) Hypertension
    2. Characteristics
        a) Slow in starting
        b) Chronic
        c) Recurrent
    3. Assessment
        a) Failure of left side of heart (pulmonary symptoms)
            (1) Dyspnea
            (2) Cough
            (3) Pulmonary edema
        b) Failure of right side of heart (systemic symptoms)
            (1) Edema of lower extremities
            (2) Collection of fluid in liver and abdominal organs (ascites)
            (3) Some mental confusion
        d) Gradual failure of both sides
            (1) Difficult breathing
            (2) Cyanosis
            (3) Edema
            (4) Orthopnea (inability to breath except in an upright position)
            (5) Irregular pulse
            (6) Anxiety
    4. Treatment
        a) Treatment of individual symptoms
        b) Bedrest during acute stages
        c) Digitalis to slow and strengthen heart beat
        d) Sedatives for rest
        e) Pain relief
        f) Diuretics to increase urinary output and to get rid of fluid
        g) Sodium-restricted diet
    5. Nursing care
        a) Position patient comfortably.
        b) Keep accurate record of intake and output.
        c) Weigh patient daily.
        d) Take rectal temperature daily.
        e) Lift patient on and off bedpan.
        f) Give passive exercise to prevent venostasis.
        g) Carefully observe vital signs.
        h) Maintain personal hygiene of patient.
        i) Prepare patient for oxygen.
        j) Feed patient.
        k) Assist with treatments, e.g., phlebotomy, rotating tourniquets.
        l) Observe for signs of pulmonary edema.
        m) Monitor for digitalis toxicity.
        n) Monitor for electrolyte imbalance from diuretics.

J. Acute Bacterial Endocarditis
   1. Causes
      a) Rapid, progressive infection of endocardium
      b) Hemolytic streptococcus, *Bacillus* influenza, pneumococcus or gonococcus
      c) Rheumatic fever or congenital defects of heart
   2. Treatment
      a) Antibiotic therapy
      b) Bedrest
      c) Symptomatic treatment

K. Subacute Bacterial Endocarditis
   1. Causes
      a) Alpha hemolytic streptococcus and nonhemolytic streptococcus are most common.
      b) Forerunners are rheumatic fever and congenital defects.
   2. Assessment
      a) Prolonged fever
      b) Chills
      c) General malaise
      d) Fatigue
      e) Anemia
      f) Embolic phenomena
   3. Treatment
      a) Antibiotics
      b) Bedrest
      c) Symptomatic treatment

L. Pericarditis
   1. Definition of **pericarditis:** Inflammation of the heart membranes
   2. Causes
      a) Viral infections
      b) Bacterial infection as complication of other infectious diseases
      c) As complication of other diseases
      d) Chest trauma
      e) Metastasis
   3. Symptoms
      a) Depend on cause
      b) May include pain and fever
   4. Treatment
      a) Treatment of underlying disease
      b) Symptomatic treatment
      c) Bedrest
      d) Antibiotics

M. Irregularities of the Heart
   1. Normal mechanism
      a) Regular contractions of heart are controlled by
         (1) Impulses arising in S-A node (also called pacemaker of heart)
         (2) Conduction system of heart
      b) Contractions are affected by extracardiac causes and cardiac causes.
   2. Types of arrhythmias
      a) Sinus arrhythmia
         (1) Variation of heart rate with respiration
         (2) Not indicative of disease

b) Extrasystoles
    (1) Premature beats followed by compensatory pause
    (2) Causes
        (a) Irritability of heart muscle from nervousness, coffee, tobacco, overdoses of digitalis
        (b) Myocardial disease
c) Paroxysmal tachycardia
    (1) Sudden onset of very rapid, regular rhythm of short duration
    (2) Not indicative of disease
d) Auricular flutter
    (1) Very high auricular rate with ventricular rate of half amount
    (2) Rapid, regular ventricular rate
e) Auricular fibrillation
    (1) Absolute arrhythmia of atrial myocardium
    (2) Irregular auricular impulses
f) Heart block
    (1) Auricles and ventricles contract independently of each other.
    (2) Block may be partial or complete.
    (3) Condition may be lethal.

3. Control of lethal arrhythmias
  a) Closed-chest cardiac massage
  b) Cardioversion (electric shock to chest wall)
  c) Cardiac pacemaking
    (1) Weak, periodic electric shocks to induce beating
    (2) Monitoring system for constant observation of rhythm

4. Nursing care relative to pacemaker implantation
  a) Preoperative
    (1) Reassure patient.
    (2) Follow preoperative orders.
  b) Postoperative
    (1) Observe for symptoms of congestive heart failure.
    (2) Monitor patient's pulse closely and record.
    (3) Teach patient to take own pulse twice daily for 1 full minute.
    (4) Urge patient to have periodic medical checkups.
    (5) Assess implantation site: watch for signs and symptoms of infection around generator and leads.

XIII. Diseases Related to the Blood Vessels

A. Peripheral Vascular Disease
  1. Varicose veins
    a) Definition of **varicose veins:** Enlarged, twisted veins with abnormally functioning valves
    b) Causes
      (1) Congenitally defective venous valves
      (2) Obesity
      (3) Pregnancy
      (4) Occupation requiring long periods of standing
    c) Symptoms
      (1) Fatigue
      (2) Swelling and heaviness in legs after prolonged standing
      (3) Pains in legs

      d) Treatment
          (1) Removal of cause
          (2) Support of veins by use of elastic stockings or elastic bandages
          (3) Surgical treatment, such as removal or tying off of affected vein

2. Varicose ulcers—occur on legs
    a) Causes
        (1) Impaired circulation
        (2) Venostasis
        (3) Injury
    b) Treatment
        (1) Elastic bandages
        (2) Unna paste boot
        (3) Surgical treatment
            (a) Debridement
            (b) Skin grafts to area

3. Thrombophlebitis
    a) Definition of **thrombophlebitis:** Inflammation of a vein associated with formation of a blood clot in the vein
    b) Assessment
        (1) Pain in calf of leg
        (2) Tenderness over region of clot
        (3) Elevated temperature
        (4) Erythema along course of the vein
    c) Treatment
        (1) Bedrest
        (2) Elevation of leg
        (3) Warmth to leg
        (4) Anticoagulant therapy (Coumarin derivatives, dicumerol, and/or heparin)
        (5) Attention to general health of patient
        (6) No massage of leg because clot may be dislodged and pulmonary embolus result

4. Arteriosclerosis of extremities
    a) Definition of **arteriosclerosis:** Disorder characterized by loss of elasticity and hardening of the walls of the arteries
    b) Symptoms
        (1) Numbness and coldness of extremities
        (2) Leg cramps at night
        (3) Fatigue of legs
    c) Treatment
        (1) Improvement of circulation by exercise
        (2) Drugs, such as Quinnam, at night to improve circulation
        (3) Elevation of legs
        (4) Amputation if gangrene occurs

5. Aortic aneurysm
    a) Definition of **aneurysim:** Localized dilatation of blood vessel
    b) Possible causes
        (1) Syphilis
        (2) Arteriosclerosis
        (3) Congenital factors
    c) Treatment—surgical

6. Peripheral arterial disease
    a) Arteriosclerosis obliterans
    b) Buerger's disease
    c) Raynaud's disease

          d) Peripheral emboli
          e) Arteriovenous fistula
          f) Arterial aneurysm
             (Note: This section is included for vocabulary purposes only.)

    B. General Nursing Care
        1. Measures to prevent constriction of blood vessels
          a) Avoidance of cold
          b) Avoidance of constricting clothing
          c) Special care for feet
          d) Avoidance of nicotine (constricts blood vessels)
          e) Avoidance of long periods of sitting with legs crossed
          f) Elevation of feet
          g) Exercises under direction of physician
          h) Frequent turning of bedrest patients
          i) Elastic stockings to give support to blood vessels in legs
          j) Reducing diet for obese patients
          k) Increase of fluids to hasten excretion of waste products
        2. Drugs
          a) Vasodilators to increase size of blood vessels and thus improve circulation
          b) Anticoagulants to thin blood and prevent formation of blood clots

XIV. Cerebrovascular Diseases

    A. Arteriosclerosis of brain
        1. Assessment
          a) Impairment of mental capacity
          b) Decrease in intelligence
          c) Psychosis
        2. Treatment—symptomatic and nonspecific

    B. Stroke (Cerebrovascular Accident)
        1. Cause—obstruction of blood flow in cerebral artery due to
          a) Formation of clot within cerebral artery
          b) Spasm of arterial artery
          c) Rupture of artery with hemorrhage into brain
        2. Assessment (symptoms vary depending upon extent of damage)
          a) Transitory dizziness and weakness
          b) Severe headache
          c) Speech disturbances
          d) Paralysis on one side of body
          e) Coma
         3. Treatment
          a) Prevention of obstruction of breathing
          b) Suctioning and maintenance of open airway
          c) Tube feeding, if necessary
          d) Intravenous fluids
          e) Proper positioning of patient
          f) Passive exercises to maintain functions of joints

XV. Heart Surgery

    A. General Principles

1. Required to correct congenital conditions, traumatic lesions, or acquired defects in children or adults
2. May be open- or closed-heart surgery
3. Requires highly trained team of which practical nurse may be a member

B. Preoperative Care
   1. Physical examination
   2. Special tests and examinations
   3. Consultations between various physicians or team members
   4. Preparation of patient for operation and for postoperative procedures by nurse
   5. Sedation given before surgery
   6. Venous cut-down done by physician
   7. Preoperative nursing care

C. Postoperative Nursing Care
   1. Check vital signs and record them every 15 minutes for the first 24 hours.
   2. Give oxygen continuously by tent, mask, or nasal catheter.
   3. Maintain closed drainage system with chest catheters.
   4. Have Levine tube connected to suction machine.
   5. Position patient according to surgeon's orders.
   6. Constantly monitor intake and output.
      a) Give oral fluids as soon as nausea has ceased.
      b) Check urinary output hourly, including specific gravity.
   7. Be aware that secretions from pulmonary system must be removed by coughing or by endotracheal suctioning.
   8. Administer antibiotics routinely.
   9. Frequently check dressing for hemorrhage.
   10. Constantly observe for abnormal reactions.
       a) Cyanosis
       b) Numbness
       c) Pain
       d) Sudden paralysis
       e) Disorientation
   11. Increase activity gradually.

XVI. Vascular Surgery

A. Types–venous ligation and stripping common

B. Care
   1. Preoperative care similar to other surgical care
   2. Postoperative care
      a) Check dressings for hermorrhage
      b) Take and record vital signs routinely.
      c) Encourage early ambulation as ordered by physician.
      d) Tighten elastic bandages as necessary.

XVII. Cardiovascular Surgery

A. Indications
   1. Trauma
   2. Pericarditis
   3. Valvular abnormalities

4. Coronary artery disease
5. Varicose veins
6. Vascular injuries
7. Aneurysms
8. Occlusive arterial disease
9. Lymphedema

XVIII. The Lymphatic System

A. Structure and Functions
   1. Structure
      a) Is a network of capillaries, vessels, ducts, nodes, and organs
      b) Comprises a circulatory system (of lymph vessels) similar to blood circulatory system
   2. Functions
      a) Collects from smaller lymphatics by thoracic duct and right lymphatic duct
      b) Empties into large veins of neck

B. Forms of Lymphoid Tissue
   1. Lymph nodes
      a) Produce lymphocytes
      b) Act as filters to remove poisonous substances, microorganisms, malignant cells, and dead blood cells
   2. Tonsils—filter pathogens from tissue fluid in upper respiratory tract
   3. Adenoids—filter pathogens from tissue fluid in upper respiratory tract
   4. Thymus gland
      a) Active during early years
      b) Essential to prenatal growth
   5. Spleen
      a) Produces lymphocytes and monocytes
      b) Produces antibodies
      c) Destroys old red blood cells
      d) Acts as reservoir for blood

C. Disorders of the Lymphatic System
   1. Lymphangitis
      a) Cause—streptococcus invasion
      b) Assessment
         (1) Chills
         (2) Elevation of temperature
         (3) Tender and swollen lymph node
      c) Treatment
         (1) Heat applications to area
         (2) Fluids
         (3) Antibiotics
         (4) Bedrest
         (5) Light diet
   2. Lymphedema
      a) Cause—accumulation of lymph fluid in tissues and obstruction of lymphatics
      b) Symptom—nonpitting edema
      c) Treatment
         (1) Warm, moist compresses
         (2) Rest

    (3) Elevation of part above level of heart
    (4) Elastic bandages
    (5) Surgery

UNIT 5: THE RESPIRATORY SYSTEM

VOCABULARY

antibiotic	substance produced by a living organism which has the power to destroy other organisms
	Broad spectrum antibiotic—acts against a wide number of bacterial organisms
	Specific antibiotic—acts against a specific organism
apnea	absence of respiration
atelectasis	lack of air in lungs; lung collapse, partial or complete
blood gases	oxygen and carbon dioxide in bloodstream
COPD	chronic obstructive pulmonary disease
hemoptysis	coughing up blood
humidity	moisture in the atmosphere
hypoxia	condition in which amount of oxygen available is inadequate to meet needs of tissues
IPPB	intermittent positive pressure breathing
lavage	washing out of a cavity or organ
lobectomy	surgical removal of a lobe of lung
orthopnea	inability to breathe when in a horizontal position
pneumonectomy	surgical removal of a lung
spirometry	measurement of air capacity of lungs
tomogram	one of a series of body-section X rays, commonly referred to as a "cut"
tomography	body-section radiography
thoracentesis	removal of fluids from chest by tapping through chest wall

  I. **Function and Structure**

      A. Function
          1. Exchange of oxygen and carbon dioxide in the body
             a) Oxygen from outside air passes through walls of alveoli into lung capillaries.
             b) Oxygen carried by blood cells in capillaries diffuses into cells.
             c) Carbon dioxide leaving cells enters tissue capillaries and is carried in blood back to alveoli of lungs.
             d) Carbon dioxide leaves blood in lung capillaries and passes through walls of alveoli to be exhaled into outside air.

      B. Structure
          1. Organs of respiration—nose, pharynx, larynx, trachea, bronchi, lungs
             a) Nose
                (1) Has two cavities (airways) separated by a septum
                (2) Is lined by mucous membrane, which has cilia that act as filters
                (3) Warms, moistens, and filters air breathed
                (4) Contains sense organs of smell (ends of olfactory nerves)
                (5) Joins with pharynx
              b) Pharynx
                (1) Is lined with mucous membrane
                (2) Contains tonsils and adenoids

        (3)   Has openings into it of nasal passages, mouth, esophagus, larynx, and eustachian tubes

        (4)   Acts as passageway for food from mouth to esophagus

        (5)   Acts as passageway for air from nose to trachea

   c) Larynx

        (1)   Has nine cartilages, largest of which is thyroid cartilage (Adam's apple)

        (2)   Has epiglottis, which covers larynx when one swallows so that food does not go into trachea

        (3)   Has vocal cords, which stretch across interior of larynx

        (4)   Produces sound

        (5)   Serves as passageway for air between outside and lungs

   d) Trachea (windpipe)

        (1)   Extends from lower part of larynx to level of upper border of fifth thoracic vertebra, where it divides into two bronchi

        (2)   Is a cartilaginous and membranous tube

        (3)   Serves as passageway for air from larynx to bronchi

   e) Bronchi (singular: bronchus), bronchioles, and alveoli

        (1)   Bronchi are composed of imperfect rings of cartilage.

        (2)   Right bronchus is wider and shorter than left.

        (3)   Bronchi divide into smaller tubes (bronchioles).

        (4)   Bronchioles end in grapelike clusters of sacs called *alveoli.*

        (5)   Bronchi and bronchioles act as passageways for air.

        (6)   Alveoli are used for exchange of gases between air and blood (functional unit of lungs).

   f) Lungs

        (1)   Lungs are located in thoracic cavity.

        (2)   Lungs are covered by pleura—a thin, lubricated membrane, which prevents friction.

        (3)   Right lung has three lobes; left lung, two.

        (4)   Lungs rest on diaphragm.

        (5)   Lungs function in respiration—exchange of oxygen and carbon dioxide.

C. Accessory Organs of Respiration

   1. Muscles

      a) Diaphragm

         (1)   Separates chest from abdomen

         (2)   Increases size of chest cavity upon inspiration

      b) External intercostal muscles, which contract to move ribs in respiration (expand size of thoracic cavity during inspiration)

   2. Thoracic cage

      a) Ribs

      b) Sternum

      c) Thoracic vertebrae

D. Physiology of Respiration

   1. Respiration may be controlled voluntarily.

   2. Respiratory center is located in brain (medulla oblongata).

   3. Carbon dioxide in blood acts as respiratory stimulant.

II. Symptoms of Respiratory Disease

A. Cough

   1. Two types

        a) Nonproductive
           (1) Is dry, harsh, and hacking
           (2) Is exhausting
           (3) Does not remove secretions from bronchi
        b) Productive
           (1) Is moist and deep
           (2) Removes secretions from bronchi
           (3) Produces sputum
    2. Preparations to relieve coughs
        a) Narcotic cough mixtures
           (1) Depress cough reflex
           (2) Are habit forming
           (3) Depress respiration
           (4) Examples
               (a) Codeine
               (b) Hycodan
        b) Expectorants
           (1) Increases secretions
           (2) Reduce hacking quality of cough
           (3) Examples
               (a) Ammonium chloride
               (b) Robitussin
        c) Demulcents
           (1) Protect mucous membrane of upper respiratory tract
           (2) Reduce cough due to irritation
           (3) Examples
               (a) Syrups
               (b) Steam

B. Respiratory Distress
    1. Abnormal types of respiration
        a) Dyspnea—difficult or labored respiration
        b) Hyperpnea—increased respiratory rate, especially with exercise
        c) Apnea—temporary absence of respiration
        d) Cheyne-Stokes—respiration gradually increases in rapidity and volume until it reaches a climax, then gradually subsides and then begins again—usually a forerunner of death
        e) Abdominal—diaphragm active but chest walls at rest

C. Chest Pain
    1. Causes
        a) Lung abscess
        b) Tuberculous cavity
        c) Pleurisy
        d) Lung mass
    2. Diagnosis—physical examination, chest X ray, and/or CAT scan needed to distinguish from nonpulmonary pain

D. Wheeze
    1. Causes
        a) Asthma
        b) Foreign body
        c) Tumor

    2. Diagnosis
      a) Pulmonary function test
      b) Chest X ray

  E. Hemoptysis
    1. Causes
      a) Pulmonary disorder
      b) Pulmonary circulation abnormality (larynx, bronchus, etc.)
      c) Granulation tissue
      d) Clotting defects
    2. Diagnosis
      a) Lung scan
      b) Chest X ray
    3. Nursing care
      a) Observe patient closely as to amount of bleeding, skin-color changes, type of breathing.
      b) Record and report to charge nurse any changes.

III. Disorders of the Respiratory System

  A. Infection
    1. Upper respiratory infections
    2. Pneumonia
    3. Pleurisy
    4. Influenza
    5. Tuberculosis

  B. Obstructive Disorders
    1. Bronchial asthma
    2. Acute bronchitis
    3. Chronic obstructive pulmonary disease (C.O.P.D.)
    4. Atelectasis

  C. Degenerative Disorders
    1. Emphysema
    2. Bronchiectasis

  D. Traumatic Disorders
    1. Stab wound
    2. Fractured ribs

  E. Lung Abscess

  F. Occupational Lung Diseases
    1. Silicosis
    2. Pneumoconiosis
    3. Occupational asthma

  G. Pulmonary Embolism

  H. Pleurisy

I. Neoplasm
    1. Squamous cell
    2. Undifferentiated small cell
    3. Undifferentiated large cell
    4. Adenocarcinoma
    5. Lymphoma
    6. Sarcoma
    7. Metastatic

IV. **Diagnostic Procedures**

A. Laboratory Procedures
    1. Complete blood count
    2. Carbon dioxide combining power—to determine the degree of acidosis
    3. Blood gases
    4. Sputum examination
        a) Smear of material coughed up from lungs
        b) Staining of material
        c) Culture and sensitivity
    5. Gastric washings (lavage)
        a) Used when tuberculosis is suspected
        b) Used to examine tumor cells

B. Radiology
    1. Chest X-ray study
        a) No special preparation is necessary.
        b) X rays may be taken in different views: A-P, lateral, oblique.
    2. Fluoroscopy—radiologist can observe lungs in motion
    3. Bronchogram
        a) X-ray study of bronchial tree outlined by radiopaque dye
        b) Fasting required until local anesthetic has worn off
    4. Tomogram
    5. Lung scan
    6. Magnetic resonance imaging (MRI)
    7. Ultrasound

C. Bronchoscopy—used to
    1. Remove foreign bodies
    2. Make biopsy
    3. Remove secretions for examination

D. Spirometry—used to measure air capacity of lungs

E. Thoracentesis
    1. Relief of respiratory restrictions due to large quantities of pleural fluid
    2. Introduction of medications into pleural space

F. Bronchial Lavage

G. Lung Biopsy

H. Tracheal Aspiration

V. Classification of Drugs for Treatment of Respiratory Diseases

A. Antipyretics
   1. Act on central nervous system to lower body temperature
   2. Act as analgesics
   3. Examples
      a) Aspirin
      b) Sodium salicylate

B. Antihistamines
   1. Help to dry up secretions of upper respiratory tract
   2. Have side effects such as extreme drowsiness
   3. Examples
      a) Pyribenzamine
      b) Chlor-Trimeton

C. Bronchodilators
   1. Relax contraction of smooth muscle in bronchioles
   2. Examples
      a) Adrenaline
      b) Aminophylline

D. Antibiotics
   1. Are used to counteract infection
   2. May be specific or nonspecific (broad spectrum)

E. Steroids
   1. Used in bronchial asthma and in some cases of carcinoma
   2. Examples
      a) Cortisone
      b) Prednisone
      c) Decadron

VI. Important Treatment Procedures

A. Nasal Irrigation
   1. Aids in removing secretions from respiratory tract
   2. Must be given gently so as not to spread infection into sinuses

B. Aerosols
   1. Aerosols are medications applied by inhalation directly into bronchial tree.
   2. Solutions may contain specific medications such as antibiotics and/or bronchodilators.

C. IPPB
   1. Delivers various drugs such as antibiotics, liquifying agents, and bronchodilators directly to bronchial tree
   2. Helps increase inspired air (expands lungs)
   3. Helps in exchange of oxygen and carbon dioxide

VII. Nursing Care

A. General Principles
   1. Observe and record vital signs.

NURSING CARE OF THE ADULT PATIENT

2. Administer medications as ordered.
3. Provide frequent mouth care.
4. Provide comfortable positions to make breathing easier (Fowler's position).
5. Recognize signs of oxygen deficiency (cyanosis, dyspnea, respiration rate).
6. Reassure patient.
7. Keep air moist to soothe mucous membranes.
8. Monitor diet.
   a) High-calorie, high-vitamin liquids at first.
   b) Gradual change to soft and then regular foods.
9. Monitor IV fluids.

VIII. **Disorders of the Upper and Lower Respiratory Tracts**

A. Upper Respiratory Tract
   1. Common cold
      a) Cause—primarily viral; bacteria may be secondary invader
      b) Occurrence—frequent
      c) Treatment—symptomatic only
   2. Acute pharyngitis
      a) Definition of **acute pharyngitis:** Inflammation of pharynx
      b) Causes
         (1) Virus or bacteria
         (2) Infection or irritation
      c) Treatment—depends on cause
   3. Tonsillitis
      a) Definition of **tonsillitis:** Inflammation or infection of a tonsil; may lead to severe complications such as rheumatic fever or glomerulonephritis
      b) Cause—may be acute or chronic bacterial infection, generally strep or staph
      c) Treatment depends on cause
   4. Laryngitis
      a) Definition of **laryngitis:** Inflammation of larynx (known as croup in children)
      b) Cause—may be irritation, infection, or neoplastic disease
      c) Treatment—depends on cause
   5. Sinusitis
      a) Definition of **sinusitis:** Infection and inflammation of lining of sinuses
      b) Cause—viral or bacterial
      c) Treatment—symptomatic

B. Lower Respiratory Tract
   1. Influenza
      a) Is caused by virus
      b) May be complicated by pneumonia
      c) May be dangerous in very young or very old
   2. Bronchitis
      a) Definition of **bronchitis:** Inflammation of bronchial mucous membrane
      b) Two types
         (1) Acute
            (a) Causes
               i) Exposure to cold
               ii) Extension of common cold
               iii) Inhalation of irritating substances
            (b) Treatment—depends on cause
         (2) Chronic

(a) Assessment
    i) Persistent productive cough
    ii) Dyspnea upon exertion
    iii) Generally no fever
(b) Treatment—antibiotics, respiratory antiseptics, expectorants, and warm climate

3. Pneumonia
   a) May be viral (primary atypical pneumonia)
      (1) Patchy infection throughout lung
      (2) Longer convalescent period needed than in pneumococcal pneumonia
   b) If bacterial, is usually caused by pneumococcus

4. Pleurisy
   a) Definition of **pleurisy:** Inflammation of membranes surrounding lung
   b) Two types
      (1) Dry pleurisy
      (2) Pleurisy with effusion—increase of serious fluid within pleural cavity
   c) Assessment
      (1) Fever
      (2) Sharp, stabbing pain in chest intensified by respiration
   d) Specific treatment and nursing care
      (1) Bedrest
      (2) Observation for signs of respiratory distress
      (3) Immobilization of chest wall by strapping
      (4) Observation for signs of pulmonary infection
      (5) Thoracentesis when effusion present

5. Pulmonary tuberculosis
   a) Definition of **pulmonary tuberculosis:** Chronic disease caused by tubercle bacillus and characterized by lesions within lung
   b) Assessment
      (1) Persistent low-grade fever
      (2) Cough
      (3) Weight loss
      (4) Night sweats
      (5) Hemoptysis
   c) Specific treatment and nursing care
      (1) Rest
      (2) Fresh air
      (3) Good nutrition
      (4) Drugs (used in combination)
         (a) Streptomycin
         (b) Isoniazid (INH)
         (c) Rimactane
         (d) Para-aminobenzoic acid (PABA)
      (5) Surgery in some cases
         (a) Thoracoplasty to collapse and rest the affected lung
         (b) Lobectomy or pneumonectomy

6. Pulmonary emphysema
   a) Definition of **pulmonary emphysema:** Permanent overdistension and dilatation of lung alveoli
   b) Characteristics—dyspnea, persistent hacking cough, loss of weight
   c) Cause—repeated infections and irritation of lungs
   d) Specific treatment and nursing care
      (1) Bronchodilators and inhalation therapy as ordered by physician

   (2) Postural drainage
   (3) Rest
   (4) Nutritious diet
   (5) Supportive nursing measures
   (6) Emotional support
   (7) Proper care of secretions
 7. Bronchiectasis
  a) Definition of **bronchiectasis:** Permanent dilatation of bronchi, resulting from chronic respiratory infections and characterized by cough with large amounts of foul-smelling sputum
  b) Specific treatment and nursing care
   (1) Postural drainage
   (2) Bronchodilators and expectorants
   (3) Aerosol therapy
 8. Chronic obstructive pulmonary disease (COPD)
  a) Definition of **COPD:** Constant respiratory distress due to long-standing pulmonary disease
  b) Assessment
   (1) Wheezing-type cough
   (2) Dyspnea upon exertion
   (3) Cyanosis
   (4) Anxiety
  c) Specific treatment
   (1) Bronchodilators
   (2) Corticosteroids
   (3) Antibiotics
   (4) Exercises
   (5) IPPB therapy
   (6) Good nutrition
   (7) Prevention of overexertion
 9. Neoplastic disease
  a) Occurence—frequent in larynx and in lung
  b) Assessment
   (1) Constant hoarseness is early symptom of laryngeal involvement.
   (2) Cough and hemoptysis are frequent in lung cancer.
  c) Treatment of both types
   (1) Surgery
   (2) Chemotherapy
   (3) Radiation

IX. Chest Surgery

Nurse's Role
1. Check and record vital signs frequently.
2. Observe closely for signs of respiratory distress.
3. Change patient's position frequently according to surgeon's order.
4. Observe drainage tubing frequently for patency and maintenance of "closed system."

X. Tracheotomy and Tracheostomy

Nurse's Role
1. Reassure patient.
2. Suction tube frequently to keep it patent.

3. Protect membranes of throat from injury while suctioning.
4. Be aware that moist air (vaporizer) may make patient more comfortable.
5. Clean tubes and change dressing routinely.

UNIT 6: THE DIGESTIVE SYSTEM

VOCABULARY

achlorhydria	absence of free hydrochloric acid in gastric juice
alimentary canal	continuous passageway for food formed by organs of digestion
ascites	fluid in peritoneal cavity
aspiration	removal of fluids or gases from cavity by suction
atresia	closure or congenital absence of normal anatomical opening
cecostomy	surgical formation of cecal fistula or artificial anus
cholecystectomy	surgical excision of gallbladder
choledochotomy	incision of common bile duct
cholelithiasis	presence of stones in gallbladder
colectomy	excision of part of colon
deglutition	act of swallowing
diverticulum	sac or pouch in walls of colon or other tubular organ
duodenitis	inflammation of duodenum
enteritis	inflammation of intestines
enteroptosis	prolapse of intestines or abdominal organs
fecal fistula	abnormal tubelike passage from rectum to outside or to another cavity containing feces
fistula-in-ano	abnormal tubelike passage near anus
gastritis	inflammation of stomach
gastroenteritis	inflammation of stomach and intestines
gastroenterostomy	surgical anastomosis between stomach and intestine
hemorrhoid	dilated blood vessel in anal region
hepatitis	inflammation of liver
jaundice	yellowing of skin due to bile pigment in blood; icterus
Laënnec's cirrhosis	atrophic cirrhosis of liver
mastication	act of chewing
melena	dark stools stained with blood and blood pigments
paracentesis	surgical puncture of cavity for aspiration of fluid
parenteral	not through alimentary canal
varicose veins	enlarged, twisted veins

I. **Components of Digestive System**

A. Main Organs of Digestion
  1. Mouth (oral or buccal cavity)
     a) Tongue
     b) Salivary glands
     c) Teeth
  2. Pharynx
  3. Epiglottis
  4. Esophagus
  5. Stomach
  6. Small intestine (small bowel)
     a) Duodenum
     b) Jejunum
     c) Ileum

    7. Large intestine (large bowel)
        a) Cecum
        b) Appendix
        c) Ascending colon
        d) Transverse colon
        e) Descending colon
        f) Sigmoid
        g) Rectum
        h) Anus

  B. Accessory Organs of Digestion
      1. Liver
      2. Gallbladder
      3. Pancreas

II. Structure and Functions of Main Organs of Digestion

  A. Mouth
      1. Receives food
      2. Contains glands that secrete amylase and ptyalin
      3. Starts the process of digestion

  B. Tongue
      1. Lies partly in floor of mouth and partly in pharynx
      2. Functions in manipulation of food in mastication and deglutition; taste
      3. Has extrinsic muscles that move it

  C. Salivary Glands
      1. There are three pairs:
          a) Parotid
          b) Submaxillary
          c) Sublingual
      2. They pour their secretions into mouth and start digestion of starches.
      3. They have an enzyme, ptyalin, that acts on starches.

  D. Teeth
      1. Are hard, bonelike organs set in sockets of jawbone (see Figure 14)
      2. Perform first step of digestion by cutting, tearing, and grinding food, and mixing it with saliva
      3. Help to form sounds of speech
      4. Help to determine facial expressions
      5. Have different shapes to perform different functions (see Data Summary 10)
      6. Appear in two sets during person's lifetime (see Data Summary 11)

Data Summary 10
Shapes and Functions of Teeth

Name of Tooth	Shape	Function
Incisor	Sharp, chisel-like edges	Bite or cut
Canine (cuspid)	Pointed	Tear and shred
Bicuspid	Double-pointed	Tear and grind
Molar	Broad, uneven edges	Grind and crush

NURSING CARE OF THE ADULT PATIENT

Data Summary 11 Dentition*		
Dentition	Number of Teeth	Age of Appearance
Primary (baby teeth, milk teeth, deciduous teeth)	20	Appear between the ages of 6 months and 2½ years
Permanent	32	Appear between the ages of 6 and 21 years

*Notes:
1) The baby is born with the beginnings of his/her baby teeth well developed within the jaws and with the buds of the first permanent molars. The permanent teeth start developing in the jaws during the early years of the child. By the time a permanent tooth is ready to replace a primary tooth, the root of the primary tooth has been absorbed by the jaw tissue.

2) Although the teeth are different in shape and perform different functions, they have the same general features.

The composition of each tooth is as follows: crown—protrudes in the mouth; enamel—hard covering; dentine—ivorylike composition; pulp chamber—center of tooth with nerves; cementum—a protective layer of material; peridontal membrane—protective layer that cushions the tooth.

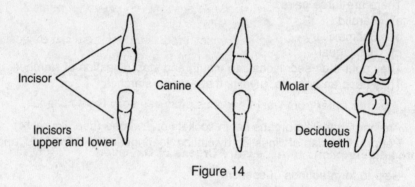

Incisor

Incisors upper and lower

Canine

Molar

Deciduous teeth

Figure 14

E. Pharynx
1. Serves as passageway for air and food
2. Extends from mouth to esophagus (in digestion)

F. Epiglottis
1. Prevents food or liquid from entering airway when swallowing

G. Esophagus
1. Is muscular canal extending from pharynx to stomach
2. Is narrowest part of digestive tract
3. Is approximately 10 inches in length in adult

H. Stomach (directly connected to esophagus)
1. Cardiac sphincter, located with cardiac orifice, relaxes to permit food to enter stomach and constricts to prevent regurgitation of food.
2. Cardiac orifice is opening between esophagus and stomach.

I. Small Intestine (Small Bowel)
1. Is divided into three sections:
    a) Duodenum
    b) Jejunum
    c) Ileum
2. Is composed of smooth muscle
3. Produces peristalsis
4. Is innervated by autonomic nervous system through vagus nerve
5. Has mucous membrane lining with glands that secrete intestinal juice
6. Has villi on surface of lining that contain blood vessels and lymph capillaries
7. Is part where most digestion and absorption occur
8. Communicates with biliary duct system through duodenum (see Figure 15)

J. Large Intestine (Large Bowel)
1. Extends from end of ileum to anus
2. Is 6 feet 5 inches long and 2½ inches wide
3. Is divided into three sections:
    a) Colon—approximately 4½ feet
    b) Rectum—approximately 5 inches
    c) Anus—approximately 1½ inches
4. Is innervated by autonomic nervous system through vagus nerve
5. Has mucous membrane lining without villi
6. Has smooth muscle in its wall which produces peristalsis and defecation
7. Has cecum, a blind pouch at beginning of large bowel
8. Has appendix, a small, blind, wormlike tube projecting from the cecum
9. Has no enzymes
10. Absorbs water from waste and thus produces solid fecal material

III. Structure and Functions of Accessory Organs of Digestion

A. Liver
1. Is largest gland in body
2. Lies mainly on right side of abdominal cavity
3. Manufactures a digestive fluid called *bile*
4. Removes sugar from blood and changes it into glycogen
5. Stores glycogen to be given out again when body needs sugar
6. Stores vitamins, minerals, and proteins
7. Manufactures albumin, globulin, fibrinogen, and prothrombin
    a) Prothrombin important in blood-clotting mechanism
    b) Fibrinogen important in blood-clotting mechanism
8. Forms urea from protein metabolism and releases it into bloodstream, where it is carried to kidneys and then excreted
9. Weighs approximately 3 pounds in adult
10. Helps in detoxification of certain drugs and poisonous substances

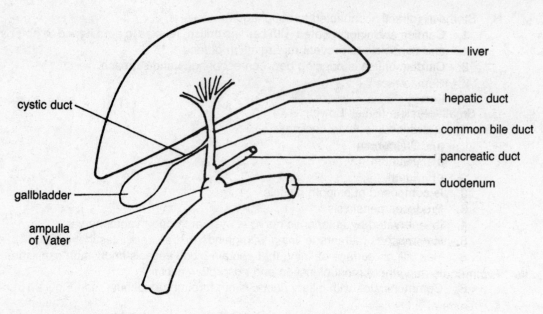

The Liver

Figure 15

B. Gallbladder
   1. Gallbladder is pear-shaped sac on undersurface of right lobe of liver.
   2. It stores and concentrates bile.
   3. It can hold about 50 cc of bile.
   4. It constricts and ejects bile into duodenum as needed for fat digestion.
   5. Cystic duct (bile duct) joins with hepatic duct to form common bile duct.
   6. Common bile duct and pancreatic duct unite and empty into small intestine at ampulla of Vater.

C. Pancreas
   1. Lies crosswise and behind stomach
   2. Consists of endocrine (ductless) and exocrine gland
      a) Endocrine function—has small islands of glandular tissue (Islets of Langerhans) that pour their secretion (insulin) directly into bloodstream
         (1) Insulin is very important in body's use of glucose circulating in bloodstream.
         (2) If not enough insulin is formed, rate of glucose transported through membranes of body cells is decreased.
         (3) Glucose accumulates in the blood and tissues.
         (4) Result is condition called *diabetes mellitus.*
      b) Exocrine function—produces pancreatic juice, which contains enzymes that are passed into duodenum during digestion
         (1) Trypsin—breaks down protein to peptides and amino acids
         (2) Amylase—breaks down carbohydrates to form disaccharides
         (3) Lipase—hydrolyzes fats into glycerol and fatty acids

IV. **Assessment of Digestive System**

   A. Esophagus, Stomach, and Small and Large Intestines
      1. Dysphagia

    2. Pain
    3. Nausea and vomiting
    4. Constipation
    5. Diarrhea
    6. Hematemesis
    7. Bloody stools
    8. Fecal incontinence

B. Liver and Gallbladder
    1. Jaundice
    2. Edema and ascites
    3. Pain
    4. Dsypnea
    5. Anorexia
    6. Weakness

V. Preliminary Nursing Care

A. General Principles
    1. Observe patient's symptoms.
    2. Withhold food and/or fluid as ordered if doctor's orders state "NPO."
    3. Reassure patient, and provide for rest and comfort.
    4. Prepare patient for specific examinations.
    5. Fill out necessary laboratory forms.
    6. Collect specimen(s) for laboratory.
    7. Accurately record intake and output.
    8. Give mouth care.
    9. Give appropriate skin care.
   10. Discourage smoking.
   11. Maintain patient's personal hygiene.
   12. Weigh patient daily.
   13. Assess nutritional status.
   14. Prevent skin breakdown.
   15. Protect perineum.

VI. Diagnostic Procedures

A. Laboratory Procedures
    1. Complete blood count
      a) Erythrocyte count
        (1) Increased in severe diarrhea, dehydration, and poisoning
        (2) Decreased in anemias and leukemias, and after hemorrhage
      b) White cell count
        (1) Increased following surgery or trauma, and in acute infectious diseases (bacterial), acute leukemia, eosinophilia, collagen diseases, allergy, and intestinal parasitosis
        (2) Decreased in aplastic anemia and agranulocytosis, and by toxic agents (important in chemotherapeutic treatment of malignancy)
    2. Erythrocyte sedimentation rate (ESR)
      a) Increased in tissue destruction (inflammations, degenerations)
      b) Increased in acute febrile diseases
    3. Gastric analysis
      a) Purposes

                (1) Assess acidity of gastric contents
                (2) Assess presence of gastric retention
                (3) Assess presence of gastric hemorrhage
            b) Significance
                (1) Presence of acid excludes diagnosis of pernicious anemia.
                (2) Retention indicates pyloric or duodenal obstruction.
                (3) Presence of cancer cells indicates carcinoma.
    4. Gastric test meals to determine
        a) Secretory response to food
        b) Acidity
    5. Stool examination to determine
        a) Ova and parasites
        b) Blood
    6. Blood chemistry
        a) SMA 12 and SMA 6 ordered on admission routinely include all necessary tests.
        b) Individual pertinent tests are as follows:
            (1) Glucose
            (2) Liver function
            (3) Cholesterol and esters
            (4) Serum amylase
            (5) Electrolytes (Na^+, K^+, Cl^-, and CO_2^-)
            (6) Alkaline phosphatase

B. Esophagoscopy, Gastroscopy, Sigmoidoscopy, Anoscopy, and Proctoscopy
    1. Are performed by physician
    2. Afford direct visual examination of mucosa

C. Rectal Examination
    1. Included in physical examination by physician
    2. Important in detecting lesions of rectum and anus
    3. Important in examination of prostate
    4. Important in examination of many intra-abdominal organs such as appendix, colon, uterus, ovaries

D. X-ray Studies
    1. Gastrointestinal series
        a) X-ray examination of esophagus, stomach, and small intestine after drinking barium solution
        b) Help in recognizing ulcers, growths, and obstructions
    2. Barium enema
        a) X-ray examination of large intestine after barium enema
        b) Help in recognizing tumors, ulcers, obstructions, and other abnormalities of bowel
    3. Gallbladder series
        a) X-ray examination of gallbladder and ducts after oral dye
        b) Help in recognizing stones and degree of function
    4. CAT scan
    5. Ultrasound

E. Liver and Gallbladder Examinations
    1. Liver biopsy
        a) Process of taking tiny amount of liver tissue by introducing biopsy needle and aspirating tiny amount of tissue
        b) Help in establishing diagnosis of liver disease

2. MRI
3. Gallbladder series
4. Liver function tests

F. Role of the Practical Nurse
   1. Allay patient's fears and apprehensions in regard to procedures.
   2. Observe and chart patient's symptoms.
   3. Prepare patient for procedure according to doctor's orders.
      a) Instruct patient regarding necessary fasting before GI series and/or other laboratory procedures.
      b) Administer enemas and/or purgatives as prescribed before specific lab tests.
      c) Provide appropriate diet preceding specific diagnostic tests.
      d) Administer oral dyes at correct times when prescribed for specific tests.
      e) Administer cleansing enemas after specific tests, e.g., barium enema.
   4. Prepare correct requisition and equipment for procedure.
   5. Assist health team members in performance of nursing and/or medical procedures.

VII. **Common Nursing Procedures**

A. Cleansing Enema
   1. Purposes
      a) To correct improper elimination
      b) To relieve gaseous distension of the lower bowel
      c) To cleanse rectum and lower bowel for proper examination
   2. Solutions used (ordered by physician)
      a) Plain tap water
      b) Saline solution
      c) Soapsuds
      d) Commercial preparations
   3. Temperature—105° F; measured by bath thermometer
   4. Pressure and rate of flow
      a) Slow rate and low pressure
      b) Regulation by elevation of irrigator and size of rectal tube
      c) Results of excessive pressure and rate of flow
         (1) Damage to tissue
         (2) Discomfort
         (3) Premature expulsion
   5. Position of patient—left Sims's
      a) Favors relaxation of abdomen
      b) Favors flow into sigmoid
   6. Procedure after administration
      a) Bed patient turned on back and placed on bedpan
      b) Ambulatory patient assisted to toilet

B. Retention Enema
   1. Purposes
      a) To soften fecal matter
      b) To give medication to yield local or systemic effect
   2. Solutions used
      a) Oil for fecal softening
      b) Solutions or medications as ordered by physician
   3. Temperature—tepid to warm
   4. Pressure and rate of flow—lower than that of cleansing enema

       a) Avoids an immediate bowel movement
       b) Ensures retention

C. Gastrointestinal Intubations
  1. Purposes
      a) To obtain stomach or duodenal specimen for laboratory analysis
      b) To lavage stomach
      c) To gavage patient
      d) To suction stomach and intestine (decompression)
         (1) Continuous drainage of fluid
         (2) Continuous drainage of gas
      e) Preoperatively, to stabilize intestine to make surgery easier
      f) Preoperatively and prophylactically, to prevent obstruction after abdominal surgery
      g) Postoperatively, to relieve vomiting after abdominal operations
  2. Types
      a) Levine tube
         (1) Is soft-walled tube
         (2) Is used for collection of gastric specimens and for lavage, gavage, and suction
      b) Stomach tube (Ewald)
         (1) Is heavy-walled tube
         (2) Has funnel attached
      c) Duodenal tube (Rehfuss)
         (1) Is rubber tube
         (2) Is used to obtain specimens of duodenal drainage
      d) Cantor tube
         (1) Is 10-foot-long, single-lumen tube
         (2) Is used for intestinal decompression
         (3) Has mercury-weighted rubber bag to help move tube down
         (4) Is radiopaque (location in stomach or intestine can be shown on X ray—helpful in treatment)
      e) Miller-Abbott tube
         (1) Is 10-foot-long, double-lumen tube
         (2) Is used for intestinal decompression
         (3) Has balloon at end to help move tube down
         (4) Is radiopaque
      f) Blakemore-Sengstaken tube
         (1) Nasogastric tube with three lumens
            (a) One lumen is used for irrigation, aspiration, and gavage; runs entire length of tube.
            (b) One lumen inflates balloon beyond cardiac sphincter.
            (c) One lumen inflates elongated balloon proximal to cardiac sphincter.
         (2) Inflated balloon used as tamponade to control esophageal bleeding by compression of veins
  3. Nursing management of intubated patients
      a) Explain treatment and purpose to patient.
      b) Assist physician to intubate.
      c) Be aware that tube is passed to desired length
         (1) Fasten to nose with small amount of tape.
         (2) Connect to suction apparatus.
      d) Give frequent attention to mouth and nose.
      e) Observe patient for signs of dehydration.

        (1)   Dryness of skin and mucous membranes
        (2)   Decreasing urinary output
        (3)   Lethargy
        (4)   Exhaustion
        (5)   Drop in body temperature
     f) Remove tube carefully.
        (1)   Deflate balloon.
        (2)   Withdraw gently.
        (3)   Do not use force.

VIII. Disorders of the Digestive Tract

   A.   Common Disorders
      1.   Esophagitis
      2.   Gastritis
      3.   Enteritis
      4.   Appendicitis
      5.   Colitis
      6.   Stones in duct system (see Figure 16)
      7.   Diverticulitis

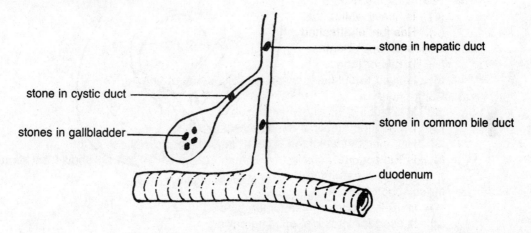

Stones in Duct System

Figure 16

      8.   Ulceration
        a) Peptic ulcer
          (1)   Gastric
          (2)   Duodenal
        b) Ulcerative colitis
      9.   Obstructions (see Figure 17)
        a) Acute (generally small bowel)
          (1)   Intussusception
          (2)   Strangulation
          (3)   Volvulus
          (4)   Foreign bodies
          (5)   Adhesions
          (6)   Tumors

(7) Strictures
(8) Gallstones in intestines
b) Chronic
(1) Stricture
(2) Inflammation
(3) Abscesses
(4) Tumors
(5) Impacted feces

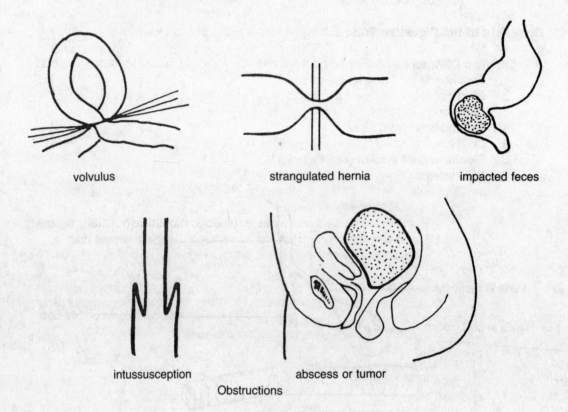

volvulus   strangulated hernia   impacted feces

intussusception   abscess or tumor
                  Obstructions

Figure 17

10. Neoplasms
a) Cancer of oral cavity
b) Cancer of throat
c) Cancer of stomach
d) Cancer of colon
e) Cancer of rectum
11. Degenerative changes

B. Common Symptoms and Signs
1. Pain
2. Bleeding—may be slight or copious
(a) Tarry stools
(b) Hematemesis (coffee-ground color or bright red blood color)
3. Difficulty in swallowing
4. Nausea and/or vomiting
5. Anorexia

6. Flatulence
7. Changes in bowel habits—constipation or diarrhea
8. Jaundice
9. Pruritis ani
10. Inflammation
11. Fever

IX. Specific Disorders of the Digestive Tract

A. Stomatitis
   1. Definition of **stomatitis:** Inflammatory condition of oral mucosa
   2. Causes
      a) Infection caused by pathogenic microorganisms (thrush, Vincent's angina)
      b) Nutritional deficiencies
      c) Excessive exposure to irritants, e.g., smoking
      d) Blood disorders
      e) Systemic infections
      f) Result of chemotherapy for cancer
   3. Treatment and nursing care
      a) Relieving underlying cause
      b) Following specific orders of physician
         (1) Maintain prescribed diet
         (2) Maintain meticulous oral hygiene (specific mouthwash usually ordered).
         (3) Administer topical medications as ordered.
         (4) Administer systemic antibiotics as ordered, e.g., penicillin.

B. Vincent's Angina (Trench Mouth)
   1. Definition of **Vincent's angina:** Ulceration of gums, mucous membrane of mouth, tonsils, and/or pharynx
   2. Cause—infection by spirochete and fusiform bacillus
   3. Assessment
      a) Painful bleeding in area
      b) Pain in swallowing
      c) Mild fever.
      d) Swelling of cervical lymph nodes
   4. Treatment and nursing care
      a) Goals
         (1) Provide for patient's comfort.
         (2) Maintain nutrition.
         (3) Control infection.
         (4) Maintain meticulous oral hygiene.
      b) Nursing care
         (1) Isolation precautions
         (2) Frequent mouth washes with 2% solution sodium perborate or diluted hydrogen peroxide
         (3) Systemic antibiotics, if ordered
         (4) Soft or liquid diet
         (5) Sterilization of dishes and eating utensils
         (6) Patient education

C. Parotitis
   1. Definition of **parotitis:** Acute inflammation of parotid gland; may be mumps caused by a virus or a complication of some systemic disease

2. Causes
   a) Virus (mumps)
   b) Staphylococcus (if focus is elsewhere)
3. Assessment
   a) Pain and tenderness in region of gland
   b) Fever
   c) Difficulty in swallowing
   d) Pain in gland caused by ingestion of sour food (pickles, etc.)
4. Complications
   a) Inflammation of testicles (orchitis)
   b) Occasionally, facial nerve palsy
5. Treatment and nursing care
   a) Meticulous oral hygiene
   b) Ice bag on face
   c) Adequate nutrition
   d) Treatment of systemic conditions

D. Fracture of Mandible
   1. Cause—trauma
   2. Treatment—surgical
      a) Jaws immobilized with mandible fixed to upper jaw
      b) Treated as compound fracture
   3. Nursing care
      a) Observe nasogastric tube carefully if present.
      b) Lubricate lips to prevent cracking.
      c) Maintain good nutrition with soft foods that will not require mastication.
      d) Maintain meticulous oral hygiene.
         (1) Warm mouthwashes
         (2) Careful use of soft toothbrush
      e) Educate patient as to care of mouth.

E. Gastritis
   1. Definition of **gastritis:** Acute or chronic inflammation of the gastric mucous membrane
   2. Assessment
      a) Pain, generally in epigastric region
      b) Nausea
      c) Vomiting, which may relieve symptoms when stomach is empty
      d) Constipation, unless intestine is involved
      e) Abdominal distension
      f) Slight fever
      g) Collapse and prostration depending upon severity
   3. Treatment and nursing care
      a) Bedrest, at first
      b) No solid or semisolid food
      c) Gastric lavage if vomiting has not occurred
      d) Antiemetic drugs (oral or rectal) for nausea as ordered, e.g., tincture of belladonna
      e) Other medications as ordered depending upon cause of gastritis
      f) Rectal tube for relief of abdominal distension
      g) Meticulous oral hygiene
      h) General nursing procedures for promoting patient's comfort
      i) Intravenous fluids as ordered to prevent dehydration

      j) Fluids by mouth as tolerated
          (1) Clear liquid—no residue, nonstimulating, nonirritating
          (2) Full liquid—foods liquefying at room temperature or at body temperature
      k) Bland diet as patient progresses
      l) Careful observation of patient, and reporting and recording of any untoward signs.

F. Peptic Ulcer
    1. Definition of **peptic ulcer:** Erosion of mucous membrane of stomach or duodenum
    2. Assessment
      a) Burning, gnawing pain, generally epigastric or left upper quadrant
      b) Heartburn
      c) Frequent belching
      d) Abdominal distension
      e) Nausea and/or vomiting food or blood
      f) Anorexia
      g) Weight loss
      h) Anemia
    3. Complications
      a) Perforation
      b) Obstruction
      c) Hemorrhage
    4. Causes
      a) Cause may not be specifically known.
      b) There may be hypersecretion of acid gastric juice.
      c) Emotional factors (stress) seem to be a predisposing cause.
    5. Diagnosis
      a) History as to pain and relief related to food intake
      b) Physical examination
      c) Laboratory and X-ray examinations
          (1) CBC—anemia may be present
          (2) Gastric analysis
             (a) Levine tube introduced
             (b) Gastric juice aspirated to test for acidity
      d) X-ray studies
          (1) GI series may show ulcer.
             (a) Ulcer crater is diagnostic for duodenal ulcers (duodenal ulcers almost never undergo malignant change).
             (b) It may be difficult to differentiate between benign and malignant ulcers of stomach.
          (2) Some ulcers are not shown on X ray.
      e) Gastroscopy
          (1) Is useful in differentiating benign from malignant lesions
          (2) May visualize ulcers not seen on X ray
      f) Esophagoscopy—useful in visualizing esophageal ulcers
    6. Treatment and nursing care
      a) Rest and elimination of stress
          (1) Sedatives (phenobarbital may be prescribed)
          (2) Tranquilizers for rest and relaxation (Compazine, Librium)
          (3) Psychotherapy if indicated
      b) Decreasing of gastric hyperacidity and intestinal spasm
          (1) Frequent feedings; Sippy diet; bland diet
          (2) Antacids—calcium carbonate, amphojel, magnesium oxide

c) Depression of gastric acid secretion and prolongation of gastric emptying time—medications usually prescribed are drugs with atropine-like effect (antispasmodics); e.g., tincture of belladonna, methscopolamine, atrophine sulphate, Banthine, Probanthine

d) Attention to tendency toward constipation
   (1) Stool softeners—Colace, Doxinate, Surfak
   (2) Bulk-increasing, mild laxatives—Agorol, Metamucil, Petrogalar

e) Reporting and recording of nature and amount of vomitus

f) Observing, reporting, and recording of symptoms and reactions to diet and medications

g) Weighing of patient periodically, and recording.

h) Diet—liquid or bland diet usually prescribed; dependent upon severity
   (1) Diet is important in healing (nonirritating chemically or mechanically).
   (2) Patient may have hourly feedings of Sippy diet during acute stage.
   (3) Protein supplements are added to in-between meal feedings.

i) Difficulties of this regimen
   (1) Alkalosis due to unsupervised self-medication of alkaline substances
   (2) Formation of renal calculi due to prolonged antacid therapy

7. Complications of peptic ulcer
   a) Hemorrhage from erosion of a blood vessel
      (1) Blood transfusions and gastric decompression may help.
      (2) Surgery may be needed for recurrent or massive hemorrhage.
   b) Perforation
      (1) This complication is more frequent in duodenal than in gastric ulcers.
      (2) It is more frequent in men.
      (3) Perforation is a major surgical emergency.
      (4) Peritonitis may ensue if surgery is delayed.
         (a) There is boardlike abdominal rigidity.
         (b) Abdominal pain is agonizing.
         (c) X rays show air in abdominal cavity if perforation exists.
   c) Obstruction due to pylorospasm and pyloric stenosis
      (1) Obstruction may be partial or complete.
      (2) Vomiting, gastric retention, foul gaseous eructations, and visible peristalsis may be present.
      (3) Condition is diagnosed by X ray.
      (4) Gastric intubation is necessary.
      (5) Surgery is advisable.
   d) Penetration of ulcer and adhesion to liver or pancreas
   e) Malignant change

8. Surgical treatment
   a) Indications that surgery is required
      (1) Ulcer is not responsive to medical treatment.
      (2) Complications (hemorrhage, perforation) must be treated.
      (3) Ulcer has recurred repeatedly.
      (4) There is progressive pyloric obstruction.
      (5) There is evidence or suspicion of malignant change.
   b) Procedures
      (1) Vagotomy
      (2) Subtotal gastrectomy
      (3) Total gastrectomy
      (4) Repair of perforation if present

9. Nursing care after gastric surgery
   a) Goals

(1) Provide relief of pain and discomfort
    (a) Periodic turning to prevent pulmonary and vascular complications; semi-Fowler position to promote gastric tube drainage
    (b) Meticulous oral hygiene and nasal care
    (c) Analgesics as ordered to control pain
    (d) Parenteral antibiotics as ordered
    (e) Maintenance of gastric decompression; observe and report nature and amount of drainage
(2) Assist in adequate nutrition
    (a) Nothing by mouth until ordered
    (b) IV fluids (observe drip rate and patency of tube)
    (c) Oral fluids when bowel sounds return
    (d) Bland diet when ordered; record amount ingested and discomfort if presented
    (e) Vitamin-iron supplementation if ordered
(3) Pay special attention to indwelling tubes (see Section VII. C, gastrointestinal Intubations)
(4) Observe for complications following gastric surgery
    (a) Observe and record vital signs frequently.
    (b) Encourage deep breathing and coughing.
    (c) Inspect dressings and binders frequently.
    (d) Encourage turning and moving frequently.

b) Patient education
  (1) Instruct patient to report any untoward symptoms.
  (2) Strengthen physician's instructions for periodic followup.
  (3) Reinforce dietician's explanations of special dietary requirements.

G. Appendicitis
  1. Definition of **appendicitis:** Bacterial infection of appendix—acute or chronic
  2. Causes
    a) Primary inflammation of appendiceal mucosa
    b) Stenosis or occlusion of lumen of appendix
  3. Assessment
    a) Pain, colicky in nature and gradually increasing in intensity
    b) Chills and fever
    c) Anorexia
    d) Nausea and vomiting
    e) Later, leukocytosis
    f) Rebound tenderness upon examination over McBurney's point, in right flank, or over umbilical region (depends on location of appendix)
    g) Tenderness upon rectal examination with movement of abdominal organs by examining finger
  4. Treatment—appendectomy
  5. Nursing care
    (1) Provide general preoperative nursing care.
    (2) Provide postoperative nursing care, and encourage early ambulation.
    (3) Observe and record any untoward symptoms and/or signs, e.g., elevated temperature, symptoms of infection.

H. Peritonitis
  1. Definition of **peritonitis:** Acute or chronic inflammation of peritoneum
  2. Cause normal bacteria of gastrointestinal tract, e.g., coliform bacillus, streptococcus, staphylococcus, proteus.

        a) Inflammation or perforation of gastrointestinal tract
        b) Traumatic penetration of abdominal wall
        c) Infection from female genital tract
        d) Accidental contamination during abdominal surgery
        e) Blood or lymph dissemination of some organisms

3. Assessment (symptoms depend upon cause and underlying disease)
        a) Severe, constant pain
        b) Intense rigidity of abdominal wall
        c) Shallow respirations
        d) High leukocytosis and pulse
        e) Chills and fever
        f) Anxiety and confusion

4. Treatment and nursing care
        a) Patient care
            (1) Bedrest
            (2) Nothing by mouth
            (3) Control of pain
            (4) Catheterization of bladder
            (5) GI suction by Levine or Miller-Abbott tube
            (6) Administration of IV fluids or blood transfusion
            (7) Accurate record of intake and output
        b) Antibiotic therapy
            (1) Antibiotics are given after samples of peritoneal fluid have been taken for culture and sensitivity.
            (2) Penicillin and streptomycin in combination may be effective.
            (3) Sensitivity tests determine antibiotic to be used.
        c) Removal of focus of infection
            (1) Draining of abscess
            (2) Removal of ruptured appendix
            (3) Removal of strangulated bowel

H. Ulcerative Colitis
1. Definition of **ulcerative colitis:** Chronic, inflammatory, and ulcerative disease of colon
2. Cause—unknown, but disease is more common in nervous, anxious individuals
3. Assessment
        a) Diarrhea containing blood, pus, and mucus
        b) Mild lower abdominal cramps
        c) Marked weight loss and anemia
        d) Possibly, dehydration and malnutrition
        e) High fever, leukocytosis, and tachycardia in some severe cases
4. Treatment and nursing care
        a) Observation and recording of number and character of stools
        b) Rest
        c) High-protein, high-vitamin diet
        d) Antidiarrheal drugs
        e) Surgery, if not responsive to medical treatment
        f) Emotional support

I. Intestinal Obstruction
1. Definition of **intestinal obstruction:** Blockage that results in failure of the intestinal contents to pass through the intestines—may be partial or complete
2. Causes

    a) Mechanical
      (1) Adhesions causing narrowing or closing of the lumen
      (2) Pressure from adjacent tumors
      (3) Impacted feces
      (4) Twisting of the gut (volvulus)
      (5) Telescoping of one part of the intestine into another (intussusception)
    b) Paralytic—paralytic ileus
  3. Assessment
    a) Intermittent, crampy abdominal pain
    b) Vomiting (may be fecal in character)
    c) Abdominal distension
    d) Visible peristalsis
    e) Low serum chlorides, and alkalosis
    f) No passage of gas or feces in some cases
  4. Treatment and nursing care
    a) Patient's anxieties and fears must be allayed.
    b) Necessary diagnostic and therapeutic procedures must be explained to patient.
    c) Abdominal decompression is obtained by use of Miller-Abbott tube.
    d) Continuous suction drainage is provided.
    e) IV fluids are given as ordered.
    f) Parenteral vitamins are given.
    g) Transfusions of whole blood or infusions of protein hydrolysate are given to supply protein requirements.
    h) Types of surgical treatment depends on cause of obstruction.
    i) Careful observation of patient and recording of signs are required.

J. Neoplasms
  1. Type—may be benign or malignant
    a) Tumors of pancreas are generally malignant.
    b) Malignancies of liver are generally metastatic.
  2. Causes
    a) Causes are not generally known
    b) Nonhealing peptic ulcers that do not respond to strict medical regimen are considered malignant.
    c) Stomach tumors are more common in males.
  3. Assessment
    a) Esophagus
      (1) Dysphagia
      (2) Pain, retrosternal or dorsal
    b) Stomach
      (1) Upper abdominal distress, worse after eating
      (2) Epigastric pain
      (3) Anorexia
      (4) Weight loss
      (5) Indigestion
      (6) Hematemesis (coffee-grounds-color vomitus)
      (7) Occult blood in stools or melena
    c) Small intestine
      (1) Intermittent pain
      (2) Melena with anemia
      (3) Weakness
    d) Colon
      (1) Change in bowel habits

      (2) Blood or mucus in stools
      (3) Intermittent cramps in lower abdomen
      (4) Unexplained anemia
  4. Diagnosis
     a) Test for achlorhydria
     b) X-ray examinations
     c) Gastroscopy, proctosigmoidoscopy
     d) Diagnostic cytology studies
  5. Treatment surgical
  6. Nursing care
     a) L.P.N. surgical.
     b) L.P.N. assists R.N. in following physician's preoperative orders.
     c) Routine pre- and postoperative nursing care is given.

K. Hernia
  1. Definition of **hernia:** Protrusion of part of gastrointestinal tract through a defect in muscles of the abdominal wall; may be
     a) Congenital (present at birth)
     b) Acquired
     c) Reducible—gentle pressure on hernia may cause it to be replaced
     d) Incarcerated—hernia cannot be replaced
     e) Strangulated—pressure causes blood supply to part to be cut off and gangrene can result
  2. Types (by location)
     a) Inguinal hernia
     b) Diaphragmatic hernia (hiatus hernia)
     c) Ventral hernia
     d) Umbilical hernia
     e) Incisional hernia
  3. Assessment
     a) Mass in area seen visually or on X ray (hiatus hernia)
     b) Pain
     c) Occasionally, symptoms of obstruction
  4. Treatment for hiatus hernia—medical first and surgical later if no relief

L. Hepatitis
  1. Definition of **hepatitis:** Inflammation of liver
  2. Types
     a) A
     b) B
     c) Non-A, non-B
  3. Causes
     a) Viruses
     b) Bacteria
     c) Toxins
     d) Alcohol
     e) Drugs
  4. Assessment
     a) Fever
     b) Tenderness over region of liver
     c) Jaundice
  5. Treatment and nursing care—varies with cause
     a) Bedrest

    b)   Diet rich in carbohydrate and protein, and restricted in fat
    c)   IV glucose if needed
    d)   Good personal hygiene
    e)   Frequent, small feedings if anorexic

M.   Hepatic Cirrhosis
   1.   Definition of **hepatic cirrhosis:** Chronic disease characterized by rapid growth of connective tissue of liver, thus destroying liver cells
   2.   Two types
      a)   Portal cirrhosis (Laënnec's cirrhosis)
      b)   Biliary cirrhosis
   3.   Causes
      a)   Chronic alcoholism (resulting in malnutrition)
      b)   Chronic poisoning
      c)   Malnutrition
         (1)   Protein deficiency
         (2)   Vitamin B deficiency
   4.   Assessment
      a)   Gastrointestinal symptoms—indigestion, nausea, anorexia, flatulence, occasional vomiting
      b)   Bleeding from esophageal varices
      c)   Melena
      d)   Ascites
      e)   Enlargement of spleen
      f)   Mild jaundice
      g)   Enlargement of liver
      h)   Constipation or diarrhea
      i)   Edema of extremities
      j)   Fever
      k)   Hemorrhagic signs—nosebleeds, petechiae, bleeding gums
      l)   Mental changes—lethargy, stupor, hallucinations, and finally hepatic coma
   5.   Treatment and nursing care
      a)   Maintain nutrition.
         (1)   Report and record when patient refuses to eat.
         (2)   Record accurate intake and output.
         (3)   Maintain meticulous oral hygiene.
            (a)   Prevents stomatitis
            (b)   Prevents parotitis
            (c)   Prevents fetid-odor of breath
         (4)   Administer vitamin supplements as ordered.
      b)   Assemble equipment for paracentesis in ascites.
         (1)   Assist physician by supporting and reassuring patient.
         (2)   Maintain strict asepsis.
         (3)   Encourage patient to void before procedure to prevent injury to bladder.
      c)   Advise patient against alcohol intake.
      d)   Support patient while physician inserts Blakemore-Sengstaken triple-lumen tube to apply hemostasis to esophagus and to decompress stomach.
      e)   Provide skin care to prevent decubitus ulcers.
      f)   Encourage permitted exercise to guard against thrombosis.
      g)   Provide patient education.
         (1)   Encourage patient to cooperate and participate in the treatments.
         (2)   Encourage patient to follow regimen for remainder of life; provide health teaching to family where indicated.

        (3)   Irrigate T-tube at physician's order.

        (4)   Observe and record amount and character of drainage from T-tube.

        (5)   Administer routine pre- and postoperative care.

N.   Cholecystitis
1.   Definition of **cholecystitis:** Inflammation of gallbladder—acute or chronic
2.   Causes
    a)   Are not generally known
    b)   May be chemical irritation or stones
3.   Assessment
    a)   Frequent indigestion
    b)   Knifelike pain radiating to scapula from right upper quadrant
    c)   Palpable gallbladder
    d)   Fever
    e)   Jaundice
    f)   Nausea and vomiting
4.   Treatment and nursing care
    a)   Medical nursing
        (1)   Maintain bedrest
        (2)   Observe nothing-by-mouth precautions.
        (3)   Observe amount and character of drainage if continuous gastric suction is in progress.
        (4)   Record intake and output accurately in order to assist physician to maintain fluid and electrolyte balance.
        (5)   Administer antibiotics as ordered.
        (6)   Administer analgesics and antispasmodics as ordered.
        (7)   Observe and record any untoward symptoms.
        (8)   Make patient as comfortable as possible, physically and mentally.
    b)   Surgical intervention (cholecystectomy) if required
        (1)   In severe attack
        (2)   In cases where stone obstructs ducts

O.   Pancreatitis
1.   Definition of **pancreatitis:** Inflammation of the pancreas—acute or chronic
2.   Causes
    a)   Gallbladder infection
    b)   Obstruction
    c)   Alcoholism
    d)   Metabolic disturbances
    e)   Trauma
3.   Assessment
    a)   Pain in area
    b)   Moderate fever
    c)   Nausea and vomiting
    d)   Constipation
    e)   Shock and circulatory collapse
4.   Treatment and nursing care
    a)   Control of pain with meperidine (Demerol); observe precautions in administration of narcotics
    b)   Blood and/or plasma for shock
    c)   Nothing by mouth
    d)   Support of nutrition and electrolytes
    e)   Observation and recording of symptoms

      f) Observation and recording of suction aspirations if used

      g) Close observation of IV infusions

      h) If surgery, routine pre- and postoperative nursing care

P. Anorectal Disorders
1. Types
    a) Anorectal abscess
    b) Proctitis
    c) Fistula-in-ano
    d) Anal fissure
    e) Hemorrhoids (piles)
    f) Pruritus ani
    g) Rectal prolapse
2. Causes
    a) Localized disorders
    b) Secondary occurrence to more serious intestinal disease
3. Treatment and nursing care
    a) Recognition and removal of cause
    b) Reduction of inflammation and pain
      (1) Application of heat
        (a) Sitz baths, 4-6 times daily
        (b) Hot soaks
      (2) Application of medications
        (a) Creams and ointments
        (b) Suppositories
        (c) Topical anesthetics
    c) Prevention of hard and/or frequent bowel movements
      (1) Dietary measures
        (a) Low-residue foods
        (b) Prohibition of iced drinks
        (c) Avoidance of eating between meals
      (2) Measures to decrease frequency of bowel movements
      (3) Medications to maintain a soft stool
    d) Promotion of necessary rest
      (1) Pain relief
      (2) Reduction in bowel activity
      (3) Facilitation of treatment
    e) Specific medical and/or surgical treatment
    f) Anesthesia of region when necessary

Q. Congenital Disorders
1. Harelip
2. Cleft palate
3. Esophageal atresia
4. Rectal atresia

UNIT 7: THE URINARY SYSTEM

VOCABULARY

anuria	urinary suppression (less than 100 ml in 24 hours)
bacteriuria	bacteria in urine
cystitis	inflammation of bladder

dysuria	painful urination
-ectomy	refers to cutting out
nephritis	inflammation of kidney (Bright's disease)
nephro-	pertaining to kidney
nocturia	excessive urination at night
oliguria	diminished urination (between 100 and 400 ml in 24 hours)
-otomy	refers to cutting into
polyuria	frequent urination (excessive secretion)
pyuria	pus in urine
-sclerosis	hard, stonelike
suppression	complete failure of urinary excretion due to renal conditions
retention	failure to expel urine from bladder
uremia	toxic condition caused by urinary waste products in blood, result of disturbed kidney function
urethritis	inflammation of urethra

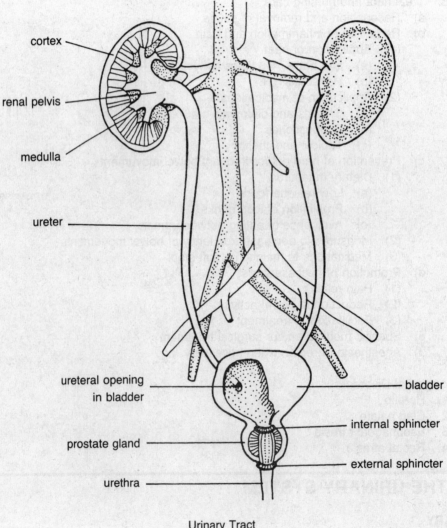

Urinary Tract

Figure 18

NURSING CARE OF THE ADULT PATIENT

I. Structure and Functions

A. Kidneys (see Figures 18 and 19)
  1. Two bilateral bean-shaped organs in region of twelfth rib
  2. Act as excretory glands
    a) Excrete waste such as urea and uric acid
    b) Have cortex—outer layer
    c) Have medulla—inner layer
      (1) Renal tubules—essential renal unit
      (2) Nephron—functional unit
  3. Are important in maintaining water and salt balance, tonicity, volume, and acid-base balance of body fluids
    a) Excrete salts, i.e., regulate amount of sodium and potassium in the blood
    b) Excrete acids or bases to regulate acid-base balance
    c) Absorb excessive amount of certain filtered substances such as glucose, water, and salts
    d) Excrete about 1200-1500 cc urine every 24 hours

B. Ureters
  1. Extend from kidney to urinary bladder
  2. Drain urine from kidney to urinary bladder

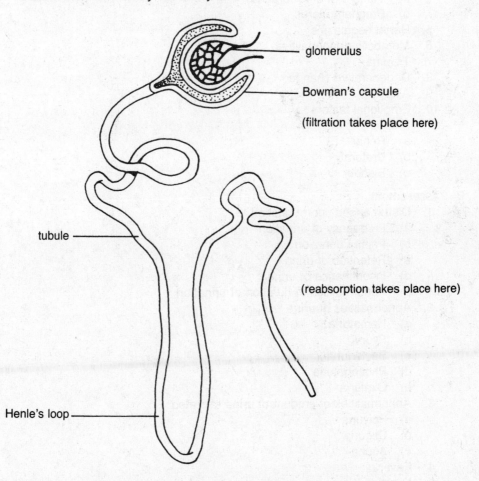

glomerulus

Bowman's capsule

(filtration takes place here)

tubule

(reabsorption takes place here)

Henle's loop

Figure 19

C. Urinary Bladder
1. Is large, muscular, distensible, hollow organ
2. Acts as reservoir for urine
3. Has normal capacity of about 500 cc in adult

D. Urethra
1. Extends from bladder to outside of body
2. Acts as passageway for urine from bladder to outside
3. Is 1–2 inches long in female and 6–8 inches long in male
4. Has opening to outside called *urinary meatus*
    a) In male, located at end of penis
    b) In female, located between vagina and clitoris
5. Is intimately connected to genital system in male

II. Disorders of the Urinary System

A. Causes
1. Congenital conditions
2. Abnormalities in vascular system, such as arterial obstruction
3. Infections caused by bacteria, e.g., streptococcus, tuberculosis
4. Intra-abdominal pressure caused by
    a) Tumors of other organs
    b) Pregnant uterus
5. Renal neoplasms
6. Metabolic abnormalities
7. Trauma
8. Degenerative change
9. Allergy
10. Emotional factors
11. Stones
    a) Renal
    b) Ureteral
    c) Bladder

B. Assessment
1. Disturbances upon urination
    a) Frequency of urination
    b) Painful urination
    c) Retention of urine
    d) Incontinence of urine
    e) Abnormalities in duration of urination
2. Abnormalities of urine
    a) Hematuria
    b) Pyuria
    c) Bacteriuria
    d) Phosphaturia
    e) Oxaluria
3. Abnormalities of amount of urine secreted
    a) Polyuria
    b) Oliguria
    c) Anuria
4. Fever
5. Uremia
6. Pain

NURSING CARE OF THE ADULT PATIENT

C. Nursing Care
    1. Understand nature of patient's urinary disturbance.
    2. Carefully observe patient during intravenous therapy.
        a) Record type and amount of fluid received.
        b) Record output.
    3. Prepare patient for catheterization (observe sterile procedure precautions while assembling equipment).
    4. Observe skin.
        a) Care to relieve itching.
        b) Frequent position changes to prevent decubiti.
        c) Protection of edematous parts of body.
    5. Observe and care for mouth.
    6. Observe breath odor.
    7. Observe and record vital signs (many renal disturbances are accompanied by hypertension).
    8. Become familiar with various procedures and equipment needed.
    9. Give general nursing care of symptoms.
    10. Report any change to R.N.

III. Diagnostic Tests and Procedures

A. Evaluation of Renal Function
    1. Routine urinalysis—usually first test done (see Data Summary 12)
        a) Preparation
            (1) Voided specimen should be collected in clean vessel after surrounding urethral area is cleansed.
            (2) Catheterized specimen may be collected if necessary.
            (3) Urine is taken immediately to laboratory.
        b) Laboratory examinations
            (1) Gross examination
                (a) Color and appearance—normal urine generally pale yellow and clear
                (b) Reaction—normal pH 4.6-8 (depending on diet)
                (c) Odor—of value only in fresh urine
                (d) Specific gravity—normal 1.015-1.030; demonstrates how the tubules are concentrating the urine.
                (e) Low or high concentration—may be symptomatic
                    i)   Low—large fluid intake; low salt intake; chronic nephritis; diabetes insipidus; primary aldosteronism
                    ii) High—diabetes mellitus; dehydration; sweating; acute glomerulonephritis; vomiting
            (2) Chemical examinations to determine abnormal substances
                (a) Protein
                (b) Sugar
                (c) Acetone
            (3) Microscopic examination to help describe disease of upper and lower urinary tracts
                (a) Casts indicate disease of tubules.
                (b) Calculi may come from ureter, bladder, or kidney.
                (c) Blood indicates inflammation, injury, or tumor.
                (d) Bacteria indicates infection.
                (e) Pus indicates infection or inflammation.

DATA SUMMARY 12
Characteristics of Normal Urine

Amount in 24 hours	1200–1500 ml
Color	Yellow (light to deep)
Specific gravity	1.015–1.030
pH	Slightly acid
Albumin	0
Glucose	0
Acetone	0

---

2. Blood chemistry studies
   a) Kidney function is evaluated by laboratory analysis of blood.
   b) Urea, nitrogen, and creatinine are generally done.
3. Concentration and dilution tests
   a) Measure ability of tubules to concentrate urine
   b) Are not necessary if specific gravity of urine is 1.025 or higher

B. X-ray Studies
   1. Intravenous pyelogram (IVP)
      a) IVP is contraindicated if patient has sensitivity to iodine.
      b) Intravenous injection of a special dye allows kidneys to be visualized by X-ray machine.
      c) Preparation is as follows:
         (1) Cathartic is administered night before.
         (2) Patient fasts after midnight until X rays are taken.
   2. Retrograde pyelogram
      a) Assesses degree, type, cause, and length of obstruction
      b) Is used when patient is allergic to IV radiopaque chemicals
      c) Allows detailed examination of pelvocalyceal collecting system, ureters, and urinary bladder
   3. Ultrasound
      a) Is noninvasive and innocuous technique
      b) Is useful in fetal and neonate examinations
   4. CAT
      a) Is useful in evaluating extent of renal masses
      b) Shows extrarenal involvement by tumor
   5. MRI
      a) Is useful when other imaging techniques fail
      b) Is useful in early transplant rejection
      c) Can distinguish between hemorrhage and infection in cyst fluid

C. Nuclear Radiography
   1. Radioactive renogram
      a) Dye containing radioactive iodine is injected intravenously.
      b) Urine specimen is scanned with Geiger counter to compute amount of dye excreted.
      c) Individual kidneys can be tested by withdrawing urine from **ureters**.
   2. Renal scan
      a) Isotopes are injected intravenously.
      b) Radioactivity in various parts of kidney is recorded.

D. Cystoscopy
    1. Direct method of bladder visualization and study by urologist
    2. Disinfection of cystoscope by use of ethylene oxide
    3. Patient preparation
        a) Explanation of procedure
        b) Administration of sedative if ordered by physician
        c) Either local bladder anesthetic, spinal anesthetic, or general anesthesia
        d) Complete aseptic technique
    4. Postcystoscopy nursing care
        a) Bedrest
        b) Sedatives if necessary and as ordered by physician
        c) Application of hot water bag to abdomen
        d) Liberal intake of fluids
        e) In cases of urinary retention, hot sitz baths and administration of bladder relaxants

E. Culture and Sensitivity of Urine
    1. Culture
        a) Laboratory examination serves to identify microorganisms in urine.
        b) Specimen may be collected by catheterization or by clean catch into sterile vessel.
    2. Sensitivity—laboratory procedure to detect which antibiotics would be bacteriocidal to organisms grown on urine culture

IV. Important Nursing Procedures

A. General Principles
    1. Carefully record fluid intake and output.
    2. Observe and record changes in urinary output.
    3. Record daily weight.
    4. Insert and care for retention catheter, which should allow urine to flow freely.
        a) Observe urethral opening for irritation, and give appropriate meatal care.
        b) Check to see that catheter is in securely.
        c) Periodically sterilize or replace catheter and drainage apparatus.
        d) Measure fluid drained at regular intervals; cup collection begins below level of kidneys and off floor.
        e) Periodically irrigate catheter.
    5. Provide care of dressed wounds.
        a) Change dressing frequently.
        b) Protect skin by appropriate care.
        c) Keep dry and free from urinary odor.
    6. Give skin-care instruction for patient using ileal bag.
        a) Use sterile technique.
        b) Observe output, changes in quality, and amount.
        c) Irrigate as ordered.
        d) Inspect area around catheter once daily.
    7. Monitor special diet as ordered by physician.
    8. Observe for symptoms of infection.
        a) Chills and fever
        b) Nausea and/or vomiting
    9. Observe for symptoms of uremia.
        a) Drowsiness
        b) Headaches

    c) Sleeplessness
    d) Nausea and vomiting
    e) Twitchings, spasms, and convulsive seizures
    f) Decrease in urinary output
       (1) Retention of metabolites
       (2) Low PSP excretion

V. Specific Genitourinary Disorders

A. Inflammations of Urinary Tract
  1. Cystitis
    a) Definition of **cystitis:** Inflammation of urinary bladder
    b) Causes
       (1) Infection
       (2) Drugs
       (3) Irrigating solutions
    c) Assessment
       (1) Pain and burning on urination
       (2) Frequency
       (3) Urgency
       (4) Hematuria
       (5) Pus and red blood cells, visible on microscopic examination of urine
    d) Nursing care
       (1) Follow orders of physician in giving drugs.
       (2) Increase fluid intake of patient.
       (3) Reassure patient in regard to color changes in urine if dyes are given.
       (4) Instruct patient about diet (no spicy foods).
       (5) Record intake and output.
  2. Pyelonephritis
    a) Definition of **pyelonephritis:** Inflammation of kidney substance and pelvis; often mistaken for glomerulonephritis
    b) Cause—infection, which may come from a distant point in body
       (1) Hematogenous route—bacteria reach kidney by bloodstream
       (2) Ascending route—bacteria spread from bladder, ureter, and renal pelvis
    c) Assessment
       (1) Fever, general malaise, headache
       (2) Dysuria and frequency
       (3) Pain in kidney region
       (4) Leukocytosis
       (5) Hematuria, pyuria, and bacteriuria
    d) Nursing care
       (1) Give medications as ordered by physician.
       (2) Maintain bedrest.
       (3) Force fluids.
       (4) Take frequent urine specimens to laboratory for diagnosis.
       (5) Observe and record vital signs.
  3. Glomerulonephritis
    a) Definition of **glomerulonephritis:** Inflammation of the glomerulus (network of blood capillaries) of the kidneys
    b) Causes
       (1) Frequently follows a streptococcus infection of respiratory system
       (2) May be a complication of scarlet fever
       (3) May occur with no recent history of infection

    c) Assessment
      (1) Decrease in amount of urine (oliguria)
      (2) Hematuria
      (3) Edema
      (4) Headaches, poor appetite, and weakness
      (5) Sometimes, high blood pressure
      (6) Abnormal urinalysis and elevated BUN
    d) Nursing care
      (1) Maintain bedrest until symptoms have subsided.
      (2) Protect patient from chills.
      (3) Isolate patient from people with respiratory infections.
      (4) Give special diet, low in protein and salt.
      (5) Restrict fluids.
      (6) Accurately record intake and output.
      (7) Accurately record daily weight.
      (8) Observe patient's condition and vital signs carefully, and note any appearance of mental confusion or drowsiness.
      (9) Accurately record blood pressure at stated intervals.
     (10) Follow physician's orders carefully.
  4. Nephrotic syndrome (nephrosis)
    a) Cause unknown
    b) Assessment
      (1) Edema
      (2) Albuminuria
      (3) Hypoproteinemia
      (4) Hyperlipemia
    c) Outcome—patient may develop complications or kidney failure, or may recover

B. Obstructions
  1. Renal stones—may be ureteral or bladder stones
    a) Small, sandlike stones are generally passed in urine.
    b) Large stones cause severe colic.
    c) Fluids should be increased to 300 ml per day, and intake and output recorded.
    d) All urine must be strained, and bedpans and urinals inspected.
    e) Surgery may be necessary.
  2. Neoplasms
    a) Tumors may be benign or malignant.
    b) Tumors occur chiefly in the bladder and the kidney.
    c) Wilms tumor occurs in young children.
    d) Treatment is generally surgical.

C. Trauma
  1. Stab wounds
  2. Gunshot wounds
  3. Crushing injuries

D. Uremia
  1. Definition or **uremia:** Retention of excessive by-products of protein metabolism in the blood and the toxic condition produced thereby
  2. Types
    a) May be acute due to sudden injury to large number of tubules
    b) May be chronic due to replacement of most of kidney tissue by fibrous tissue
  3. Symptoms

        a) Nausea
        b) Vomiting
        c) Lethargy
    4. Specific nursing care—should be immediate
        a) Accurately observe, record, and report signs.
        b) Maintain alkaline reserve by administration of sodium chloride if ordered by physician.
        c) Encourage fluids.
        d) Carefully record intake and output.
        e) Protect against infections.
        f) Observe and report cerebral irritation.
        g) Protect patient against self-injury.
        h) Record onset of convulsions, duration, extent, and general effect.
        i) Institute suitable therapy as ordered by physician.
        j) Prepare for injections of magnesium sulfate.
        k) Prepare setup for lumbar puncture if ordered.

VI. Drug Therapy for Urinary Disorders

  A. Diuretics
    1. These drugs increase flow of urine.
    2. They reduce edema by decreasing water from tissues.
    3. Different diuretics act in different ways.
        a) Water
        b) Acid-forming salts (ammonium chloride)
        c) Xanthine diuretics (not in much use now)
            (1) Caffeine
            (2) Theophylline
        d) Mercurial diuretics
            (1) Action on kidney tubule
            (2) Example—Mercuhydrin
            (3) Side effects—renal damage, mercury poisoning
        e) Thiazide diuretics
            (1) Action—on kidney tubule
            (2) Examples—Diuril, Hydrodiuril
            (3) Side effects—acidosis, muscle cramps, dizziness, weakness, nausea
        f) Carbonic anhydrase inhibitors
            (1) Action—on kidney tubule; they decrease formation of aqueous humor (important in glaucoma and other eye diseases)
            (2) Example—Diamox
            (3) Side effects—acidosis, numbness of skin, drowsiness
        g) Sulfonamide diuretics—Lasix (furosemide)

  B. Urinary Antiinfectives (Urinary Antiseptics)
    1. Azo dyes
        a) Use—more for relief of symptoms
        b) Action—acidify urine and thus are antibacterial
        c) Examples—Mandelamine (effective in acid urine), Pyridium (acts also as local anesthetic)
    2. Sulfonamides
        a) Use—mostly against gram-negative organisms
        b) Examples—Gantrisin, Gantanol
        c) Side effects—nausea, renal disturbances, blood dyscrasia

NURSING CARE OF THE ADULT PATIENT

      3. Antiinfectives
         a) Antibiotics—specific according to culture/sensitivity tests
         b) Chemotherapeutics—sulfonamides

  C. Antispasmodics—belladonna-like Drugs
      1. Action—relax spastic bladder
      2. Examples—belladonna, Donnatal, Urecholine

  D. Analgesics
      1. Drugs chosen by physician according to condition
      2. Examples—aspirin, opium derivatives

VII. Surgical Intervention

  A. Purposes
      1. To remove a kidney (nephrectomy)
         a) Neoplasm
         b) Large calculus
      2. To incise a ureter (ureterotomy)
         a) To correct stricture
         b) To remove calculus
         c) To repair injury
      3. To remove a bladder (cystectomy)
         a) Ureters are transplanted.
         b) Usual reason is malignancy.
      4. To incise bladder
         a) Done in suprapubic prostatectomy
         b) Done to remove neoplasm or calculus
      5. To repair uretheral stricture
         a) May be congenital
         b) May be of infectious origin
         c) May be residual of prior surgery or manipulation

VIII. Dialysis

  A. Types
      1. Acute dialysis, used for acute reversible conditions that cause acute renal failure
         a) To maintain acid-base equilibrium of blood
         b) To gain time for acute conditions to heal
      2. Chronic dialysis, used to
         a) Extend life of patients in whom renal function cannot be improved
         b) Prepare selective patients for kidney transplants
      3. Peritoneal dialysis
         a) Blood is filtered through sterile peritoneal fluid to remove wastes.
         b) Complete dialysis requires 36 hours.
      4. Hemodialysis, used in chronic kidney failure
         a) Poisons are removed from blood by diffusion.
         b) Machine outside of body is known as artificial kidney.
         c) Artificial kidney works on same principles as normal functioning kidney.
         d) Special diet is needed to keep waste products at low level.
         e) Hemodialysis may be home or clinic procedure if several treatments per week are needed.

B. Nursing Management in Peritoneal Dialysis
1. Explain procedure to patient, and make him/her comfortable.
2. Weigh patient before dialysis and daily.
3. Take vital signs before dialysis.
4. Take blood pressure and vital signs at stated intervals.
5. Observe patient for respiratory difficulty, severe pain, hemorrhage, shock.
6. Maintain accurate records of procedure and administration of drugs.

UNIT 8: THE ENDOCRINE SYSTEM

VOCABULARY

basal metabolism	energy consumption of body at complete rest
BMR	basal metabolic rate; measurement of metabolic rate of body at complete rest (in terms of calories produced)
cortisone	hormone from cortex of adrenal gland
ductless	having no duct, secreting only internally
dysphagia	inability to swallow
electrolyte	chemical substance that conducts electricity when it is dissolved or melted
exophthalmos	abnormal bulging of eyeball caused by dysfunction of thyroid gland
gland	secreting organ
hormone	secretion of ductless glands; chemical substance secreted by an organ, and conveyed through blood to another part of body, stimulating it to increased activity or secretion
polydipsia	excessive thirst
polyuria	excessive secretion and discharge of urine
secretion	product resulting from activity of gland; can be internal or external

I. **Types, Characteristics, and Functions of Endocrine Glands**

    A. Types and Characteristics
       1. Types
         a) Ductless glands
         b) Glands of internal secretion
           (1) Secretions are poured directly into bloodstream.
           (2) Internal secretions contain active principles (hormones) that regulate body functions.
       2. Characteristics
         a) Nine in number
           (1) Thyroid
           (2) Parathyroids—4
           (3) Adrenal (suprarenal)—2
           (4) Pituitary (master gland)
           (5) Thymus
           (6) Pineal
           (7) Testes—2
           (8) Ovaries—2
           (9) Islands of Langerhans
         b) Interrelated
           (1) Action of secretion of one has influence on actions of other glands.
           (2) Secretions are carried by blood.
         c) Abnormal if either overactive or underactive

    B. Functions—*see* Data Summary 13

DATA SUMMARY 13 Functions of the Endocrine Glands		
Gland	Secretion	Function
PITUITARY		
Anterior lobe	Thyrotrophic hormone	Stimulates thyroid gland
	Somatotrophic hormone	Stimulates growth
	Gonadotrophic hormones	Affect growth, maturity, and functioning of primary and secondary sex organs
	Adrenocorticotrophic hormone (ACTH)	Stimulates cortex of adrenal glands
Posterior lobe	Antidiuretic hormone (ADH)	Decreases production of urine
	Oxytocic principle	Stimulates uterine contractions
THYROID	Thyroxine	Stimulates metabolism
PARATHYROIDS	Parathormone	Regulate calcium level in body fluids
ADRENAL		
Cortex	Three main groups of hormones:	
	Glucocorticoids	Tend to increase amount of sugar in blood
	Mineralocorticoids	Tend to increase amount of blood sodium and decrease amount of potassium in blood
	Androgens (male hormones)	Govern certain secondary sex characteristics
		All corticoids important for defense against stress or injury to body tissues—reduce efficiency of body defense mechanisms and should be used judiciously.
Medulla	Epinephrine (adrenaline)	Elevates blood pressure
		Converts glycogen to glucose when needed by muscles for energy
		Increases heartbeat rate
		Dilates bronchioles
THYMUS		Prevents autoimmunity
OVARIES	Estrogen and progesterone	Stimulate development of secondary sex characteristics
		Prepare endometrium for implantation of fertilized ovum
		Effect repair of endometrium after menstruation
TESTES	Testosterone	Is essential for normal functioning of male reproductive organs
		Stimulates development of male secondary sex characteristics
ISLANDS OF LANGERHANS (pancreas)	Insulin	Promotes metabolism of carbohydrates

NURSING CARE OF THE ADULT PATIENT

II. **Thyroid**

   A. Structure and Function
     1. Is composed of two lateral lobes joined by transverse isthmus
     2. Is situated over larynx and trachea
     3. Is covered by capsule and infrahyoid muscles
     4. Secretes thyroxine, which influences BMR
     5. Needs iodine to form thyroxine (without it an abnormal colloid fills follicles of gland)

   B. Diagnostic Tests
     1. Laboratory examinations
       a) CBC
       b) Sedimentation rate
       c) BMR
         (1) BMR measures metabolism at complete rest.
         (2) Normal value is −20 to +20.
         (3) Value is decreased in hypothyroidism and increased in hyperthyroidism.
       d) Blood cholesterol
       e) PBI
         (1) PBI measures amount of protein-bound iodine in blood.
         (2) Normal value is 4-8 μg.
         (3) Value is decreased in hypothyroidism and increased in hyperthyroidism.
       f) ^{131}I uptake
       g) TSH stimulation test
     2. X-ray studies
       a) Chest films
       b) Bone-age films
       c) Barium swallow to show substernal goiter
     3. Physical examination—important to correlate thyroid function with clinical findings

   C. Disorders of the Thyroid
     1. Simple goiter
       a) Enlargement of gland
       b) No increase in thyroxine
       c) Cause—a decrease in iodine intake
       d) Assessment
         (1) Enlargement of gland
         (2) Dysphagia
       e) Treatment
         (1) Administration of iodine in either diet or medications
         (2) Removal of gland may be necessary if dyspnea and dysphagia present
     2. Hypothyroidism (cretinism in children, myxedema in adults)
       a) Assessment
         (1) Retardation, both mental and physical, in children
         (2) Lethargy
         (3) Excessive weight gain
       b) Treatment—thyroid extract
     3. Hyperthyroidism (Graves's disease, toxic goiter)
       a) Assessment
         (1) Extreme nervousness
         (2) Weight loss
         (3) Excessive appetite
         (4) Increase in metabolism

          (5)   Emotional disorders
          (6)   Exophthalmos
          (7)   Sensitivity to heat
     b) Treatment—reduce thyroid activity
          (1)   Propylthiouracil
          (2)   Iodine
          (3)   Thyroidectomy if medical treatment fails
          (4)   High-calorie diet (high in carbohydrate and protein)
     c) Postoperative nursing care
          (1)   Support head, neck, and shoulders with pillows.
          (2)   Place patient in semi-Fowler's position.
          (3)   Carefully observe for vital signs, swelling, edema, and tremors.
          (4)   Administer humidified oxygen if breathing labored.
          (5)   Check dressing for pressure.
          (6)   Check back of neck for bleeding.
          (7)   Keep tracheostomy set at bedside and have suction equipment available.
     d) Postoperative complications
          (1)   Respiratory distress
          (2)   Change of voice quality and/or loss of voice
          (3)   Tetany (parathyroids may have been removed); note reflexes
          (4)   Hoarseness (may be due to laryngeal edema)
          (5)   Thyroid crisis

III. Parathyroids

  A. Structure and Function
     1. There are four glands, embedded in capsule of thyroid.
     2. Hormone regulates use of calcium in body.

  B. Disorders of the Parathyroids
     1. Hyperparathyroidism
        a) Definition of **hyperparathyroidism:** Excessive secretion of parathyroid hormone; depletion of calcium from bones yields spontaneous fractures and/or kidney stones
        b) Treatment—surgical removal of all but one of the glands
     2. Hypoparathyroidism
        a) Definition of **hypoparathyroidism:** Underactivity of the parathyroid glands, causing a lowering of calcium levels in the blood
        b) Assessment—tetany and/or muscular spasms
        c) Treatment—administration of vitamin D and calcium

IV. Adrenal Glands

  A. Structure and Function
     1. A gland is situated at apex of each kidney.
     2. The gland is essentially a double organ.
        a) Cortex secretes corticoid hormones (steroids).
        b) Medulla secretes epinephrine (adrenaline).

  B. Disorders of Adrenal Glands
     1. Addison's disease
        a) Cause—underactivity of adrenal cortex due to
          (1)   Infection

        (2) Tumor
        (3) Inflammation
        (4) Drug therapy suppressing gland
     b) Assessment
        (1) Fatigue
        (2) Weight loss
        (3) Nausea and vomiting
        (4) Dehydration
        (5) Circulatory failure
     c) Treatment—cortisone on lifetime basis
  2. Cushing's syndrome
     a) Cause—increase in production of hormones from adrenal cortex
     b) Assessment
        (1) "Moon face"
        (2) Occasional mental disturbances
        (3) Abnormal sexual development, e.g., hirsutism
        (4) Weight gain
     c) Treatment
        (1) Adjustment of electrolytes
        (2) Low-sodium, high-potassium diet
        (3) Treatment of depression

V. Pituitary (Master) Gland

  A. Structure
    1. Located on underside of brain
    2. Divided into three lobes
     a) Anterior
     b) Intermediate
     c) Posterior

  B. Function
    1. Anterior lobe—six hormones
     a) Adrenocorticotrophic (ACTH)
        (1) Regulates adrenal activity
        (2) Increases excretion of nitrogen, potassium, phosphorus, and uric acid
        (3) Increases retention of sodium, chloride, and water
        (4) Elevates blood sugar
        (5) Lowers serum cholesterol
        (6) Is used in treatment of Addison's disease and others
     b) Growth hormone
        (1) Excess causes gigantism.
        (2) Deficiency causes dwarfism.
     c) Thyrotrophic hormone—regulates thyroid gland
     d) Two gonadotrophic hormones
        (1) Stimulate growth of ovarian follicles (FSH)
        (2) Promote growth of corpus luteum (LH)
     e) Lactogenic hormone—stimulates lactation in postpartum women
    2. Intermediate lobe—important in pigment metabolism
    3. Posterior lobe
     a) Vasopressin (pitressin)
        (1) Regulates blood pressure
        (2) Decreases water excretion (antidiuretic hormone)

      b) Oxytocin—causes smooth muscle contractions
         (1) Stimulates contractions in walls of milk ducts in lactating women
         (2) Stimulates contractions of muscles of uterus
         (3) Induces labor in obstetrical patients
     c) Disorders of the Pituitary Gland
        1. Gigantism
        2. Acromegaly
        3. Hypertension
        4. Diabetes insipidus

VI. Islands of Langerhans

A. Structure and Function
    1. The endocrine gland consists of small, interlobular masses in the pancreas.
    2. Beta cells secrete insulin, which regulates carbohydrate metabolism.

B. Diabetes Mellitus
    1. Definition of **diabetes mellitus:** Complex and chronic disorder of metabolism
    2. Cause—insufficient production of insulin by beta cells in Islands of Langerhans results in disturbance in carbohydrate metabolism.
    2. Diagnostic tests
       a) Urinalysis—glucose spills over into urine from blood when blood glucose level is high
       b) Blood glucose—normal value is 80–120 mg/100 ml
       c) Glucose tolerance
         (1) Large amounts of glucose are given to a fasting patient at regular intervals.
         (2) Thereafter blood glucose levels are measured to determine how long it takes the body to handle the extra glucose.
         (3) If glucose remains in blood for excessive period of time, it is an indication of disorder in carbohydrate metabolism.
         (4) The test is valuable in calculating diet and amount of insulin needed.
         (5) Two-hour postprandial test is a modification.
    3. Assessment
       a) Polyuria
       b) Polydipsia
       c) Polyphagia
       d) Disturbances in vision
       e) Elevation of blood glucose
       f) Glycosuria
    4. Treatment—combination of diet, exercise, insulin or oral hypoglycemics, and education to
       a) Keep diabetes under control
       b) Prevent the complications of diabetes
    5. Nursing care
       a) Give special skin care.
       b) Provide general hygienic care.
       c) Administer insulin (see Data Summaries 2, 14, and 15).
       d) Report any untoward symptoms immediately.
       e) Collect, test, and record urinary specimens.
       f) Guard against complications—hypoglycemia, hyperglycemia.
       g) Serve prescribed diet and observe patient intake.
       h) Assist in teaching patient personal hygiene care.
       i) Assist in educating patient concerning disease.

6. Diet
   a) Diet is the most important factor in treatment (may be only therapy).
   b) Caloric values of foods are important
   c) Weighing and measuring of diet are necessary in some cases.
7. Complications of diabetes mellitus
   a) Diabetic coma (diabetic acidosis)
   b) Circulatory disturbances, such as arteriosclerosis, which may lead to gangrene
   c) Deterioration of vision; retinitis common
   d) Affections of peripheral nerves (polyneuritis)
   e) Infections—meticulous care of skin is essential
   f) Insulin reactions
8. Prevention of complications
   a) Good nutrition
   b) Immediate treatment of glycosuria
   c) Freedom from hypoglycemic reactions
   d) Freedom from diabetic acidosis by careful observation and immediate treatment
   e) Periodic ophthalmic examinations and examinations of arterial system
   f) Assist patient in blood glucose monitoring

	DATA SUMMARY 14 Characteristics of Oral Hypoglycemic Agents			
Name	Size of Tablet or Capsule (mg)	Daily Dosage Range (mg)	Duration of Action (hours)	Frequency of Administration
Sulfonylureas				
Orinase	500	500–3000	6–10 (short)	Usually divided doses, 1–3 times daily
Diabinese	100 250	100–500	20–60 (prolonged)	Single dose
Dymelor	250 500	250–1500	10–16 (medium)	Single or divided doses
Tolinase	100 250	100–1000	10–16 (medium)	Single or divided doses
Biquanides				
DBI	25	25–50	6–7 (short)	Divided doses
DBI–TD	50 100	50–200	12–14 (medium)	Divided doses

DATA SUMMARY 15
Differences between Diabetic Coma and Insulin Reaction

Factor	Diabetic Coma (Acidosis)	Insulin Reaction (Shock)
Onset	Gradual; may be rapid in children	Sudden
Skin	Hot and dry	Cold and clammy
Respiration	Labored	Shallow
Appetite	Nausea	Hunger
Vision	No change	Double vision
State of con-sciousness	Loss (late)	Loss
Urine	Heavily positive for glucose	Generally negative
Blood sugar	High	Low

Emergency treatment for insulin reaction (shock):
1. Immediate treatment (warning symptoms appear):
   a. patient should take a drink containing sugar or eat a candy bar.
   b. carbohydrates stop this reaction within a few minutes.
2. Unconscious patient:
   a. patient should be given an intravenous injection of glucose.
   b. subcutaneous injection of epinephrine 1:1000 in a dose of 0.5 cc may restore patient to level of consciousness to enable him/her to take a drink of orange juice or of sweetened water.

VII. Gonads

A. Testes (primary male sex organs—male gonads)
   1. Location—in scrotal sac
   2. Functions
      a) Secrete hormone called testosterone
      b) Produce spermatozoa
      c) Secrete seminal fluid

B. Ovaries (primary female sex organs—female gonads)
   1. Two parts—cortex and medulla
   2. Location—in pelvis
   3. Functions
      a) Secretion of estrogen from follicles
         (1) Is primary female sex hormone
         (2) Develops and maintains female secondary sex organs
         (3) Causes most of cyclic endometrial growth
      b) Secretion of progesterone from corpus luteum
         (1) Prepares uterus for implantation of ovum
         (2) Restrains contractility of uterus
         (3) Stimulates the endometrium
      c) Interaction of hormones with those of anterior pituitary to control menstrual cycle

UNIT 9: THE REPRODUCTIVE SYSTEM

VOCABULARY/Male Reproductive System

cryptorchidism	undescended testes
impotence	inability (partial or complete) to perform sexual act
orchitis	inflammation of testes
prostatitis	inflammation of prostate gland
spermatogenesis	process of sperm development
testosterone	hormone responsible for masculine characteristics (also used for treatment of cryptorchidism)
urethritis	inflammation of the urethra (frequently a symptom of gonorrhea)

I. **Structure and Function**

   A. Structure
      1. Primary sex organs
         a) Testes (male gonads)
            (1) Small oval glands
            (2) Located in scrotum
      2. Secondary sex organs
         a) Ducts
            (1) Epididymis—lies coiled along top and sides of each testicle
            (2) Seminal duct
            (3) Ejaculatory duct—inside prostate gland
         b) Prostate gland—lies just below bladder, surrounds urethra, and is traversed by ejaculatory duct
         c) Scrotum—double pouch containing the testes and part of spermatic cord
         d) Penis
            (1) Is suspended from front and sides of pubic arch
            (2) Consists of glans penis, body, and root
            (3) Is traversed by urethra, which opens at extremity of glans
            (4) Has a head (glans penis), which contains opening of urethra
            (5) Has prepuce of foreskin, which covers glans penis

   B. Functions
      1. Testes
         a) Production of sperm
         b) Production of testosterone, male hormone
         c) Production of seminal fluid to fertilize female ovum
      2. Prostate gland—adds secretion to seminal fluid
      3. Penis—has dual function
         a) Urination
         b) Copulation

II. **Disorders of the Male Genital Tract**

   A. Congenital Malformations
      1. Hypospadias
         a) Definition of **hypospadias:** Opening of urethra on undersurface of penis
         b) Correction—by plastic surgery
      2. Epispadias
         a) Definition of **epispadias:** Opening of urethra on dorsum of penis

   b) Correction—by plastic surgery
3. Phimosis
   a) Definition of **phimosis:** Contraction of orifice of prepuce so that foreskin cannot be pushed back over glans penis
   b) Correction—by circumcision
4. Undescended testes (cryptorchidism)
   a) Definition of **cryptorchidism:** Failure of one or both testes to descend into the scrotum as the fetus develops; testes remain in abdomen
   b) Treatment
      (1) Medical—injection of chorionic gonadotrophin three times weekly
      (2) Surgical in some cases
5. Hydrocele
   a) Definition of **hydrocele:** Condition in which fluid accumulates in the scrotum
   b) Treatment—surgical

B. Inflammations and infections
   1. Urethritis, prostatitis, seminal vesiculitis
      a) Causes
         (1) Gonococcus (most frequent cause)
         (2) Infection from other foci
         (3) Benign prostatic hypertrophy if normal drainage is obstructed
      b) Assessment
         (1) Frequency, urgency, and burning on urination
         (2) Urethral discharge
      c) Treatment
         (1) Antibiotics
         (2) Bedrest
         (3) Local applications of heat
   2. Orchitis
      a) Definition of **orchitis:** Inflammation of one or both testes
      b) Causes
         (1) Trauma
         (2) Metastasis
         (3) Mumps
         (4) Infection from other foci
      c) Assessment
         (1) Pain in scrotal area
         (2) Fever
         (3) Fatigue
         (4) Swelling
      d) Treatment
         (1) Bedrest until fever subsides
         (2) Suspension of scrotum
         (3) Medication for pain
         (4) Treatment of primary focus
   3. Epididymitis
      a) Definition of **epididymitis:** Inflammation of epididymis—acute or chronic
      b) Causes
         (1) Specific or nonspecific infection
         (2) Trauma
      c) Assessment
         (1) Local pain
         (2) Fever

          (3)   Swelling
          (4)   Redness
      d) Treatment
          (1)   Bedrest
          (2)   Antibiotics
          (3)   Suspension of scrotum
  4. Syphilis
      a) Definition of **syphilis:** Contagious disease leading to many structural and cutaneous lesions and transmitted by direct intimate contact or *in utero.*
      b) Cause—spirochete (pathogenic microorganism)
      c) Three stages
          (1)   Initial stage—chancre develops 2–6 weeks after inoculation
          (2)   Secondary stage—rash appears 6–7 weeks after chancre
          (3)   Tertiary stage—appears years later and may attack cardiovascular system and/or brain (neurosyphilis); also termed *latent stage*
      d) Diagnosis
          (1)   Physical examination
          (2)   Serological tests
          (3)   Dark-field examination
  5. Neoplasms
      a) Benign prostatic hypertrophy
          (1)   Is benign enlargement of prostate tissue
          (2)   Begins under posterior urethra
      b) Carcinoma of prostate—unrelated to benign hypertrophy of gland but may exist with it
          (1)   Malignant growth that metastasizes to adjacent tissues and bones
          (2)   Assessment
              (a) Urinary difficulty
              (b) Bladder infection
              (c) Hypertension
          (3)   Treatment
              (a) Treatment of coexisting bladder infection
              (b) Surgery
                 i)   Transurethral prostatic resection
                 ii) Suprapubic prostatectomy
                 iii) Retropubic prostatectomy
                 iv) Radical prostatectomy
      c) Neoplasm of testes—most common form of malignant disease in 25–35 year age group

III. Nursing Management after Prostatic Surgery

Note: This surgery is among most common procedures referrable to male reproductive tract and is, therefore, used as an example. Also note that pre- and postoperative care are under the supervision of an R.N.

  A. Preoperative
    1. Help patient adjust to conditions.
    2. Encourage fluid intake; monitor intake and output.
    3. Monitor high-protein diet.
    4. Carefully observe and record symptoms and signs.
    5. Gradually remove urine if retention is present.
    6. Follow preoperative orders as left by surgeon.

B. Postoperative
1. Immediately check pulse and blood pressure.
2. Carefully observe for hemorrhage at site.
3. Frequently inspect indwelling catheter for signs of blockage.
4. Encourage high fluid intake.
5. Change dressing daily, using aseptic technique.
6. Take temperature orally if perineal resection done.
7. Follow physician's orders regarding pain and sedation medication.

VOCABULARY/Female Reproductive System

agglutination	clumping of cells
amenorrhea	absence of menstruation
benign	not malignant
curettage	scraping of a cavity
dilatation	expansion of an opening by a dilator
dilation	expansion of an organ, orifice, or vessel
dysmenorrhea	painful menstruation
endometrium	lining of uterine cavity
gestation	period of intrauterine fetal development
Graafian follicle	vesicle of any ovary that contains an ovum
gyneco-	pertaining to woman
hystero-	pertaining to uterus
leukorrhea	white or yellowish mucous discharge from cervical canal or vagina
malignant	cancerous; harmful
mammary glands	breasts
menorrhagia	excessive bleeding at time of menstrual period
metrorrhagia	uterine bleeding at times other than menstrual period
myometrium	muscle wall of uterus
oophoro-	pertaining to ovary
Papanicolaou smear	smear of cervical scrapings to be examined for cancerous cells
parturition	childbirth
pessary	device inserted into vagina to hold uterus in place
-rraphy	repair
-rrhea	discharge

I. Structure and Functions

A. Structure
1. Primary sex organs—ovaries
a) Are oval-shaped glands located on either side of uterus
b) Contain Graafian follicles
2. Secondary sex organs—uterus, breasts, and series of supporting organs
a) Uterus
(1) Is hollow, muscular organ about 3 inches long
(2) Is located in abdominal cavity between bladder and rectum
(3) Is composed of a cervix, a body, and a fundus
(4) Has mucous membrane, called *endometrium*, lining its cavity
(5) Has thick, muscular wall called *myometrium*
(6) Has eight ligaments that anchor it in place

        b) Uterine tubes (fallopian tubes)
- (1) Extend from superior angle of uterus to ovary
- (2) Have no direct connection to ovary
- (3) Have fingerlike processes, *fimbria,* which overhang ovary
- (4) Have mucous membrane lining with moving cilia

        c) Vagina
- (1) Is situated behind bladder and in front of rectum
- (2) Surrounds vaginal portion of cervix

        d) External genitalia
- (1) Mons pubis
  - (a) Lies over symphysis pubis
  - (b) Is covered by hair at puberty
- (2) Labia majora—two prominent cutaneous folds
- (3) Labia minora—two small cutaneous folds between labia majora
- (4) Clitoris—erectile structure similar to penis, partially hidden by labia minora
- (5) Vaginal orifice—median slit below urethra and above rectum
- (6) Perineum—pelvic floor

        e) Breasts (mammary glands)
- (1) Lie over pectoral muscles
- (2) Are composed of glands in grapelike clusters
- (3) Have nipples surrounded by pigmented area

B. Functions
1. Ovaries
   - a) Production of ova
   - b) Production of sex hormones
2. Uterus—has three functions
   - a) Menstruation
   - b) Housing fetus during pregnancy
   - c) Expulsion of fetus (labor) at end of pregnancy
3. Fallopian tubes—act as shelter for fertilization of ovum
4. Vagina
   - a) Serves as passageway for menstrual flow
   - b) Receives seminal fluid during copulation
   - c) Is birth canal
5. Breasts—secrete colostrum from beginning of pregnancy

II. Menstruation

A. Physiology
1. Is caused by decrease in secretion of estrogen and progesterone
2. Starts at puberty (11-15 years)—menarche
3. Generally occurs regularly at 28-, 21-, 26-, or 30-day intervals
4. Lasts 2–8 days
5. Gives off about 60 cc of blood

B. Synopsis of Menstrual Cycle
1. Postmenstrual state (repair)
   - a) Lining of uterus returns to its normal state.
     - (1) Estrogen titer rises to accomplish this.
     - (2) Progesterone prepares lining for reception of ovum.
   - b) Stage is about 5 days in length.

2. Estrogen stage
   a) Estrogen is secreted.
   b) Ovulation occurs about 14th day of 28-day cycle.
3. Premenstrual stage
   a) Lining of uterus thickens and becomes congested with blood.
   b) Stage begins about 5 days before menstruation.
4. Menstruation
   a) Epithelium of lining is expelled.
   b) Capillary hemorrhage occurs.
   c) Duration is 2–8 days.

III. Diagnostic Tests

Procedures
1. History and physical examination
2. Laboratory tests
   a) Urinalysis
   b) Complete blood count
   c) Serology
   d) Papanicolaou smear (cytological test for cancer)
   e) Other smears
      (1) Bacteria
         (a) Gonococcus
         (b) Pneumococcus
      (2) *Trichomonas vaginalis*
         (a) Usually "hanging drop" examination is done.
         (b) If present, the organism can be seen in Pap smear.
      (3) *Candida albicans*
      (4) Nonmotile intracellular parasite
      (5) Endocrine balance
   f) Schiller's test
      (1) Test guides gynecologist in doing biopsy.
      (2) Exact areas for biopsy of cervix are indicated by nonstaining.
   g) Huhner test—sterility test to determine viability, and motility of spermatozoa
   h) Cultures and sensitivity for bacteria
      (1) Gonorrhea
      (2) *Bacterium coli*
      (3) Streptococcus
   i) Pregnancy tests
      (1) Chorionic gonadotrophin, detectable in urine on gonads of various animals
         (a) There are three of these tests:
            i) Aschheim-Zondek test
            ii) Friedman's test
            iii) Frog test (rana pipiens)
         (b) These tests are cumbersome, time consuming, and largely obsolete.
      (2) Rapid immunodiagnostic tests, which can be interpreted within 2 hours
         (a) Have diagnostic accuracy of 95% in normal pregnancy
         (b) Have diagnostic accuracy of 98.5% in absence of pregnancy
         (c) Can detect pregnancy as early as 4 days after the missed menstrual period
      (3) DAP (Direct Agglutination Pregnancy) test
         (a) Is 2-minute test
         (b) Can detect pregnancy as early as 4 days after missed menstrual period

      j) Rubin test
- (1) Tubal insufflation is done to determine patency of tubes.
- (2) Test is important in diagnosing sterility problems.

      k) Hysterosalpingogram
- (1) X-ray study of uterus and tubes is made after instillation of radiopaque oil.
- (2) Test is important in diagnosing sterility problems.

      l) HIV examination for AIDS virus (with patient's permission)

  3. Surgical procedures
- a) Biopsy
- b) Culdoscopy
  - (1) Definition of **culdoscopy:** Visualization of pelvic structures through vaginal vault
  - (2) Hospital procedure
- c) Colposcopy—for detection of suspicious and early malignancies
- d) Dilatation and curettage
  - (1) Definition of **D&C:** Expansion of opening of cervix by dilator, and scraping of uterine cavity to remove lining
  - (2) Generally a diagnostic procedure
  - (3) Therapeutic procedure in incomplete abortion and for removal of polyps
- e) Laparoscopy—examination of interior of abdomen by means of laparoscope

B. Preparation for Pelvic Examination
1. The following equipment is necessary:
- a) Vaginal speculum
- b) Gloves
- c) Lubricant
- d) Pap smear materials
- e) Light

2. Procedure is explained to patient.
3. Patient is put in lithotomy position and draped.
4. Patient should empty bladder just before examination.

IV. Disorders of the Female Genital Tract

A. Malposition of Uterus
1. Symptoms
- a) Pelvic pain
- b) Backache
- c) Menstrual abnormalities
- d) Infertility

2. Types
- a) Anteflexion—uterus bent forward
- b) Retroflexion—uterus bent backward
- c) Retroversion—uterus tilted backward without bending
- d) Retrocession—uterus displaced backward without bending
- e) Prolapse—uterus lowered into vagina

3. Diagnosis
- a) Hysterography
- b) Uterine sound—direction will give indication

4. Treatment
- a) Pessary
- b) Surgery

B. Cystocele and/or Rectocele
  1. **Definitions:** Relaxation of vaginal walls allows bulging of bladder **(cystocele)** or rectum **(rectocele)** into vaginal canal (through walls)
  2. Symptoms
     a) Incomplete voiding of urine (cystocele)
     b) Urinary frequency (cystocele)
     c) Urinary incontinence (cystocele)
     d) Urinary tract infection (UTI)
     e) Constipation (rectocele)
     f) Distension of introitus (cystocele and rectocele)
  3. Treatment—surgery

C. Inflammations of the Female Genital Tract
  1. Vulvovaginitis
     a) Definition of **vulvovaginitis:** Inflammation of the vulva and vagina
     b) Types
        (1) Monilial vaginitis
           (a) Cause—*Candida albicans*
           (b) Assessment
              i) Pruritus
              ii) Vulval inflammation
              iii) Cottage-cheese-appearing discharge
           (c) Treatment—local applications of certain drugs
              i) Betadine
              ii) Gentian violet
              iii) Mycostatin
        (2) *Trichomonas vaginalis*
           (a) Cause—*Trichomonas* parasite
           (b) Assessment
              i) Pruritis
              ii) Persistent white vaginal discharge
              iii) Inflammation of vaginal mucosa
           (c) Treatment
              i) Local applications to change pH of vagina (vinegar douches); must continue during menstruation
              ii) Specific treatment—Flagyl orally; acidic vaginal suppositories—Floraquin, Diodoquin
        (3) Gonorrheal infection   See Section V, Sexually Transmitted Diseases.
        (4) Chlamydia   See Section V.C.
        (5) Atrophic vaginitis
           (a) Cause—endocrine deficiency
           (b) Treatment—hormone administration
        (6) Nonspecific inflammation—no specific pathogen identified; other forms of vaginitis excluded
  2. Cervicitis
     a) Definition of **cervicitis:** Inflammation of the uterine cervix—acute or chronic
     b) Etiology
        (1) Gonorrhea and/or secondary invading organisms
        (2) Poor hygiene (anal-vaginal contamination)
        (3) Irritation caused by pessaries or other foreign bodies
     c) Assessment
        (1) Leukorrhea
        (2) Pain

        (3) Dyspareunia
        (4) Urinary abnormalities
        (5) Abortion
        (6) Sterility
  3. Pelvic inflammatory disease
     a) Salpingitis
        (1) Definition of **salpingitis:** Inflammation or infection of a fallopian tube—acute, subacute, or chronic
        (2) Causes
           (a) Gonococcus (75% of cases)
           (b) Staphylococcus
           (c) Streptococcus
           (d) Colon bacillus
           (e) Tubercle bacillus (8% of cases)
        (3) Assessment
           (a) Pain in lower abdomen
           (b) Chill
           (c) Nausea
           (d) Fever
           (e) Backache
           (f) Loss of appetite
           (g) Dysuria
           (h) Leukorrhea
           (i) Dysmenorrhea
           (j) Sterility
        (4) Diagnosis
           (a) Physical examination
           (b) White blood count of 15,000–20,000
           (c) Smears
           (d) Cultures and sensitivity
        (5) Treatment
           (a) Absolute bedrest
           (b) Ice bag to abdomen
           (c) Local treatment
           (d) Systemic antibiotics
           (e) Fowler's position
     b) Oophoritis
        (1) Definition of **oophoritis:** Inflammation of one or both ovaries—acute, subacute, or chronic
        (2) Assessment
           (a) Pain
           (b) Swollen ovary
           (c) Leukorrhea
           (d) Occasional amenorrhea
        (3) Treatment
           (a) Bedrest
           (b) Generally surgery

D. Tumors of the Uterus
  1. Benign tumor—fibromyoma of uterus
     a) Location—muscle wall or surface beneath endometrium
     b) Assessment

             (1)   Menorrhagia and/or metrorrhagia
             (2)   Pressure symptoms
       c) Treatment
             (1)   Myomectomy or hysterectomy, depending upon other factors
             (2)   Occasionally radiation therapy

  2. Cancer of uterus
       a) Occurrence—cervix is most common site of malignancy in reproductive tract
       b) Classification of cancer
             (1)   Stage 0—not visible to naked eye
             (2)   Stage I—confined to mucosa
             (3)   Stage II—visible lesion but confined to cervix
             (4)   Stage III—cancer spread beyond cervix but not beyond pelvis
             (5)   Stage IV—malignancy spread to bladder and/or rectum
       c) Assessment
             (1)   Bleeding after intercourse
             (2)   Slight vaginal discharge
             (3)   Positive Pap smear
       d) Treatment
             (1)   Surgery
             (2)   Radiation therapy before or after surgery

  3. Cancer of vulva
       a) Assessment
             (1)   Pruritus
             (2)   Leukoplakia
       b) Treatment
             (1)   Surgery (vulvectomy) with removal of lymph glands
             (2)   Radiation therapy
       c) Nursing care
             (1)   General nursing care—same as for abdominal surgery
             (2)   Special nursing care referrable to radiation
                  (a) Protection of nurse—must be constantly aware of dangers of **overexposure** and take necessary precautions; amount of radiation received by nurse depends on distance between nurse and patient (source), **amount** of time spent with patient, and degree of shielding provided
                 (b) Nursing measures—emotional support of patient, reassurance of **patient,** providing sufficient rest, encouraging nourishing meals
       d) Additional measures because of type of surgery
             (1)   Low-residue diet
             (2)   Retention catheter
             (3)   Long-term analgesics
             (4)   Low Fowler's position in bed if indicated
             (5)   Active or passive exercises of extremities
             (6)   Heat lamp to promote healing

E. Tumors of the Ovaries
  1. Ovarian cyst—may contain fluid or other material such as hair (dermoid cyst)
       a) Symptoms
             (1)   May be silent or acutely painful
             (2)   May exert pressure on surrounding structures
             (3)   May cause heavy feeling in pelvis
             (4)   May cause variable changes in secondary sex characteristics

       b) Treatment—surgical
       c) Nursing care—similar to that for other abdominal surgery
          (1) Emotional support of patient
          (2) Education of patient as to necessary care
          (3) Efforts to restore patient to reasonable health before specific cancer therapy
          (4) Daily acetic acid douches
          (5) Antibiotics when necessary for concurrent infection
          (6) Surgery and/or radiation
  2. Ovarian cancer
       a) Assessment
          (1) Backache
          (2) Abdominal pressure
          (3) Edema of extremities
          (4) Abdominal enlargment
          (5) Specific findings on examination
       b) Treatment
          (1) Surgery
          (2) Radiation
          (3) Chemotherapy

F. Carcinoma of Endometrium
  1. Occurrence—second most common female genital malignancy
  2. Assessment
       a) Abnormal uterine bleeding
       b) Occasional malodorous vaginal discharge
       c) Pain, late in disease
  3. Diagnosis
       a) Laboratory tests
          (1) Sedimentation rate
          (2) Cancer cells visible in vaginal smears
       b) X-ray study—hysterosalpingogram
       c) Special examinations
          (1) Dilatation and curettage
          (2) Aspiration biopsy of endometrium
          (3) Search for extension of cancer by other tests: chest X ray, cystoscopy, proctoscopy, IVP
  4. Complications
       a) Rupture of uterus
       b) Perforation of uterus during curettage
       c) Metastatic spread

G. Menstrual Disorders
  1. Amenorrhea—absence of menstruation
       a) May be primary (pregnancy)
       b) May be secondary (caused by factors other than pregnancy)
  2. Dysmenorrhea—painful or difficult menstruation
       a) Mild discomfort may be relieved by rest, moderate exercise, heat, and simple analgesics.
       b) Severe pain may be caused by underlying pathology and should be investigated by the gynecologist.
  3. Menorrhagia—excessive menstruation
  4. Metrorrhagia—bleeding or spotting between menstrual periods (most common gynecological symptom next to leukorrhea)

H. Endometriosis
    Etiology
    a) Patches of endometrium are present in ovaries and throughout pelvis.
    b) Misplaced endometrium functions under hormonal control in same manner as endo-
        metrium of uterus.
    c) Bleeding takes place, and chocolate-colored cysts of ovary are formed.
    d) Inflammation, pelvic pain, adhesions, and, at times, sterility are present.

V. **Sexually Transmitted Diseases**

Note: These are infectious diseases usually transmitted through direct sexual contact, although there
       have been *rare* cases of nonsexual infection. The incidence of venereal infection and disease is
       on the increase at the present time.

A. Gonorrhea
    1. Infecting organism—gonococcus *(Neisseria gonorrhoeae)*
    2. Assessment
        a) Gonorrhea may be asymptomatic in female.
        b) Vaginal discharge is usual symptom.
    3. Diagnosis
        a) Smear
        b) Culture
    4. Characteristics
        a) Disease is highly contagious (mucous membranes and eyes must be protected).
        b) Nurses must be extremely careful—hand washing after patient contact is essen-
            tial.
        c) Gonorrhea can infect eyes; it causes blindness of infant during birth if mother has
            disease.
    5. Treatment
        a) Penicillin is drug of choice.
        b) Instillation of 1% silver nitrate or appropriate antibiotic is given to prevent ophthalmic
            neonatorum.
        c) Other drugs may also be used, especially in persons who are allergic to penicillin or
            who are infected by organisms resistant to penicillin.
        d) Nurse should be careful while handling pads, etc., containing discharge; pads
            should be either disinfected or burned.
        e) Short- and long-term patient education is important.

B. Syphilis
    1. Infecting organism—a spirachete, *Treponema pallidum*
    2. Assessment of early syphilis
        a) Chancre
        b) Positive serology
        c) Skin rash
        d) Presence of organism in cerebrospinal fluid
        e) Unexplained pain in bones
    3. Assessment of late syphilis
        a) Gumma (soft tumor)
        b) Symptoms of nervous system disease and/or disease of circulatory system
    4. Treatment
        a) Penicillin is drug of choice.
        b) Other antibiotics may be used in persons allergic to penicillin or in drug-resistant
            disease.

c) Nurse must follow physician's orders carefully.

d) In early syphilis, lesions are infectious and patients therefore should be isolated.

e) Isolation precautions are needed until 24 hours after initiation of effective therapy.

C. Chlamydial Infection
1. Infecting organism—*Chlamydia trachomatis*
2. Assessment
   a) Mild dysuria
   b) Clear to mucopurulent discharge
   c) Pelvic pain
   d) Dyspareunia
   e) Cervicitis
3. Treatment
   a) Tetracycline
   b) Erythromycin in pregnant women

D. Trichomoniasis
1. Infecting organism—*Trichomonas vaginalis* (protozoa)
2. Assessment
   a) Copious, greenish yellow, frothy vaginal discharge
   b) Dysuria and dyspareunia
3. Treatment—Metronidazole

E. Genital Candidiasis
1. Assessment
   a) Vulval irritation
   b) Vaginal discharge (white, cheesy material)
2. Treatment
   a) Nystatin
   b) Clotrimazole

F. Chancroid
1. Assessment
   a) Small papules
   b) Ulcers
2. Diagnosis—mostly on clinical findings
3. Treatment—erythromycin

G. Hepatitis
1. Assessment
   a) Abdominal pain
   b) Nausea
   c) Diarrhea
   d) Fever
2. Prevention—hepatitis B vaccine (see Table 1 of the Appendix)
3. Treatment
   a) Symptomatic treatment of hepatitis
   b) Immune globulin
   c) Removal of cause

H. Acquired Immune Deficiency Syndrome (AIDS)
   1. Definition of **AIDS:** Serious, often fatal condition in which the immune system breaks down and does not respond normally to infection
   2. Assessment
      a) Generalized lymphadenopathy
      b) Weight loss
      c) Intermittent fever
      d) Malaise
      e) Chronic diarrhea
      f) Lymphopenia
      g) Anemia
      h) Thrombocytopenia
      i) Immunologic abnormalities
      j) Opportunistic infections

Note: Many other symptoms and signs can also appear.

   2. Treatment
      a) The specific treatment for AIDS has not as yet been established; therefore the treatment is symptomatic, the symptoms being treated as they appear.
      b) A few drugs, e.g., AZT, ddC, and ddI, originally developed for cancer treatment, are legally available for AIDS patients in the United States.
   3. Test for HIV—can be given only with the patient's permission

Note: There are several more sexually transmitted diseases that have not been listed here. However, the practical nurse should be familiar with their names:
Lymphogranuloma Venereum (LGV)   Genital Herpes
Granuloma Inquinale   Genital Warts

VI. **Surgery of the Female Reproductive System (excluding obstetrical procedures)**

A. Cauterization of the Cervix
   1. Chronic cervicitis
   2. Eversion of cervix
   3. Obliteration of Nabothian cysts

B. Removal of Cervical Polyps (Polypectomy)

C. Cervical Biopsy

D. Conization of Cervix (cancer study)

E. Cervical Repair (Trachelorrhaphy)

F. Endometrial Biopsy
   1. Diagnosis of endometrial cancer
   2. Identification of causes of abnormal uterine bleeding
   3. Evaluation of gynecological hormone therapy
   4. Evaluation of infertility problems

G. Dilatation and Curettage (used in diagnosis and in abortion)

H. Myomectomy
   1. Definition of **myomectomy:** Removal of tumor from uterus, leaving uterus in place

I. Hysterectomy
   1. Subtotal—removal of body of uterus leaving cervix in place
   2. Total—removal of entire uterus
   3. Panhysterectomy—removal of uterus, tubes, and ovaries
   4. Vaginal hysterectomy—removal of uterus through vagina
   5. Abdominal hysterectomy—removal of uterus through abdominal incision

J. Colporrhaphy
   1. Definition of **colporrhaphy:** Repair of vaginal walls
   2. Types
      a) Anterior colporrhaphy—repair of cystocele
      b) Posterior colporrhaphy—repair of rectocele

K. Culdoscopy

L. Laparoscopy

VII. Drugs Used for Female Genital Tract Disorders

A. Antibiotics (use is according to culture and sensitivity tests)

B. Analgesics

C. Hormones
   1. Relieve menopausal symptoms due to deficiency of ovarian function
   2. Treat atrophic vaginitis
   3. Treat menstrual abnormalities
   4. Treat sterility problems
   5. Prevent conception
   6. Treat habitual abortion

D. Antispasmodics

E. Uterine Stimulants

VIII. Nursing Care of the Gynecological Patient

A. Adequate and Proper Draping Procedures

B. Care to Protect Self and Others from Infections

C. Postoperative Care
   1. After abdominal surgery of reproductive organs, nursing care is same as for any other abdominal surgery.
   2. To prevent bladder distention, Foley catheter may be necessary for several days.
   3. Early ambulation and exercises are needed to prevent phlebitis.
   4. Deep breathing exercises and coughing should be encouraged.
   5. Medication for pain is administered as necessary.
   6. Perineal care is given as directed by physician.
   7. Special procedures after perineal surgery are given as ordered by gynecologist.

NURSING CARE OF THE ADULT PATIENT

D. Care after Radiation Therapy
1. Inspect all linens and dressings so that radium applicator is not discarded by mistake.
2. Inspect contents of each bedpan so that the tube which encloses radium will not be lost.
3. Report lost radium applicators to supervisor immediately.
4. Protect yourself from radiation exposure.

IX. Diseases of the Breast

Note: The breasts are part of the female reproductive system. Estrogens initiate the growth of the breasts and the breasts' milk-producing apparatus. Progesterone promotes their secretory function and prolactin promotes lactation during pregnancy.

A. Mastitis
1. Definition of **Mastitis:** Inflammation of the breast
2. Etiology
a) Mastitis usually occurs in lactating women
b) Pathogens enter through a lesion or abrasion of the nipple.
3. Assessment
a) Erythema below breast
b) Fever
c) Pain
4. Treatment
a) Interrupt nursing if postpartum.
b) Administer antibiotics
c) Apply heat to affected area (review nursing principles regarding application of heat).
d) Incise and drain if abscess forms (soiled dressings are highly infectious; observe isolation precautions).

B. Chronic Cystic Mastitis (Fibrocystic Disease of Breast)
1. Etiology—hormonal imbalance
2. Assessment
a) Uncomfortable feeling in breast
b) Presence of small nodules
c) Occasional shooting pains
3. Treatment
a) Administration of hormones
b) Incision and drainage in acute mastitis

C. Cancer
1. Assessment
a) Small lump in breast—distorted breast contour
b) Dimpling of skin over lump
c) Bloody discharge from nipple
d) Retraction of nipple
e) Edema of skin of breast
f) Enlarged axillary lymph nodes
g) Slow growth, except inflammatory carcinoma
2. Treatment
a) Examination of biopsy by pathologist, and diagnosis
b) Mastectomy (treatment of choice) or, in some clinics, lumpectomy if specimen is malignant

        (1)   Simple mastectomy involves removal of breast only as palliative measure to make patient more comfortable.

        (2)   Radical mastectomy involves removal of
- (a) Entire breast
- (b) Overlying skin
- (c) Pectoralis major and minor
- (d) Axillary lymph nodes

        (3)   Modified radical mastectomy involves
- (a) Total mastectomy
- (b) Axillary dissection with pectoralis major and minor left intact.

        (4)   Radiation therapy may be used pre- and postoperatively

        (5)   Hormone therapy may be instituted in some cases; i.e., estrogens, androgens, adrenocortical hormones.

3. Complications of radical mastectomy
   a) Edema of arm in 10-30% of cases due to lymphatic obstruction
   b) Local recurrence of the disease
4. Nursing care
   a) Follow pre- and postoperative nursing care procedures.
   b) Do not take blood pressure on affected side.
   c) Provide psychological support.
5. Preoperative care
   a) Emotional care of patient is important.
   b) Normal preoperative surgical care is given.
6. Postoperative care
   a) Apply pressure dressing over operative site.
      (1) Reduces chances of hemorrhage
      (2) Reduces seepage of lymphatic fluid between skin and chest wall
   b) Frequently observe dressings on ventral and dorsal aspects of chest.
   c) Observe and report circulatory abnormalities.
      (1) Numbness of fingers or lower arm
      (2) Swelling of arm—elevate arm on pillow
      (3) Severe pain—give ordered medication
   d) Encourage patient to take exercises as ordered by physician.
      (1) Brushing hair
      (2) Wall climbing
   e) Encourage patient to cough and breathe deeply.
   f) Encourage patient to be fitted with prosthesis after healing has taken place.

Nursing Care of the Obstetrical Patient

UNIT 1: OBSTETRICS AND NORMAL PREGNANCY

VOCABULARY

antepartum	referring to period between conception and onset of labor
areola	dark ring around nipple
chloasma	mask of pregnancy; brown discoloration of face during pregnancy; usually appears across nose and on cheeks
conception	fertilization of ovum
fetus	product of conception after third month of development
gestation	development of new life within uterus, from conception to birth
maternity	motherhood
menopause	period when menstruation ceases permanently; change of life; reduction in production of hormones, causing cessation of menstruation
obstetrician	medical doctor who specializes in obstetrics
obstetrics	science of care of women during pregnancy, childbirth, and puerperium
pregnancy	condition of being with child
prenatal care	care given to mother before delivery in order to teach her and help ensure safe delivery of healthy baby
puerperium	period after third stage of labor until complete involution of pelvic organs
quickening	feeling of life or movement of fetus
virgin	girl or woman who has had no sexual intercourse

I. **Principles of Obstetrical Nursing**

    A. Introduction
        1. Purpose of obstetrical care is to reduce maternal and infant mortality associated with childbirth and ensure delivery of healthy baby.
        2. Despite many advances in modern medicine, both women and children still die at child-birth.
        3. Infant mortality rates are not as low as they should be.
        4. Other western nations have lower maternal and infant mortality rates than the United States.

    B. Obstetrical Care
        1. Used to be provided by midwives and family members
        2. Became more effective after discovery of aseptic techniques, anesthesia, and antibiotics

    C. Public Education

1. Public is more aware today of need for adequate medical supervision during pregnancy and after delivery.
2. Federal, state, and city governments have sponsored many maternal and child care programs.
   a) School health programs
   b) Hospital-run prenatal clinics and well-baby clinics
   c) Visiting nurse services
   d) Immunization programs

D. Responsibilities of Practical Nurse
   Must have knowledge of
   1. Normal functioning of reproductive organs
   2. Normal processes of gestation and delivery
   3. Physical and emotional demands of mother and child before, during, and after birth

II. Normal Pregnancy

A. Length
   1. Is approximately 280 days
   2. Is equivalent to 10 lunar (9 calendar) months

B. Physiological Changes Associated with Pregnancy
   1. Circulatory changes
      a) Cardiac output increases 20–40%.
      b) Blood pressure and pulse remain normal.
      c) Tissues retain excess fluid (about 3 quarts).
   2. Breasts
      a) Become enlarged
      b) May become painful
      c) Have increased pigmentation of nipples
      d) Form colostrum
   3. Uterus (cavity where implantation of fertilized ovum takes place)
      a) Is organ most affected by pregnancy
      b) Enlarges to almost five times its normal size
      c) Is softer between cervix and its body (Hegar's sign)
   4. Vagina—changes to bluish color (Chadwick's sign)
   5. Cervix
      a) Contains mucous plug to protect fetus from bacteria
      b) Softens to permit delivery of child (Goodell's sign)
      c) Becomes bluish
   6. Abdomen
      a) Becomes enlarged
      b) Occasionally shows appearance of striae
   7. Digestive tract—slowing of peristaltic action leads to nausea and constipation
   8. Urinary tract
      a) Urination is more frequent because of pressure of uterus on bladder.
      b) Kidneys must do more work.
   9. Respiration—rate increases during last trimester to supply needed oxygen
   10. Weight gain—total of approximately 20–25 pounds is considered normal
   11. Skin—striae gravidum appear
       a) Are caused by stretching and rupture of internal tissue
       b) Occur on breasts, thighs, and abdomen
       c) Usually disappear after delivery

12. Metabolism—accelerates

C. Assessment of Pregnancy
1. Presumptive signs
   a) Morning sickness—nausea and vomiting
   b) Absence of menstruation—amenorrhea for 1 week or more
   c) Breast changes—enlargement, some pain and tenderness
   d) Frequent urination, common during early months
   e) Fatigue
   f) Leukorrhea—increased vaginal secretions caused by stimulating effect of estrogen
2. Probable signs
   a) Chadwick's sign—vagina turns bluish to purple
   b) Ballottement—rebounding occurring when doctor taps floating fetus within uterus
   c) Pigmentation—increasing deposits in skin of breasts, face, and abdomen
   d) Goodell's sign—softening of cervix
   e) Contour of abdomen—change in contour due to changes occurring in uterus
   f) Striae gravidarum (striation of the skin)—occurs over the lower abdomen and the upper portion of the thighs and breasts
   g) Laboratory tests—HCG, Gravidex, and UGG (probable because only 96% accurate)
   h) Braxton-Hicks contractions—painless, intermittent uterine spasms
   i) Uterine souffle—a muffled, swishing pulse heard over pregnant uterus; sound is in unison with the mother's heart beat and is due to rush of blood through large uterine vessels (same sound can be heard over large vascular tumors)
3. Positive signs
   a) Fetal movements, felt by the physician
   b) Fetal cardiac motion at 6 weeks by ultrasound
   c) Fetal heart tones, heard by the physician or recorded
      (1) 10–12 weeks with ultrasound
      (2) 18–20 weeks by stethoscope
   d) Doubling of HCG levels
   e) Delivery of a fetus

D. Laboratory Tests to Determine Pregnancy
1. Early tests
   a) A–Z (Aschheim-Zondek test)—used immature female white mice
   b) Friedman's test—used adult female rabbits
   c) Berman test—used immature female rats
   d) HCG—human chorionic gonadotrophin injected into female animals
2. Since 1960, simpler and quicker tests—Gravidex and UGG—
   a) Take 2 minutes to perform; given 13 days after missed period
   b) Are based on immunological principle involving clumping HCG-coated animal red blood cells

III. **Prenatal Care**

A. Medical Supervision
1. First visit to doctor or prenatal clinic should be made as soon as pregnancy is suspected.
2. Physical examination is performed to determine general state of health of mother-to-be; included are abdominal and vaginal examinations and the taking of pelvic measurements.

B. Important Aspects of Examination, Laboratory Tests, and Danger Signals
   1. Medical history
      a) Previous diseases including communicable diseases
      b) Operations
      c) Menstrual history
      d) Past pregnancies
         (1) Number of pregnancies, including abortions and miscarriages
         (2) Duration of pregnancies
         (3) Labor—prolonged, complications, etc.
         (4) Delivery—spontaneous, breech, section, etc.
         (5) Health of living children
      e) Present pregnancy
      f) Blood transfusions
   2. Family history
   3. Patient's attitudes toward pregnancy and childbearing
   4. Complete physical examination
      a) Height and weight
      b) Skin and hair
      c) Eyes, ears, nose, and throat (including mouth and teeth)
      d) Thyroid
      e) Cardiovascular system
      f) Lungs
      g) Abdomen
      h) Pelvic exam to determine adequacy of pelvic inlet
      i) Cervical smear (for Pap test and for chlamydia)
      j) Extremities
      h) Vital signs, including blood pressure
   5. Laboratory tests
      a) CBC
      b) Serologic test for syphilis
      c) Urinalysis
         (1) Urine examined for protein, sugar, and bacteria
         (2) Tests done at every prenatal visit
      d) Rh factor blood typing, antibody screening, sickle-cell-trait screening (for blacks)
      e) A, B, O compatibility
      f) Papanicolaou test and for chlamydia
   6. Calculation of estimated date of delivery (EDC)—count back 3 months from the first day of last menstrual period and add 1 year and 7 days
   7. Subsequent visits—doctor decides how often they will be necessary; usually scheduled every 3–4 weeks until eighth month of pregnancy, then every week during ninth month
   8. Danger signals to report to doctor
      a) Frequent headache
      b) Edema of face, hands, or legs
      c) Vomiting and nausea that persist beyond first trimester
      d) Constipation
      e) Vaginal bleeding
      f) Weight loss
      g) Shortness of breath
      h) Severe pain in lower abdomen or lumbar regions
      i) Nervousness, sleeplessness, and apprehension
      j) Escape of fluid from vagina
      k) Chills and fevers

l) Any infection or illness
m) Failure to feel fetal movements after fourth month
n) Visual disturbances
o) Rapid weight gain

C. Maternal Hygiene during Pregnancy
1. Clothing—lightweight clothing should be worn; comfortable shoes with low, solid heels; maternity girdle; no constricting clothes
2. Breasts—brassiere needed; bathing for cleanliness
3. Posture—maintenance of good posture is necessary to lessen strain on muscles of back and thighs; this will prevent aches and cramps of back and leg muscles
4. Abdominal support
5. Douches—permitted as advised by physician
6. Personal hygiene—daily baths or showers
7. Dental checkup
8. Sleep and rest—necessary to avoid fatigue and irritability; rest periods should be taken periodically
9. Moderate (not strenuous) exercise to
   a) Maintain strength
   b) Improve body functions (circulation, digestion, elimination)
   c) Assure good muscle tone
10. Elimination—increased urinary output, tendency toward constipation, increased perspiration
11. Diet
    a) Regulate weight gain (3 pounds per month)
    b) Meet nutritional needs of mother and child
    c) Aid in elimination

D. Minor Discomforts of Normal Pregnancy
1. Constipation—control by adding bulk to diet, exercising daily, and taking mild laxatives as suggested by physician
2. Nausea and vomiting after first trimester—practice emotional control and eat high-carbohydrate diet
3. Pruritus—bathe frequently; use of lotion or sodium bicarbonate and increased fluids give relief
4. Varicose veins—eliminate constricting clothes such as garters; rest with elevation of hips and legs; have regular bowel movements; avoid crossing legs
5. Backache—wear well-fitted, low-heeled shoes and a good, comfortable girdle
6. Hemorrhoids
   a) Definition of **hemorrhoids:** Dilated blood vessels in anal region of body
   b) Cause—interference with venous circulation caused by pressure; condition aggravated by constipation
   c) Relief measures
      (1) Relieving constipation
      (2) Cold applications
      (3) Ointments or suppositories
7. Leg cramps
   a) Cause
      (1) Pressure on nerves by uterus
      (2) Fatigue
      (3) Tense posture
      (4) Low-calcium intake
   b) Relief measures

        (1)   Drinking adequate amount of milk daily
        (2)   Not crossing legs
        (3)   Avoiding restrictive clothing
        (4)   Avoiding fatigue
        (5)   Wearing proper shoes

   8. Flatulence
      a) Definition of **flatulence:** Abnormal amount of gas in digestive tract, causing a feeling of distension
      b) Causes
        (1)   Bacteria in intestinal tract
        (2)   Pressure exerted by growing uterus
      c) Relief measures
        (1)   Avoiding gas-forming foods
        (2)   Chewing foods well
        (3)   Daily regulation of elimination

   9. Heartburn
      a) Causes
        (1)   Worry, fatigue, nervous tension, emotional trauma
        (2)   Improper diet
        (3)   Pressure on the stomach by enlarging uterus.
      b) Relief measures
        (1)   Frequently eating small meals
        (2)   Omitting fried, highly seasoned or undigestible foods

  10. Vaginal discharges
      a) Possible causes
        (1)   Yeast infection
        (2)   Gonorrhea
        (3)   Increased glandular activity of reproductive tract
      b) Treatment
        (1)   Good hygienic practices
        (2)   If discharges are caused by venereal disease, treatment of the disease
        (3)   Medications as ordered by the physician

  11. Insomnia
      a) Cause—shortness of breath due to pressure of uterus on the diaphragm
      b) Relief measures
        (1)   Abdominal breathing
        (2)   Relaxation exercises
        (3)   Warm drink at bedtime

E. Social Life
   1. Outside interests should be included; crowded places should be avoided.
   2. Alcoholic drinks should be avoided.
   3. Smoking should be avoided; smaller babies are delivered by smokers.
   4. Drugs should be used only as prescribed by physician.
   5. Sexual relations should be discussed frankly with doctor, who will advise patient.
   6. Mental attitude should be one of confidence, calmness, and happy expectation; patient should be free from worry.
   7. Father should see that mother receives proper care; he should be encouraged to share equal degree of responsibility for future welfare and health of child.

IV. Physiology of Normal Pregnancy

A. Cardiovascular Changes

      1. Cardiac output increases.
      2. Blood volume increases.
      3. WBC count increases.
      4. Iron requirements increase (supplemental iron needed).

B. Pulmonary Changes
      1. Volume and respiratory rate increase.
      2. There is no change in vital capacity.
      3. Mild dyspnea occurs upon exertion.
      4. There is mild edema of respiratory tract.
         a) Nasal stuffiness
         b) Voice changes

C. Renal Changes
      1. Glomerular filtration rate increases.
      2. BUN and creatinine decrease.
      3. Urination is frequent at night due to sleeping position.

D. Gastrointestinal Changes
      1. Constipation may occur.
      2. GI motility decreases (heartburn and belching).
      3. Incidence of gallbladder disease increases.
      4. HCl production decreases.

E. Endocrine Changes
      1. There is an increase in glandular function.
      2. Estrogens, progesterone, glycocorticoids are produced in greater amounts.

F. Skin
      1. Increased pigment of mammary areola (melanocyte stimulating hormone)
      2. Melasma (brown color) over forehead
      3. Spider angiomas above waist

V. Fetal Development

A. First Month
      1. Early development of eyes, ears, and nose
      2. Length of embryo—approximately ¼ inch
      3. Pumping of heart by day 20

B. Second Month
      1. Formation of head and body
      2. Development of extremities
      3. Length of embryo—approximately 3 inches

C. Third Month
      1. Appearance of downy hair (lanugo) on back and shoulders
      2. Nail growth on fingers and toes
      3. Obvious sex differentiation
      4. Length of fetus—approximately 6 inches
      5. Complete organ formation except for central nervous system

D. Fourth Month

1. Detectable fetal heart beat
2. Hair development on head
3. Length and weight of fetus—approximately 10 inches and 10 ounces

E. Fifth Month
1. Appearance of eyebrows and eyelashes
2. Wrinkled, transparent skin
3. Cheesy material (vernix caseosa) covering body
4. Length and weight of fetus—approximately 12 inches and 1½ pounds

F. Sixth Month
1. Wrinkled, reddish skin, covered with vernix caseosa
2. Length and weight of fetus—approximately 14 inches and 2 pounds

G. Seventh Month
1. Fetal movements are evident.
2. Fetus is approximately 16 inches long and weighs 3–4 pounds.
3. Fetus may be viable at 28 weeks

H. Eighth Month
1. Fetus doubles weight.
2. Fetus is approximately 18 inches long.
3. Fetus has good chance of surviving if born at this stage.

I. Ninth Month
1. Skin unwrinkles.
2. Fine body hair disappears.
3. Baby is fully developed.
4. Weight is approximately 7 pounds.

Note: Most malformations occur during first 12 weeks.

UNIT 2: DISORDERS AND COMPLICATIONS OF PREGNANCY

VOCABULARY

ascites	accumulation of serous fluid in peritoneal cavity
craniotomy	perforation of fetal head to facilitate delivery
cystocele	hernial protrusion of urinary bladder into vagina
eclampsia	toxic disturbance of late pregnancy, marked by convulsions and followed by coma
edema	collection of fluid in tissue
euphoria	feeling of well-being and absence of mental anxiety or pain
gavage	tube feeding into stomach
HIV	human immunodeficiency virus
mastitis	inflammation of breast
quadruplet	any one of four persons born at one birth
quintuplet	any one of five persons born at one birth
rectocele	hernial protrusion of part of rectum into vagina
triplet	any one of three persons born at one birth

NURSING CARE OF THE OBSTETRICAL PATIENT

I. **Complications Due to Pregnancy**

A. Ectopic Pregnancy
1. Definition of **ectopic pregnancy:** Implantation of fertilized ovum outside uterus—within fallopian tube, abdomen, ovary, or cervix, or combined extra- and intrauterine
2. Symptoms—similar to those of early pregnancy, but
   a) Intense pain may be felt on affected side.
   b) Vaginal bleeding or concealed bleeding may occur.
   c) Signs of shock may be present.
3. Early diagnosis and treatment—absolutely necessary
4. Operative intervention—mandatory
5. Nursing care
   a) Keep patient warm and quiet.
   b) Prepare for operation.
   c) Observe and record vital signs.
   d) Prepare for blood transfusions.
   e) Give treatment for shock.
   f) Give emotional support.

B. Placenta Previa
1. Definition of **placenta previa:** Condition of pregnancy in which placenta is attached to lower uterine segment and partially or completely covers the outlet from the uterus to the vagina
2. Most characteristic symptom—painless hemorrhage during last trimester without cause
3. Treatment—depends on status of cervix, parity, degree of previa, presence or absence of labor, and amount of bleeding
   a) Blood replacement therapy
   b) Treatment for shock
4. Nursing care
   a) Keep patient absolutely quiet.
   b) Check vital signs, and report and record.
   c) Elevate foot of bed.
   d) Give intravenous fluids as ordered.
   e) Check fetal heart often.
   f) Observe amount of blood loss, and report and record.

C. Abruptio Placentae (Premature Separation of Normally Implanted Placenta)
1. Occurrence—during late pregnancy or at onset of labor
2. Primary cause—unknown, but may be precipitated by
   a) Overdistension of uterus
   b) Toxemia of pregnancy
   c) Trauma
3. Assessment
   a) Intense abdominal pain without contractions and relaxation of uterus
   b) Vaginal bleeding
   c) Boardlike consistency in uterus
   d) Absence of fetal heart sounds
   e) Symptoms of shock
4. Treatment
   a) Blood replacement therapy
   b) Emptying of uterus either by vaginal delivery or by cesarean section
   c) Hysterectomy if uterus fails to contract
5. Nursing care

    a) Check vital signs, and report and record.
    b) Assist in preparation of patient for immediate delivery, either vaginal or operative.
    c) Prepare for IV or blood transfusion.

D. Spontaneous and Habitual Abortion
  1. Definition of **spontaneous abortion:** Expulsion of fetus before viability (28 weeks); no death certificate is required
  2. Causes
    a) Ovular defects (50–60%)
    b) Maternal factors (15%)
    c) Unknown factors
  3. Treatment
    a) Absolute bedrest for threatened abortion
    b) Sedatives to quiet uterus
    c) Endocrine therapy
    d) If abortion incomplete, dilatation and curettage if necessary
    e) Blood replacement therapy if necessary
  4. Nursing care—same as for any clean surgical case
  5. Postpartum care if abortion is complete

E. Hydatid Mole
  1. Definition of **hydatid mole:** Benign neoplasm of utereus that destroys embryo
  2. Occurence—early in pregnancy
  3. Assessment
    a) Hemorrhage in patient whose uterus is enlarged beyond normal size for stage of pregnancy
    b) Brownish vaginal discharge
    c) Absence of embryo on X ray
  4. Treatment—immediate emptying of uterus
  5. Nursing care—same as for any surgical (gynecological) case

F. Hyperemesis Gravidarum
  1. Definition of **hyperemesis gravidarum:** Abnormal condition of pregnancy characterized by excessive nausea and vomiting after first trimester
  2. Assessment
    a) Persistent vomiting
    b) Acetone and diacetic acid in urine
    c) Weight loss
    d) Dehydration
    e) Low-grade fever
    f) Rapid pulse
    g) Scanty urine
  3. Treatment
    a) Parenteral fluids to combat dehydration
    b) Measures to relieve starvation—intravenous glucose, vitamins, and possibly tube feeding of high-vitamin, high-calorie diet
    c) Sedation and possibly psychotherapy
    d) Therapeutic abortion if following ensue:
      (1) Jaundice
      (2) Delirium
      (3) Fever above 101° F in spite of fluid intake
      (4) Steadily rising pulse rate above 130
      (5) Retinal hemorrhages

II. **Toxemias of Pregnancy**

   A. Acute Hypertensive Disease of Pregnancy (Hypertension)
      1. Occurence—generally in last trimester
      2. Assessment—generalized edema and proteinuria

   B. Preeclampsia
      1. Occurrence—in latter half of pregnancy, during labor or puerperium
      2. Assessment
         a) Nausea and vomiting
         b) Edema and weight gain (caused by fluid retention)
         c) Hypertension
         d) Albuminuria
         e) Visual disturbances
         f) Apprehension and depression
      3. Forms—mild and severe
      4. Treatment
         a) Early delivery
         b) Normal salt intake, water
         c) Bedrest
         d) Sedation
      5. Nursing care
         a) Accurate fluid intake and output record
         b) Fetal heart rate every 4-6 hours
         c) Blood pressure every 4-6 hours
         d) Daily urinalysis
         e) Sedatives for rest and for lowering blood pressure (phenobarbital)
         f) Checking and recording of vital signs as ordered
         g) Quiet room, soft lights
         h) Medication as ordered
         i) Antihypertension medication
         j) Daily weight (same time each day)

   C. Eclampsia
      1. Occurrence—mostly in primigravidas (80%)
      2. Assessment (symptoms appear in last trimester)
         a) Convulsions and coma
         b) Edema
         c) Albuminuria
         d) Elevated blood pressure
      3. Prevention
        (1) Vigilant prenatal care
        (2) Early diagnosis and treatment of preeclampsia
        (3) Immediate reporting of any symptom
      4. Treatment
         a) Sedation
         b) Protection of patient from self-injury
           (1) Patient must never be left alone.
           (2) Tongue blade is used to prevent tongue from being bitten
         c) Protection of patient from external stimuli
         d) Turning of head to prevent aspiration of mucus and/or vomitus
         e) Intravenous administration to promote urination

      f) Close observation and recording of signs to guard against complications (cerebral hemorrhage, congestive heart failure, respiratory paralysis, etc.)

      g) Administration of oxygen as needed

      h) Termination of pregnancy—only real cure

  D. Chronic Hypertensive Vascular Disease
    1. Occurrence
      a) Hypertension predates pregnancy.
      b) Condition occurs generally in obese multiparas.
    2. Outlook for fetus—poor
    3. Assessment
      a) Hypertension
      b) Headache
    4. Treatment
      a) Hypotensive drugs
      b) Rest
      c) Low-sodium diet
      d) Observation for signs of toxemia
      e) Interruption of pregnancy if symptoms become very severe

  E. Unclassified Toxemias
    1. Symptoms and signs are not sufficient to make a diagnosis.
    2. Treatment is of predominating symptoms.

III. Coincidental Complications

  A. Heart Disease (mainly rheumatic)
    1. Importance—regarded as fourth major cause of maternal death
    2. Treatment
      a) Adequate rest
      b) Avoidance of infection
      c) Observation for early signs of heart failure (edema, shortness of breath, etc.)
      d) Digitalis
      e) Complete bedrest in hospital if needed

  B. Diabetes Mellitus
    1. Reasons why disease is difficult to control in pregnant women
      a) Changes in glucose tolerance
      b) Increased tendency to ketosis
    2. Complications
      a) Excessively large fetuses
      b) Slightly increased abortion rate
      c) Increased incidence of toxemia
      d) Increased incidence of fetal death *in utero*
      e) Congenital defects
      f) Inhibition of lactation
      g) Neonatal complications
        (1) Anoxia
        (2) Immaturity
        (3) Pulmonary problems
        (4) Hypoglycemia
    3. Treatment
      a) Strict medical supervision

  b) Termination of pregnancy before term if clinical course complicated
  c) Avoidance of infection
  d) Proper rest regimen
  e) Hospital admissions for supervision before term, if needed

C. Infectious Diseases
  1. Syphilis
    a) Routine serology during pregnancy is now legislated.
    b) Intensive treatment is necessary for those diagnosed as positive.
    c) Untreated cases result in fetal deformity, prematurity, and fetal death, depending upon time of infection.
  2. Rubella (German measles)
    a) Disease causes severe maldevelopment in fetus.
    b) Infection after first trimester is not dangerous.
    c) Generally therapeutic abortion is indicated in proven cases.
  3. Gonorrhea
    a) Disease can cause blindness in fetus who contracts disease during birth.
    b) One percent silver nitrate or antibiotic is dropped into baby's eyes immediately postpartum.
  4. Chlamydia
    a) Importance
      (1) Causes a number of sexually transmitted diseases, including pelvic inflammatory disease in women
      (2) Causes neonatal conjunctivitis and pneumonia
    b) Treatment—tetracyclines and erythromycin
    c) Nursing care
      (1) Counseling of patients
      (2) Observation of untoward symptoms in infants
  5. Acquired immunodeficiency syndrome (AIDS) (Human immunodeficiency virus, HIV)
    a) Cause is retrovirus.
    b) Immune deficiency results in
      (1) Opportunistic infections (pneumonia)
      (2) Malignancies (Kaposi's sarcoma)
      (3) Neurologic lesions
    c. Syndrome is characterized by
      (1) Weight loss
      (2) Intermittent fever
      (3) Lethargy
      (4) Chronic diarrhea
      (5) Oral thrush
      (6) Lymphadenopathy
      (7) Anemia
      (8) Leukopenia
    d. Treatment is nonspecific and symptomatic.
    e. HIV is transmitted *in utero*.
      (1) Counseling for women carrier and high-risk persons
      (2) Testing for HIV for high-risk women
      (3) Education for drug users concerning risk of sharing needles

D. Drugs in Pregnancy
  1. Types
    a) Heroin and methadone (opioids)
      (1) These drugs cross placental barrier.

        (2)   Fetus is easily addicted.

        (3)   These drugs precipitate labor if there is sudden withdrawal in third trimester.

        (4)   Withdrawal symptoms appear in neonates.

        (5)   Breast feeding is not contraindicated.

   b)   Cortisone and sex hormones

        (1)   Are teratogenic

        (2)   Cause masculinization of external female genitalia

   c)   Diethylstilbesterol (DES)—may result in adenocarcinoma of vagina of female children

   d)   Thyroid drugs

        (1)   Cross placental barrier

        (2)   Can cause destruction of thyroid in fetus

   e)   Sedatives and analgesics

        (1)   Cross placental barrier

        (2)   Result in blood-coagulation abnormalities

   f)   Fetal alcohol syndrome

        (1)   Results when mother is heavy drinker

        (2)   Causes following signs and symptoms:

            (1)   Prenatal growth retardation

            (2)   Microcephaly

            (3)   Borderline mental deficiency

            (4)   Cardiovascular defects

            (5)   Failure to thrive

   g)   Tranquilizers

        (1)   Cross placental barrier

        (2)   May produce retinopathy in fetus

2.   Drug-withdrawal syndrome

   a)   Appearance

        (1)   Within 72 hours of birth if mother addicted to narcotics

        (2)   Within 7–10 days of birth if mother addicted to barbiturates

   b)   Results—symptoms of vomiting, diarrhea, sweating, irritability, convulsions, hyperventilation

   c)   Evaluation of home situation necessary before infant is discharged from hospital

   d)   Nursing care

        (1)   Try to discover what drugs mother has been taking so that withdrawal symptoms will be recognized.

        (2)   Be sure that infant has had prophylaxis against ophthalmia neonatorum.

        (3)   Collect urine for diagnosis within 24 hours.

        (4)   Monitor symptoms of withdrawal and treat appropriately.

            (a)   Tremors

            (b)   High-pitched crying

            (c)   Restlessness

            (d)   Inadequate feeding

               i)   Give small, frequent feedings.

               ii)   Maintain caloric and fluid intake for infant's desired weight.

            (e)   Vomiting/diarrhea

               i)   Position infant to prevent aspiration.

               ii)   Provide good skin care to prevent breakdown.

            (f)   Nasal stuffiness

               i)   Provide frequent nose and mouth care.

               ii)   Record respirations and infant's color.

            (g)   Respiratory distress

               i)   Place infant in semi-Fowler's position.

        ii)   Use respiratory monitor if necessary.
    (5)   Monitor results of drug therapy.
    (6)   Encourage parents to seek help and to be involved in care of child.

UNIT 3: LABOR AND DELIVERY

VOCABULARY

abortion	termination, spontaneous or induced, of pregnancy before 28th week of gestation
analgesia	insensibility to pain
colostrum	fluid secreted by mammary glands before onset of true lactation
contraction	shortening of muscle in normal response to nervous stimulus
delivery	extraction or expulsion of child at birth
dilation	stretching beyond normal dimensions
dry labor	one in which liquor amnii escapes too soon
dystocia	slow or painful delivery or birth
episiotomy	surgical incision of perineum at end of second stage of labor
expulsion	forcing out
fundus uteri	body of uterus above fallopian tubes
involution	return of uterus to its normal size after parturition
labor	function of female organism by which product of conception is expelled
lactation	secretion of milk by mammary glands
lochia	vaginal discharge after delivery
massage	systematic therapeutic friction, stroking, and kneading of the body
meconium	dark green fecal matter discharged by newborn
multipara	woman who has borne more than one child
neonatal	pertaining to the newborn
nullipara	woman who has never borne a child
perineum	area between anus and genital organs
placenta	oval structure in uterus through which fetus derives its nourishment
postpartum	occurring after delivery or childbirth
primipara	woman who has borne or who is giving birth to her first child
puerperium	period from delivery to completion of involution
stillbirth	birth of dead fetus

I.   **Important Goals of Obstetrical Nursing**

    A.   Primary Objectives of Nursing Care
        1.   Safety of mother and baby
        2.   Satisfaction of mother's physical and emotional needs

    B.   Secondary Objectives
        1.   Maintain asepsis.
           a)   Perineal shave
           b)   Enema
        2.   Check and record vital signs at regular intervals.
        3.   Encourage frequent voiding.
        4.   Encourage rest and relaxation to help avoid fatigue.
        5.   Offer fluids (unless contraindicated) to prevent dehydration.

6. Check fetal heart rate every half-hour during first stage of labor, check fetal heart rate after every contraction during second stage; check fetal heart rate immediately after rupture of membranes.
7. Time contractions and record patient's progress.
   a) Duration of contractions
   b) Interval between contractions
8. Watch for and report signs of fetal distress.
   a) Rapid, irregular, slow or absent fetal heart rate
   b) Meconium-stained vaginal leakage
   c) Hyperactivity
9. Watch for and report signs of maternal danger.
10. Record all important data pertaining to mother's care throughout labor.

II. Labor

A. Introduction
   1. Definition of **labor:** Process by which fetus, placenta, and membranes are expelled from woman's body
   2. Cause—medical science still does not know exact cause of labor; believed to be due to action of hormones
   3. Important facts
      a) Fetus, placenta, and membranes are expelled from pregnant woman's body after 38 to 40 weeks or 266 to 280 days' gestation
      b) Most desirable labor is a normal one in which termination occurs naturally without artificial aid or complications
      c) In case of premature labor, management of delivery and labor is same as in full-term labor; however, premature infant is susceptible to shock and other complications and must be handled with special precautions

B. Signs of Labor
   1. Lightening
      a) Infant descends into pelvis.
      b) Lightening may occur 2 weeks before labor.
      c) This is first sign of labor.
   2. Contractions (Braxton-Hicks sign)
      a) Are false contractions that are irregular and intermittent
      b) May occur 2 weeks before labor in primiparas and immediately before labor in multiparas
   3. Show
      a) Is release of mucous plug from cervix
      b) Has reddish tinge
   4. Rupture of membranes ("bag of waters")
      a) Is gush of water from vaginal tract
      b) May occur days or weeks before labor
   5. Regular contractions
      a) Occur closer together
      b) Are stronger

C. Stages of Labor
   1. First stage
      a) Cervix uteri dilates.
      b) First stage usually lasts 12–18 hours for first baby.
      c) Contractions occur every 10–15 minutes.

      d) Membranes rupture.

      e) Contractions begin to last longer.

  2. Second stage

      a) Fetus passes through birth canal.

      b) Second stage lasts from dilation of cervix to delivery of baby.

      c) Duration is 1–2 hours for first baby.

      d) Mother should be encouraged to relax between contractions.

  3. Third stage

      a) Placenta separates and is expelled.

      b) Duration is a few minutes.

      c) Third stage lasts from birth of baby to expulsion of placenta and membranes.

      d) Contraction of uterus controls bleeding.

D. Anesthetic Drugs Used During Labor and Delivery

  1. Anesthesia is generally ordered during labor and delivery, if mother does not wish to deliver by "natural birth."

  2. Type of anesthesia depends upon needs and condition of patient.

  3. Anesthetic may be given by inhalation, low spinal, saddle block, or caudal.

E. Admission of Patient in Labor

  1. Patient usually checks with doctor before reporting to hospital

  2. Physical preparation of patient varies with hospital; therefore, nurse must be familiar with routine of individual hospital.

  3. Practical nurse has the following responsibilities:

      a) Assist patient in undressing and getting into bed.

      b) Obtain necessary information concerning duration of pain, when pain began, whether membranes have ruptured, and previous labors if multipara.

      c) Follow doctor's orders concerning T.P.R., enemas, shaving of patient, fluid intake and output.

      d) Keep accurate record of pains and duration.

      e) Keep patient in bed after rupture of membranes.

      f) Calm and reassure patient.

      g) Observe patient closely.

      h) Provide emotional care, which includes assessing that all is progressing well.

F. Role of the Practical Nurse During Labor

  1. Take vital signs and record; report all unusual symptoms to R.N. immediately.

  2. Administer perineal prep.

  3. Check fetal heart and record.

  4. Observe for rupture of membrane.

  5. Note contractions—duration and frequency.

  6. Observe patient for any of the following unusual symptoms, and record:

      a) Change in vital signs

      b) Excessive bleeding

      c) Meconium in vaginal discharge

      d) Prolapsed cord

      e) Shock

      f) Exhaustion

      g) Dehydration

      h) Long, painful contractions

      i) Change in fetal heart rate

G. Complications of Labor and Delivery

1. Difficult labor (dystocia)
   a) Causes
      (1) Insufficiently strong contracting force
      (2) Abnormal position of fetus in uterus
      (3) Baby's being too large for birth canal
   b) Treatment—caesarean section if indicated
2. Abnormal presentation
3. Prolapsed umbilical cord
   a) This rare condition causes distress for baby.
   b) Patient's hips may be elevated to try to relieve pressure on cord.
4. Postpartum hemorrhage
   a) Cause—improper uterine involution (return to normal size) due to
      (1) Lacerations of cervix, vagina, or perineum
      (2) Retained fragments of placenta
   b) Lacerations—either first, second, or third degree
5. Multiple pregnancy
   a) Definition of **multiple pregnancy:** Condition in which two or more embryos develop at same time in uterus
   b) Types of twins
      (1) Fraternal or dizygotic—develop from two fertilized eggs; each embryo has its own placenta, amnion, and umbilical cord
      (2) Identical or monozygotic—develop from a single fertilized egg; one placenta exists, but there are two amnions and two umbilical cords
6. Abruptio placentae (premature separation of normally implanted placenta)
   a) Separation is complete or incomplete.
   b) Condition occurs in late months of pregnancy or at onset of labor.
   c) Cause is unknown
   d) Evident or concealed bleeding occurs.
7. Puerperal sepsis (infection in genital tract)
   a) Causes
      (1) Pathologic change in normal bacteria
      (2) Stretched, ruptured membranes
      (3) Prolonged labor
      (4) Traumatic delivery
      (5) Repeated examinations
      (6) Retention of placental fragments
      (7) Postpartum hemorrhage
   b) Diagnosis
      (1) Continuous high fever
      (2) Chills, headaches, malaise
      (3) High leucocytosis
      (4) Tachycardia
      (5) Soft, tender uterus
   c) Treatment
      (1) Antibiotics
      (2) Closely supervised physician followup
8. Placenta previa   See Unit 2, Section 1.B.

III. **Routine Delivery (Practical nurse may assist doctor or R.N. in delivery room)**

A. Nursing Procedure in Delivery Room
   1. Patient is placed in modified lithotomy position; sterile strict asepsis is adhered to.
      a) Preparation of pudendum: vulva and perineum shaved aseptically

    b) Sterile draping of patient, exposing only introitus
2. Patient is catheterized to prevent distension of bladder.
3. Patient is urged to push with her contractions.
4. Anesthesia, if administered by inhalation, is given; vital signs are checked.
5. Episiotomy, if necessary, is performed as head crowns.
6. Baby's mouth and nose are suctioned after delivery of head in order to remove mucus.
7. Anesthesia is discontinued; mother is given oxygen to stimulate baby's breathing.
8. After respiration is established, delivery is completed.
9. Baby is placed on mother's abdomen.
10. Cord is clamped and cut.
11. Baby is wrapped in sterile garment and placed in incubator.
12. Physician expresses placenta as it begins to separate from uterus.
13. Physician examines placenta to determine if any has remained in uterus.
14. Injection of pituitary extract is given to mother to stimulate tight contractions of uterus.
15. Nurse should examine fundus to note any changes in size or consistency.
16. If episiotomy has been performed, it is repaired.
17. Nurse cleans vulva and perineal area; a sterile perineal pad is applied.
18. Mother is returned to her room when she is out of danger.

B. Immediate Care of Mother
    1. Allow mother to rest.
    2. Check blood pressure, pulse, and respiration often until they are stabilized.
    3. Check fundus for firmness and level.
    4. Encourage mother to void.
    5. Offer fluids; if patient complains of hunger, a light diet may be given.
    6. Reassure mother that she and her baby are in good condition (if they are); fathers are permitted to visit.
    7. Report any change in patient's condition.
    8. Record vital signs and all other pertinent information concerning patient.

C. Immediate Care of Newborn Following Delivery
    1. Use proper method for identification of new baby (method used depends on hospital).
    2. Take care of baby's eyes—1% solution silver nitrate or penicillin drops instilled into each eye to prevent blindness caused by gonorrhea (required by law in most states).
    3. Check umbilical cord for bleeding.
    4. Appraise newborn 1 minute after delivery and again at 5 minutes—Apgar score (see Data Summary 17, Chapter VI, Unit 1).
    5. Place infant in supine position with head slightly lowered.
        a) Administer vitamin K if physician orders it.
        b) Aspirate mucus from nose and throat.
    6. Transfer infant to nursery.

D. Drugs Used during Labor
    1. Uses
        a) To prevent complications
        b) To treat emergencies following instrumental vaginal delivery
    2. Types
        a) Sedatives—secobarbital may be given early in labor, followed by meperidine or morphine when progress is more advanced
        b) Inhalant analgesics—Trilene and nitrous oxide
        c) Narcotic analgesics—Demerol (meperidine), Trilene, secobarbital
        d) Pitocin—for hemorrhage

e) Ergotrate—in vertex presentations
f) Oxygen p.r.n.
g) I.V. fluids—have available
h) Ready source of cross-matched or O-negative blood

IV. **Surgical Procedures Used in Connection with Delivery**

A. Use
1. Some type of surgery may be necessary.
2. Doctor determines whether surgery is necessary and whether delivery will be normal or abnormal.

B. Episiotomy and Repairs
1. Perineum is cut in order to permit delivery of baby without lacerations.
2. Episiotomy is sutured following delivery.

C. Forceps Delivery
1. Doctor assists baby through birth canal, using obstetrical forceps.
2. Forceps (and episiotomy) are often used for primaparas.
3. Forceps may harm baby if applied incorrectly.

D. Caesarean Section
1. The abdomen and uterus are opened in order to deliver baby.
2. After removal of placenta, uterus and abdomen are sutured.
3. Delivery by cesarean section requires special care of baby.

E. Version
1. Baby is turned in uterus from undesirable to desirable position.
2. Version may be external or internal.

UNIT 4: POSTPARTUM CARE

VOCABULARY

abnormal	deviating from normal
afterpains	pains that follow childbirth
apprehension	fear or anxiety
diminution	act of lessening; making smaller
distend	to stretch or spread in all directions; to dilate; to enlarge
embryo	human organism in first 3 months after conception; thereafter called a *fetus*
gynecology	branch of medicine dealing with the study and treatment of women's diseases
hypnosis	artificially induced state resembling a trance or sleep
hypnotic	any medicine causing sleep
incise	to cut
laceration	wound caused by tearing of tissues

I. **Puerperium**

A. Introduction
1. Definition of **puerperium:** Time from end of labor to return of genital organs to normal
2. Duration—varies from 6 to 8 weeks

NURSING CARE OF THE OBSTETRICAL PATIENT

    B. Physiological Changes

        1. Breasts

            a) Breasts secrete colostrum during first few days after delivery.

            b) Lactation begins between second and fourth day.

            c) Medication can be given to dry up breasts if mother cannot or does not wish to nurse.

        2. Uterus

            a) Involution, i.e., process by which uterus returns to its normal state, occurs.

            b) Uterus decreases to normal size in approximately 6 weeks.

            c) Involution entails the following:

                (1) Firming of uterus

                (2) Descent of uterus into pelvis

                (3) Normal lochia (see Section 1.6 below)

        3. Vagina—returns to normal within 4–6 weeks

        4. Perineum—returns to normal within 1 week

        5. Abdomen

            a) Striae on abdominal walls do not usually remain.

            b) Abdominal muscles regain tone.

        6. Lochia

            a) Definition of **lochia:** Discharge from uterus after childbirth

            b) Character

                (1) Lochia rubra—bright red because of blood from placental site, mucus, and decidua

                (2) Lochia serosa—brownish red because of serum from healing surfaces

                (3) Lochia alba—yellowish white

        7. Afterpains

            a) Cause—contractions and relaxations of uterus

            b) Occurrence

                (1) More frequent in multiparas

                (2) Frequent in mothers who are breast feeding

            c) Treatment

                (1) Administering analgesics

                (2) Explaining cause of pains to mother and reassuring her

        8. Return of menstruation

            a) Occurs in 6–8 weeks if mother is not breast feeding

            b) Occurs in 4–5 months if mother is breast feeding

II. Nursing Care

    A. Hospital Care

        1. Daily observation of

            a) Uterus—for height, consistency, and size

            b) Lochia—for amount, color, and consistency

            c) Perineum—observed to monitor healing process and to detect infection

            d) Mother's emotional attitude

        2. Perineal care

            a) Purpose is to keep mother clean and to prevent infection.

            b) Procedure is determined by hospital.

        3. Bladder care

            a) Patient is encouraged to void regularly.

            b) Catheterization is used only if patient is unable to void.

            c) Urine output is greater than normal.

        4. Elimination

      a) Constipation is likely to occur.

      b) Elimination should be regulated by diet, fluid intake, and establishing regular pattern of elimination.

   5. Activity

      a) Bed activity is encouraged.

      b) Activities out of bed are regulated by physician.

B. Education of Mother

   1. Purpose—to enable her to care for herself and her baby

   2. Emphasis placed on

      a) Cleanliness

         (1) Daily shower should be taken for comfort.

         (2) Tub baths are permissible after a few weeks' time.

         (3) Daily perineal care should be administered.

         (4) The hair should be shampooed as needed.

         (5) All aspects of personal hygiene, including care of the hands and feet, are important.

      b) Diet

         (1) Patient is advised on proper diet.

         (2) Well-balanced diet is essential to promote healing and ensure good health.

         (3) Green leafy vegetables, lean meats, citrus fruits, liquids, and milk are absolutely essential.

         (4) Vitamin and mineral supplements may be prescribed by physician.

      c) Rest and exercise

         (1) Quiet room and clean, dry bed are essential

         (2) Rest periods during day are necessary.

         (3) Adequate sleep is needed; at least 8 hours recommended.

         (4) Daily exercise in form of walking is recommended.

         (5) Special exercises to promote muscle tone of abdomen may be prescribed by doctor.

      d) Elimination

         (1) Cleansing enema may be ordered on third day after delivery.

         (2) Patient is encouraged to void to prevent distended bladder.

      e) Breast care

         (1) Breasts are bathed when bath is given (breasts are first part of body washed).

         (2) Doctor may order special ointment for nipples (if indicated).

         (3) A good, well-fitted brassiere will give necessary support and prevent muscle stretching.

         (4) Postpartum examination is scheduled by doctor, usually 6 weeks after delivery.

III. Postpartum Complications

A. Infection

   1. Infection is caused by bacteria generally located in lower genital tract and rectum.

   2. Puerperal infection is often caused by staphylococcus and streptococcus.

   3. Hospital personnel working in maternity wards must be free from infections.

B. Mastitis (Inflammation of Breast Glands)

   1. Cause—bacteria that enter through cracks or fissures in nipples

   2. Occurrence—most frequent during third to fourth week after delivery

    3. Assessment
       a) Temperature is elevated.
       b) Breasts become red and hard.
    4. Treatment
       a) Discontinuation of breast feeding
       b) Application of ice packs
       c) Antibiotics
       d) Incision if abscess forms

C. Thrombophlebitis—usually occurs in leg
    1. Assessment—affected area turns white and becomes swollen and painful
    2. Treatment
       a) Treatment is according to doctor's orders.
       b) Affected part should not be rubbed or massaged.

D. Depressed Mental State of Mother
    1. If mother is insecure about ability to care for infant, report concerns to R.N.
    2. Assist in providing necessary information as to infant care.
    3. Reassure mother that she is capable of caring for infant.

E. Postpartum Hemorrhage
    1. Proper monitoring of fundus during hours immediately after delivery will ensure that early symptoms, which should be reported immediately, are noted.
    2. Uterine and vaginal packing may be necessary.

F. Puerperal Sepsis
    1. Prevention is best defense against puerperal infection.
    2. Asepsis techniques during labor and throughout puerperium will prevent puerperal infection.
    3. The following symptoms of infection must be reported immediately:
       a) Fever (temperature over 100.4° F or 38° C)
       b) Local tenderness or pain
       c) Green or yellow lochia
       d) Unusual foul odor
    4. Antibiotics and sulfonamide therapy may be necessary, depending upon type of organism causing infection.

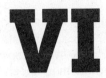

VI

Nursing Care of the Pediatric Patient

UNIT 1: THE FULL-TERM NEWBORN

VOCABULARY

birth canal	vagina
circumcision	surgical removal of foreskin of penis
cleft lip	fissure or opening in upper lip
cleft palate	fissure in midline of roof of mouth
fontanel	unossified spot in cranium of a newborn infant
heredity	transmission of physical or mental traits from parents to their progeny; hereditary material is in nucleus of sperm and ovum
immunize	to render immune to particular disease by promoting specific antibody formation in body
impetigo	infectious disease of skin caused by staphylococci or streptococci
ophthalmia neonatorum	acute conjunctivitis in newborn, caused by gonococci or gonorrhea
pediatrician	physician who specializes in treatment of infants and children
pediatrics	branch of medical science concerned with hygienic care of infants and children and treatment of diseases peculiar to them
resuscitation	measure used to promote adequate oxygenation
spina bifida	congenital defect: imperfect closure of spinal canal
vernix caseosa	cheeselike substance that covers skin of newborn

I. **Care of the Newborn**

  A. Introduction
    1. Most critical period for newborn is immediately after birth.
    2. Change from life within uterus to independent life outside uterus is traumatic.

  B. Immediate Care
    1. Purpose—to assist newborn in meeting basic needs
    2. Measures included
      a) Cord stump—inspected frequently for bleeding; dressing may or may not be applied
      b) Eyes—silver nitrate or antibiotic drops instilled
      c) Airway—nose and mouth suctioned to remove accumulated mucus and amniotic fluid
      d) Inspection
        (1) Weight—average at birth 7–7½ lbs.
        (2) Length—average at birth 19–21 inches

    (3) Temperature—rectal 98°–99°F

    (4) Recording of Apgar score (see Data summary 16)

   e) Birth registration—mandatory in all hospitals; handprints or footprints are made and name bracelets attached (method depends on hospital)

  3. Transfer to nursery or to mother's room (rooming-in) if mother is to care for her newborn baby at her bedside

   a) Special units are available for rooming-in babies with their mothers.

   b) Newborn infant receives specialized, individualized attention from parents.

   c) Mother is relieved of worry about care her child is receiving.

   d) Parents can learn many techniques of baby care from hospital staff through rooming-in.

DATA SUMMARY 16
Apgar Score of Newborn Infant

		Score		
	Item	0	1	2
A	Appearance (color)	Blue, pale	Body pink, extremities blue	Completely pink
P	Pulse (heart rate)	Absent	Below 100	Over 100
G	Grimace (irritability reflex in response to stimulation of sole of foot)	No response	Grimace	Cry
A	Activity (muscle tone)	Limp	Some flexion of extremities	Active motion
R	Respiration (respiratory effort)	Absent	Slow, irregular	Strong cry

---

II. General Characteristics of the Newborn

 A. Weight

  1. Range is 6½–9½ pounds (2,900-4,000 grams).

  2. Ten percent of this weight is lost in a few days; regained in next 10 days.

 B. Length—18–22 inches (45–55 cm)

 C. Temperature—98°–99°F (97°–100° F at birth)

 D. Skin

  1. Body is covered by vernix caseosa.

  2. Part of body is covered with lanugo.

  3. Thinness of skin may result in peeling on the trunk and the extremities.

  4. Skin becomes normal within 2 weeks.

 E. Body Color

   a) Prominence of superficial veins

   b) Mottled look

   c) Ruddy complexion

   d) Poor circulation in extremities, making them appear cyanotic

NURSING CARE OF THE PEDIATRIC PATIENT

F. Head
  1. Circumference of head is 12½–14 inches.
  2. Head accounts for one-fourth of total body length.
  3. Two soft spots anterior and posterior fontanels, are due to skull bones not having united yet.
     a) Anterior fontanel ossified within 12–18 months
     b) Posterior fontanel ossified at 2 months

G. Face
  1. Eyes
     a) Are expressionless; closed most of the time
     b) May seem to be crossed because of weak muscles
     c) Are blue-gray in color
  2. Nose—flat, pudgy
  3. Lower jaw—appears to be receding
  4. Tongue—extends only as far as gums

H. Neck
  1. Is short
  2. Has weak muscles that cannot support head

I. Chest
  1. Chest is round.
  2. Breasts may be engorged because of hormones transmitted from mother via placenta.

J. Abdomen
  1. Is round
  2. Protrudes because of size of enclosed organs
  3. Moves when baby breathes

K. Extremities
  1. Arms and legs are in fetal position (flexed).
  2. Hands are semiclosed.
  3. Legs are bowed.
  4. There are continuous, purposeless movements of extremities when baby is awake.

L. Bones—are soft

III. **Newborn's Responses to Internal and External Stimuli**

A. Sight
  1. Turns eyes to light
  2. Cannot focus until after 3 months

B. Pressure: soothing effect produced by stroking and patting

C. Hearing: delayed for several days

D. Taste: aware of strong tastes (bitter, sweet)

E. Thirst: present from beginning and demands satisfaction

F. Hunger: not always present at birth, but soon experienced

    G. Temperature: sensitive to cold and warmth

    H. Comfort: wants to be warm, fed, and unhampered in movements

    I. Discomfort: dislikes being cold, hungry, or restricted in movements

IV. Newborn's Sleep Needs and Development

    A. Sleep: newborn sleeps 20 out of 24 hours

    B. Development
       1. Builds new movements and perfects those he/she already has
       2. Finds more meaning in the world about him/her
       3. Makes connection between what he/she sees and what he/she does
       4. Later modifies his/her actions by intentional responses

V. Physiological Aspects

    A. Reflexes
       1. Has sucking and rooting reflexes
       2. Can cough, sneeze, cry, and yawn

    B. Elimination
       1. Newborn can void and pass stools.
       2. First stools are called meconium.
          a) Dark green
          b) Thick
          c) Sticky

    C. Respiration
       1. 40-60 minute
       2. Irregular

    D. Pulse
       1. 100-150 per minute
       2. Irregular

    E. Body Temperature
       1. Body temperature is normally 1° higher than that of an adult.
       2. Newborn's unit must be kept at constant temperature in order to maintain body heat.

    F. Body Movements
       1. Body movements are disorganized.
       2. Muscle tone is good.
       3. Constant, aimless moving is due to rapid growth of nerve center or to other internal stimuli.

VI. Daily Care

    A. Daily Bath
       1. Bath serves to clean skin and stimulate circulation.
       2. Routine varies according to hospital.
          a) Wash head with mild cleansing agent.

   b)   Use only water to cleanse eyelids—wipe from inner canthus outward.
   c)   Cleanse cord base with 70% alcohol—report unusual characteristics.
3.   Sponge baths are given until cord heals—tub baths usually not permitted until after navel heals.
4.   Safety precautions must be observed when giving bath.
   a)   Prepare all equipment beforehand; protect baby from drafts.
   b)   Have room temperature at 75°–80°F.
   c)   Check water temperature with thermometer; should be 90°–100°F.
   d)   Support baby's head.
   e)   Use soft towel and washcloth.
   f)   Completely rinse and dry newborn.
   g)   Cleanse area around foreskin of males; if newborn has been circumcised, follow hospital procedure.
   h)   Observe carefully for skin irritation or skin abnormalities; report any such observations immediately.

B.   Weight
   1.   Baby is weighed daily while in hospital.
   2.   Ten percent of birth weight is usually lost by end of 3–4 days; loss is regained by end of second week.
   3.   Weight is reported and recorded daily.

C.   Elimination
   1.   Urine is usually pale yellow; newborn usually voids 12–15 times daily.
   2.   Stool (meconium) is passed 4–5 times daily.

D.   Feedings
   1.   Breast feeding
   a)   Baby is taken to mother for nursing unless contraindicated
   b)   Breast feeding is easiest, simplest, and most inexpensive way to feed baby.
   c)   Mother's milk and colostrum provide substances that protect baby from disease.
   d)   Breast feeding is emotionally satisfying experience for mother and child.
   e)   Putting baby to breast during period that colostrum is secreted stimulates milk secretion.
   f)   Mother must be comfortable during nursing.
   g)   Mother must be instructed in care of breast and provided with appropriate equipment.
   2.   Bottle feeding
   a)   Formula prescribed by doctor is determined by weight and condition of baby
   b)   Formula is fed for 3 or 4 months
   c)   Formula and all utensils used in preparing formula are sterilized before they are given to newborn.
   d)   Newborn should be held during bottle feeding just as if he/she were being breast-fed.

E.   Recording of All Observations
   1.   Respirations—rate and rhythm
   2.   Stools—color and consistency, number of movements
   3.   Voiding—frequency and color
   4.   Alignment of body
   5.   Sound of cry
   6.   Reactions to noises and movements
   7.   Weight loss and/or weight gain

8. Color of body, extremities, face
9. Color and moistness of mouth

F. Nursing Care of the Neonate
   1. Delivery room
      a) Mucus is wiped or suctioned out of mouth.
      b) Apgar scoring is done by physician at 1 minute and 5 minutes.
      c) Identification procedures are carried out.
      d) One percent silver nitrate or ophthalmic antibiotic solution is dropped in eyes.
   2. Nursery
      a) Bland oil bath is given to remove vernix caseosa.
      b) Temperature is taken rectally.
      c) Neonate is measured: length, circumference of head and chest.
      d) Neonate is dressed.
      e) Neonate is placed in incubator for a few hours.
      f) Neonate is observed closely for cyanosis.

VII. Disorders of the Newborn

A. Atelectasis
   1. Definition of **atelectasis:** Incomplete expansion of lungs
   2. Causes
      a) Obstruction of bronchi
      b) Aspiration of mucus or amniotic fluid
   3. Assessment
      a) Shallow, rapid respirations
      b) Mostly abdominal respirations
      c) Cyanosis
      d) Respiratory grunt
   4. Nursing care—follow treatment ordered by physician

B. Asphyxia Neonatorum
   1. Definition of **asphyxia neonatorum:** Obstruction of air passages by mucus or amniotic fluid
   2. Type—may be mild or severe
   3. Assessment
      a) Congested appearance
      b) Cyanosis
      c) Slow pulse
      d) Symptoms of asphyxia—blue lips, pale appearance, weak rapid heart beat
   4. Treatment
      a) Stimulation of respiration
      b) Application of principles of resuscitation
   5. Nursing care—follow treatment ordered by physician

C. Cephalhematoma
   1. Definition of **cephalhematoma:** Hemorrhage beneath the periosteum; occurs most often under parietal bones
   2. Causes
      a) Birth injury
      b) Injury from forceps delivery; occurs frequently after forceps delivery
   3. Symptoms—swelling of scalp
   4. Treatment—no specific treatment since swelling usually disappears in 6–8 weeks

5. Nursing care—close observation of infant

D. Facial Paralysis
   1. Causes—usually, force exerted by forceps during delivery
   2. Symptoms—paralysis of face muscles on one side that is most noticeable when baby is crying or feeding, and usually disappears within a few days

E. Hemorrhagic Disease of the Newborn
   1. Types—internal and external bleeding
   2. Assessment
      a) Increased bleeding and clotting time
      b) Decreased number of platelets
      c) Vomitus with blood stains
      d) Bleeding from cord stump or skin
      e) In severe cases, fever, anemia, cyanosis, and convulsions
   3. Treatment—Newborn usually responds quickly to blood transfusions and dosages of vitamin K

F. Hemorrhaging from Cord
   1. Cause—slipping of cord tie or clamp
   2. Treatment—application of new ligature or clamp

G. Ophthalmia Neonatorum
   1. Definition of **ophthalmia neonatorum:** Any conjunctivitis in newborn
   2. Causes
      a) Chemical conjunctivitis due to silver nitrate
      b) Infectious conjunctivitis due to staphylococci, pneumococci, or gonococci (appears during 2nd-5th day postpartum)
      c) Inclusion conjunctivitis (appears during 5th-10th day postpartum)
   3. Assessment
      a) Inflammation of eyes
      b) Redness or swelling of lids
      c) Discharge
   4. Procedure—isolation precautions are taken, and appropriate treatment is given

H. Icterus Neonatorum
   1. Definition of **icterus neonatorum:** Physiologic jaundice
   2. Cause—immature liver functions and increased destruction of red blood cells during first 2 weeks of life
   3. Symptom—jaundice appearing on 3rd–5th day of life
   4. Duration—usually only a few days; jaundice continuing beyond 2 weeks indicates abnormality

I. Erythema Toxicans
   1. Definition of **erythema toxicans:** Newborn rash
   2. Cause—unknown
   3. Symptom—blotchy rash appearing on back, shoulders, or buttocks
   4. Duration—usually only a few days

J. Thrush (Candidiasis)
   1. Definition of **thrush:** Infection caused by a *Candida* species of fungus
   2. Transmission—by nipples, vagina, or poor hygienic procedures
   3. Diagnosis—by laboratory test

4. Preventive measures
   a) Immediate postpartum care of mouth
   b) Adequate cleaning of mother's nipples (or bottle nipples) before feeding
   c) Washing hands before handling baby
5. Treatment
   a) Observe and inspect neonate's mouth daily.
   b) Take adequate precautions when using feeding apparatus or touching neonate.
   c) Give medications ordered by physician.

K. Erythroblastosis Fetalis
   1. Definition of **erythroblastosis fetalis:** Hemolytic disease of newborn, characterized by excessive destruction of red blood cells; becomes apparent late in fetal life or soon after birth
   2. Cause—incompatibility between mother's blood and fetus's blood
      a) Rh-negative mother who
         (1) Has had more than one previous pregnancy resulting in an Rh-positive child
         (2) Has been previously transfused with Rh-positive blood
      b) Rh-positive fetus
   3. Prevention
      a) Typing of mother's blood
      b) Administration of anti-Rh gamma globulins (Rho-gam) to mother 72 hours postpartum to protect future Rh-positive children
      c) Amniotic fluid spectrophotometry—small amount of amniotic fluid withdrawn for analysis
      d) Intrauterine transfusion as preventive measure
   4. Assessment
      a) Pathologic jaundice—evident within 24 hours
      b) Anemia
      c) Enlarged liver and spleen if untreated
      d) Extensive edema if untreated
   5. Treatment
      a) Exchange transfusions administered by physician
      b) Repeated small transfusions at later time
      c) Antibiotics to prevent infection
   6. Nursing care
      a) Observe newborn's color, vital signs, urine, skin—report all changes immediately.
      b) Report any evidence of jaundice during first and second day.
      c) Apply sterile, wet compresses to umbilicus to maintain I.V. access.

L. Phenylketonuria (PKU)
   1. Definition of **PKU:** Metabolic defect due to lack of development of hepatic enzyme phenylalanine
   2. Incidence—affects approximately 0.004% of population
   3. Assessment
      a) Progressive failure of mental development observed by age 5-6 months (infant appears normal at birth)
      b) Neurological disturbances
      c) Altered skin pigmentation
      d) Eczema susceptibility
      e) Musty-odored urine
      f) Tremor and seizures in later stages if untreated
      g) Severe retardation if untreated
   4. Diagnostic tests

      a) Newborn blood sample is taken to determine phenylalanine level.

      b) Special paper is used to test urine to determine phenylalanine level.

  5. Treatment

      a) Special diet is begun soon after birth—prepared commercially low in phenylalanine.

      b) Blood levels of phenylalanine are monitored.

UNIT 2: THE PREMATURE INFANT

VOCABULARY

aspiration	withdrawing of fluid from a cavity by suction
assimilate	to absorb digested food
gestation	period of intrauterine fetal development
immature	not fully developed
incubator	apparatus with regulated temperature for premature babies to live in
lanugo	fine hair on body of fetus
regurgitation	return of food from stomach soon after eating without effort of vomiting
resuscitation	act of bringing an individual back to full consciousness
thrush	fungal infection of mucous membranes of mouth
twitch	simple, quick, spasmodic contraction of a muscle

I. **Introduction**

  A. Criteria for Prematurity
    1. Birth before 37–38th week of gestation
    2. Birth weight of less than 5½ pounds (2,500 grams)

  B. General Principles
    1. Prematurity is leading cause of death in newborn period.
    2. Of premature babies, 12–20% do not survive.

  C. Causes
    1. In many cases, unknown factors
    2. Numerous predisposing causes
    3. Multiple births
    4. Illness of mother—heart disease, infectious conditions, malnutrition, diabetes mellitus, and hazards of pregnancy

  D. Physical Characteristics of Premature Infant
    1. Physical characteristics depend upon age in weeks.
    2. Lanugo may cover entire body; vernix caseosa is absent.
    3. There is poor control of body temperature.
    4. Organs of body are immature.
    5. Body system is not functioning to capacity.
    6. Respiration is impaired
    7. Sucking and swallowing are weak.
    8. Kidneys are not functioning to capacity.
    9. Skin is thin and transparent, and may be red.
    10. Skin and mucous membranes are not functioning well.

NURSING CARE OF THE PEDIATRIC PATIENT

    11. The infant is more susceptible to infection.
    12. Cry is a weak whine.

II. Nursing Care

A. General Principles
    1. Practical nurse assists in care of premature infants.
    2. Care must be skillfully and carefully planned by health team.
    3. All observations must be included on nurse's notes.
    4. Care is supervised by R.N. with special training.

B. Specific Measures
    1. Handle infant as little as possible.
    2. Maintain body temperature in range of 97°–99° F.
    3. Maintain constant temperature 80°–90° F and humidity 40%–60% in the incubator.
    4. Record temperature of incubator each time temperature of baby is taken.
    5. Give oxygen only when ordered by doctor, and give prescribed concentration.
    6. Take care that feeding is careful and unhurried; use sterile equipment.
    7. Be aware that formula and method of feeding are ordered on individual basis.
    8. If necessary, gently suction mucus from throat between feedings.
    9. Check carefully after feeding to see that no formula, which might be aspirated, is left in mouth or throat.
    10. Usually, give oil baths 2–3 times weekly (this reduces handling).
    11. Cleanse diaper area daily with oil as necessary.
    12. Provide psychosocial support to parents.

III. Prevention of Infections

A. Procedures
    1. Wash hands (scrub).
    2. Wear cap, gown, and mask to enter nursery.
    3. Follow modified form of isolation technique each time you enter nursery.
    4. Sterilize all linen and equipment before use.
    5. See that formula is prepared properly and stored for use.
    6. Dispose of waste and soiled linen immediately.
    7. Keep nursery meticulously clean.
    8. Observe regulations of individual nursery.
    9. Enforce rules of your nursery.
    10. Wash hands before and after procedures or treatments given to infant.

IV. Discharge

A. Time of Discharge
    1. Depends on regulations of individual nursery
    2. Depends on general condition of infant

B. Usual Weight on Discharge from Premature Unit—between 5½ and 6 pounds

UNIT 3: THE INFANT

VOCABULARY

acute   appearing suddenly and lasting a short time
allergic   hypersensitive to substances that are usually innocuous

chronic	occurring frequently and lasting a long time
convalesce	to recover one's health after illness
cramp	painful, involuntary spasmodic muscle contraction
deciduous teeth	temporary teeth
deformity	physical distortion or malformation of any part of body
immune	not susceptible to specific disease
immunization	process of acquiring immunity; introduction of specific antigens to stimulate antibody production in body
infant	child in first year of life
inhalator	device used to aid breathing
malaise	sense of discomfort that accompanies onset of disease
nutrition	processes involved in utilization of food
pasteurize	to kill pathogenic microorganisms and inhibit other bacterial growth in food substances by exposure to temperatures of 60°C (140°F) for 30 minutes
sleep	natural periodic suspension of consciousness during which body regenerates itself
superficial	affecting surface only
symptom	subjective change indicative of body disorder or disease
treatment	medical and nursing management and care of patient
ulceration	necrotic inflammation of skin or mucous membranes and suppuration of surrounding area
vaccine	preparation of killed or attenuated microorganisms used to develop immunity to specific disease
virus	microscopic agent that causes disease

I. Introduction

    A. General Characteristics
        1. Infancy is a time of rapid growth and development.
        2. Infant is at oral stage of personality development, that is, sucking is important action that gives comfort and relief.
        3. Deciduous (milk) teeth erupt.
            a) Develop during fifth month of intrauterine life
            b) Appear between 4-6 months and 30 months of age
            c) Must not be neglected
        4. Permanent teeth develop just before birth and up to age 1.
        5. Development of teeth is influenced by proper diet.
            a) Mother—adequate balanced diet is essential during pregnancy.
            b) Infant—daily diet must meet growth and development needs.

    B. Nursing Care
        1. Infant should be held during feedings; if fed intravenously, infant needs extra attention.
        2. Infant's needs should be met promptly; promotes development of sense of trust.
        3. Wet or soiled diapers should be changed as soon as possible.
        4. The manner in which infant is fed or bathed is more important than exactness of procedure.

    C. Factors Influencing Rate of Growth and Development
        1. Heredity
        2. Sex
        3. Diet
        4. Manner in which basic and secondary needs are met

    5. Prenatal care
    6. Social conditions

II. Infant Development

  A. Stages and Care Required
    1. One month
      a) Weight—approximately 8 pounds
      b) Height—grows approximately 1 inch per month
      c) Can lift head slightly when lying on stomach; head should be supported when holding infant
      d) Clenches fists and stares
      e) Cries when hungry or uncomfortable; needs should be met immediately
      f) Sleeps most of the day and night; should sleep on stomach without pillow
      g) Should be fed when hungry; each infant establishes his/her own pattern
      h) Should have fresh air and sunshine as often as possible
    2. Two months
      a) Soft spots begin to disappear (posterior fontanel closes).
      b) Infant can hold a rattle briefly.
      c) Legs are active
      d) Individualized sleeping pattern develops.
      e) Infant may begin to eat solid foods; food should be placed on back of tongue (follow advice of pediatrician or pediatric nurse practitioner).
      f) Infant needs to have a place to exercise and move about.
      g) Physical examination is indicated
      h) Inoculations against diphtheria, whooping cough, tetanus, and polio are usually given (see Data Summary 17 and Table 2 of the Appendix); DPT and polio schedule vary with individual doctors.
    3. Three months
      a) Weight—10–13 pounds
      b) Can move hand to mouth
      c) Can support head steadily
      d) Takes spontaneous naps and will nap in someone's arms
      3) Enjoys being talked to
      f) Needs short play periods
    4. Four months
      a) Weight—10–14 pounds
      b) Has eye-to-body coordination
      c) Can lift head and shoulders when lying on stomach
      d) Is able to sit with support
      e) Responds to people, laughs aloud
      f) Is able to sleep despite presence of noises
      g) May have egg yolk added to diet
      h) Plays with dangling toys and rattles
      i) Needs second DPT and polio immunizations.
    5. Five months
      a) Weight—12–15 pounds
      b) Is capable of grasping objects handed to him/her
      c) Seems to put everything in mouth
      d) Seems to distinguish between familiar and strange people and things
    6. Six months
      a) Weight—double birth weight; gains 3–5 ounces each week
      b) Height—grows about ½ inch each month

    c) Is able to sit alone momentarily
    d) Has an increased interest in activities around him/her
    e) Enjoy splashing during tub baths
    f) Receives third DPT immunization
7. Seven months
    a) Cuts first deciduous teeth
    b) Begins to crawl
    c) Changes moods easily
    d) May sleep restlessly because of teething discomfort
    e) Sleeps about 12 hours at night

DATA SUMMARY 17 Immunization Schedule Recommended by New York State Department of Health							
Immunization	2 Months	4 Months	6 Months	15 Months	18 Months	4–6 Years	Every 10 Years
Polio* OPV	√	√		√		√	
Diphtheria*- tetanus- pertussis DTP (Whooping Cough)	√	√	√	√		√	
Measles*- mumps*- MMR rubella*				√		√†	
Tetanus- diphtheria Adult booster Td							√
Haemophilus* influenzae Hib (type b)					√		

*Required for school attendance. Hib vaccine required as of January 1, 1990, for children 18 months to 5 years in daycare or any preschool program.
†As of September 1990 kindergarten children are required to demonstrate receipt of TWO doses of measles vaccine (MMR vaccine preferred for both doses). Thereafter, children born on or after January 1, 1985, will be required to have two doses for school attendance. Measles (two doses), mumps, and rubella vaccines are required for college attendance as of August 1, 1990.

    f) Needs finger foods added to diet
    g) Needs second polio vaccine if not previously received (see Table 2 of the Appendix)
8. Eight months
    a) Can sit steadily if unsupported
    b) Can use thumb and index finger like pincers
    c) Can amuse him-/herself for longer time periods

        d)   Fusses when sleepy; takes two naps a day

        e)   Can ride in a stroller

        f)   Likes to play with stuffed, squeaky, or rattling toys

  9. Nine months

        a)   Begins to favor use of one hand

        b)   Can hold a bottle

        c)   Tries to imitate sounds, but not words

        d)   Should have chopped and mashed foods introduced into diet

  10. Ten months

        a)   Can stand holding onto playpen

        b)   Knows own name

        c)   Can play simple games

        d)   Can drink from a cup

        e)   Tolerates solid foods well

  11. Eleven months

        a)   Can stand upright when holding onto someone's hand

        b)   Understands simple directions

        c)   Enjoys gross motor activity and playing with toys

  12. Twelve months

        a)   Weight—approximately three times birth weight

        b)   Height—approximately 29 inches

        c)   Vital signs

            (1)   Pulse—100-140 per minute

            (2)   Respirations—20-40 per minute

        d)   Has six teeth

        e)   Can eat with a spoon and drink from a cup; plays with food

        f)   Can stand alone for short periods

        g)   Will repeat actions that receive a favorable response

        h)   Shows emotions—fear, jealousy

        i)   Takes a long nap each day

  13. Fifteen months—polio, DTP, and MMR (measles, mumps, rubella) vaccines may be given

III. Hospitalization of the Infant

  A. Very Frustrating Experience for Infant
    1. Infant is not used to being separated from parents.
    2. Infant is used to receiving a lot of attention.
    3. Infant must readjust daily routine.

  B. Nurse's Responsibility and Interventions
    1. Make hospitalization as easy as possible for both infant and parents.
    2. Give infant attention, warmth, and affection.
    3. Coax infant into eating and sleeping.
    4. Make parents feel that they are still needed by their child.
    5. Do not take over mother's role and become overattached to infant.
    6. Encourage mother to stay and care for baby.
    7. Help parents to work through their anxieties.
    8. Attempt to adjust hospital schedule to home routines.

IV. Infant Disorders

  A. The Common Cold

1. Definition of **cold:** Infection of nasal passages and upper respiratory tract
2. Cause—viruses, spread from one person to another by
    a) Coughing
    b) Sneezing
    c) Direct contact
    d) Contaminated materials or items
3. Susceptibility to infection—determined by
    a) General health
    b) Fatigue
    c) Nutritional health
    d) Age
    e) Emotional health
4. Assessment
    a) Fever
    b) Nasal discharge
    c) Cough
    d) Sore throat
    e) Vomiting and diarrhea
    f) General discomfort
5. Complications
    a) Ear infections
    b) Bronchitis
    c) Pneumonitis
6. Prevention
    a) Avoid exposure to others with colds.
    b) Get sufficient rest.
    c) Eat nutritious foods.
7. Relief of symptoms
    a) Rest
    b) Fluids
    c) Diet
8. Consultation with physician if fever is present and continuous

B. Vomiting
    1. Definition of **vomiting:** Reflex action of ejecting the stomach contents through the mouth, due to sudden contractions of the stomach muscles and diaphragm
    2. Causes
        a) Improper feeding techniques
        b) Ear, nose, and throat infections
        c) Communicable diseases
        d) Other disorders
            (1) Strangulated hernia
            (2) Bowel obstructions
            (3) Intracranial pressure
            (4) Pyloric stenosis (leads to surgery; needs special attention; see Section L)
    3. Results
        a) Electrolyte imbalance and dehydration
        b) Possibly, alkalosis due to loss of hydrochloric acid and sodium chloride from stomach
    4. Complications
        a) Aspiration
        b) Dehydration
        c) Aspiration pneumonia

      d) Electrolyte imbalance
  5. Prevention
      a) Maintain NPO; resume fluids slowly.
      b) Feed baby carefully.
      c) Feed baby in pleasant, comfortable surroundings.
      d) Prevent aspiration of vomitus by placing child on stomach or right side following feedings.
  6. Treatment
      a) When child vomits, turn head to one side; support head firmly.
      b) When vomiting ceases, rinse out infant's mouth, bathe face and hands, change bed linen and gown.
      c) Administer drugs prescribed by physician.
      d) Estimate amount and character of vomitus, report to R.N., and chart.
      e) Institute isolation techniques.
      f) Keep accurate record of weights.
  7. Administering fluids
      a) Orally
         (1) Encourage sick child to drink enough fluids.
         (2) Offer liquids frequently and in small amounts.
         (3) Keep accurate record of fluid intake and output.
      b) Parenterally
         (1) Fluids are administered parenterally when
            (a) Child is unconscious
            (b) Digestive tract needs rest
            (c) Child is vomiting frequently
         (2) Subcutaneous infusion is given on outer thigh and back (clysis)
         (3) Intravenous infusion is dangerous when administered to infants and small children.
            (a) Monitor drip rate as prescribed, and maintain patency of tubing.
            (b) Observe closely for untoward symptoms.
            (c) Chart hourly.
            (d) Maintain intake and output record.

C. Infantile Eczema
  1. Definition of **eczema:** Inflammation of the skin that produces
      a) Skin rash characterized by itching and scaling
      b) Cause—unknown; may indicate allergic reaction to allergen
  3. Assessment—lesions on skin that can form vesicles, which form dry crusts after "weeping"
  4. Treatment and nursing care
      a) Applications of specific prescribed ointments or solutions
      b) Wet soaks applied to remove crusts and to relieve itching
      c) Emollient baths
      d) Medication prescribed to relieve itching
      e) Isolation to protect against infection
      f) Restraints to keep from scratching
      g) Medicated baths
         a) Check water temperature to prevent burns.
         b) Stay with baby at all times.

D. Nutritional Deficiencies
  1. Cause—lack of nutrients necessary for bodily growth and development
  2. Occurrence—rare in children of advanced countries; marginal in poor families

3. Causes
   a) Poverty
   b) Dietary restrictions
   c) Allergic disorders
   d) Metabolic disorders
   e) Systemic disease
   f) Distortion in sense of taste
   g) Ignorance regarding proper nutrition
4. Frequent deficiencies
   a) Iron-deficiency anemia
      (1) Incidence—most common anemia
      (2) Cause—insufficient iron intake in diet for rapid growth
   b) Infantile scurvy
      (1) Cause—lack of supplementary vitamin C
      (2) Occurrence—between 6th and 12th months of life
      (3) Characteristics
         (a) irritability
         (b) anorexia
         (c) failure to thrive
         (d) pain from subperiosteal hemorrhages
         (e) anemia
         (f) fever
      (4) Diagnosis—by X ray
      (5) Prevention—early ingestion of orange juice
      (6) Treatment—administration of ascorbic acid
   c) Rickets
      (1) Causes
         (a) Inadequate exposure to sunlight
         (b) Poor diet
         (c) Deficient calcium and phosphorus metabolism
      (2) Characteristics
         (a) Knock-knee or bowleg
         (b) Beaded ribs
         (c) Chest deformities
         (d) Improperly formed teeth
      (3) Treatment—vitamin D from
         (1) Sunlight
         (2) Vitamin-D-enriched milk
         (3) Fish-liver oils

E. Otitis Media
   1. Definition of **otitis media:** Inflammation of middle ear
   2. Causes
      a) Extension of throat infection
      b) Secondary infection
      c) Various organisms
   3. Assessment
      a) Severe ear pain
      b) Poor hearing
      c) Irritability
      d) Headache
      e) Fever
      f) Vomiting and diarrhea

       g) Febrile convulsions

       h) Purulent discharge from ear

  4. Complications

       a) Deafness

       b) Chronic otitis media

       c) Meningitis

       d) Mastoiditis

       e) Rupture of eardrum

  5. Nursing care

       a) Administer antibiotics or sulfonamides (parenteral and/or local as ordered by physician).

       b) Administer aspirin to relieve pain.

       c) Administer nose and ear drops.

       d) Give local heat applications.

       e) Care for skin around ear to protect it from drainage irritation.

       f) Observe for signs of complications, and report them.

       g) Position the infant with affected ear down to make drainage easier.

       h) Assess for signs of hearing loss.

       i) Prepare for myringotomy.

          (1) Give ordered antibiotics.

          (2) Instill decongestants and nose drops as ordered.

F. Umbilical Hernia

  1. Definition of **umbilical hernia:** Protrusion of intestine through umbilical ring; bulges when infant cries or strains

  2. Prognosis—most small hernias will disappear during first year of life; do not usually cause complications

  3. Treatment

       a) Sometimes strapping

       b) No treatment if defect is small

       c) Surgical repair if hernia is large and does not disappear during first 2 years

G. Inguinal Hernia

  1. Definition of **inguinal hernia:** Protrusion of parts of intestines through inguinal canal

  2. Types

       a) Reducible—can be put back in place with gentle pressure

       b) Irreducible—cannot be put back in place with gentle pressure

       c) Strangulated—occurs when blood supply is cut off to intestine

  3. Assessment

       a) No symptoms in reducible hernia

       b) Constipation

       c) Irritability and fretfulness

       d) Vomiting and severe abdominal pain in strangulated hernia

  4. Treatment

       a) Application of truss by physician before surgery, when necessary

       b) Replacement of truss when soiled or out of place

       c) Surgical treatment—herniorrhaphy

       d) Postoperative care

          (1) Keep wound clean; leave diapers open.

          (2) Check vital signs.

          (3) Measure total intake and output.

          (4) Change position frequently.

          (5) Maintain diet that will meet child's growth needs.

NURSING CARE OF THE PEDIATRIC PATIENT

        (6)   Avoid strain on suture line.

        (7)   Prevent coughing; give cough suppressants.

H. Cleft Palate

   1. Definition of **cleft palate:** Congenital anomaly, often accompanied by cleft lip, in which fissure forms passageway between nasopharynx and nose (in midline of roof of mouth)

   2. Serious childhood disorder—complicates feeding, leads to respiratory tract and middle-ear infections, and causes speech difficulties

   3. Treatment

      a) Expert health-team work is required for a long time.

      b) A special feeding method is required (see Section I.4.c) 5.

      c) Cleft palate clinic may be required.

      d) Dental speech appliance is used if surgery is postponed.

      e) Surgery is performed once child reaches age of 1 to 5 years

I. Cleft Lip (Harelip)

   1. Definition of **cleft lip:** Congenital deformity in which there is one or more fissures opening in upper lip

   2. Cause—failure of embryonic structures of face to unite during pregnancy

   3. Occurrence—more frequent in boys

   4. Treatment

      a) Preoperative treatment

         (1)   Maintain adequate nutrition for growth and development.

         (2)   Prevent infection.

         (3)   Support respiratory efforts.

         (4)   Support parents.

      b) Surgery—within first few months of life

      c) Postoperative treatment

         (1)   Prevent injury to suture line of lip.

         (2)   Maintain adequate nutrition and fluid intake for weight gain and growth.

         (3)   Prevent dehydration.

         (4)   Use restraints to keep patient from scratching lip.

         (5)   Use special feeding method.

            (a)   Be aware that feeding procedure is long.

            (b)   Have required equipment ready—sterile medicine dropper with rubber tip or Asepto syringe with rubber tip, warmed formula, cover gown for yourself, and bib.

            (c)   Leave restraints on during feeding.

            (d)   Hold baby in sitting position.

            (e)   Draw formula into syringe or dropper.

            (f)   Place rubber tip of feeder just inside lips and on side of mouth opposite cleft or repaired area.

            (g)   Prevent sucking motions.

            (h)   Burp frequently.

            (i)   Cleanse mouth with sterile water, if ordered.

            (j)   Return baby to crib and place on right side; support back with small pillow.

            (k)   Report and chart required information

J. Congenital Heart Defects

   1. Definition of **congenital heart defect:** Defect, present at birth, in structure of heart or one or more large blood vessels

   2. Cause—improper development during fetal life

3. Assessment
    a) Dyspnea
    b) Cyanosis
    c) Abnormal (very high) pulse rate
    d) Clubbed fingers and toes
    e) Poor physical development
    f) Feeding problems
    g) Heart murmurs
    h) Cerebrovascular accidents
    i) Anoxic attacks and choking spells
    j) Recurrent respiratory infections
4. Treatment
    a) Surgical correction, if possible
    b) Supportive measures
        a) Prevent infection.
        b) Improve and maintain child's general health.
5. Nursing care
    a) Supply sufficient nutritional and fluid intake to maintain growth and developmental needs of the infant.
    b) Inhibit infection.
    c) Prepare infant for diagnostic and treatment procedures.
    d) Clarify processes to parents.
    e) Relieve respiratory distress.
    f) Relieve hypoxia associated with cyanosis.
    g) Improve oxygenation.
    h) Observe for symptoms of infection.
    i) Observe for thrombosis.
    j) Refer parents to Social Services for planning and home regimen.

K. Hydrocele
    1. Definition: Excessive amount of fluid around testicles
    2. Assessment—swelling of scrotum
    3. Treatment
        a) Treatment may not be required.
        b) Surgery is needed if sac is large.

L. Pyloric Stenosis
    1. Definition of **pyloric stenosis:** Congential blockage of pyloric opening into stomach due to increase in size of pyloric muscle; pylorus becomes abnormally large and food cannot pass properly out of stomach
    2. Occurrence
        a) More frequent among males than females
        b) Most common surgical disease of intestinal tract in infancy
    3. Assessment
        a) Vomiting—generally projectile after 14th day of life
        b) Hunger
        c) Decrease in amount and frequency of bowel movements
        d) Failure to gain weight
        e) Dehydration
        f) Distension of abdomen
        g) Gastric waves noticeable
        h) Palpation of mass during feeding
        i) Metabolic acidosis

4. X-ray findings
    a) Enlarged stomach
    b) Marked narrowing and elongation of pyloris
5. Treatment—surgical
6. Preoperative nursing intervention
    a) Assist in restoring hydration and electrolyte balance.
    b) Try to decrease vomiting.
        (1) Small feedings
        (2) Frequent burping
        (3) Observation of drainage from nasogastric tube if inserted
    c) Prop infant in upright position, slightly on right side
    d) Frequently observe infant's condition, and record.
    e) Prevent infection.
    f) Comfort infant; use pacifier.
    g) Support parents.
7. Postoperative nursing care
    a) Observe for complications.
    b) Monitor parenteral fluids to maintain hydration.
    c) Help in oral feedings.
    d) Help parents to assume care of their infant.

M. Additional Gastrointestinal Anomalies the Name of Which the Practical Nurse Should Know
1. The disorders listed below are all subject to surgical procedures.
2. The postoperative nursing care, except for prescribed medications, is similar.
3. Some of the conditions have been described previously.
    a) Esophageal atresia
    b) Tracheoesophageal fistula
    c) Diaphragmatic hernia
    d) Duodenal obstruction
    e) Intussusception
    f) Meconium ileus
    g) Hirschsprung's disease (Megacolon)
    h) Imperforate anus

UNIT 4: THE TODDLER

VOCABULARY

aspirate	to remove by suction
behavior	response to external or internal stimuli
booster	supplementary dose of an immunizing agent, given to increase immunity
convulsion	sudden, violent involuntary contraction of a group of muscles, sometimes with loss of consciousness
guidance	act of guiding and advising
hernia	protrusion of an organ through wall or cavity that normally contains it
hygiene	study of good health and its maintenance
peer	belonging to same age group or having same status
posture	position of body
punish	to impose a penalty for a fault or violation of rules of behavior or conduct
toddler	young child between the ages of 1 and 3 years
toxic	poisonous: of, relating to, or caused by poison

I. Introduction

A. General Characteristics
   1. Child is between 1 and 3 years old.
   2. Child can do things for him-/herself.
      a) Is no longer completely dependent upon care of another person
      b) Has control of hands, feet, and head movements
   3. Child is three times heavier than at birth.
   4. Child has progressed from period of rapid growth and development that characterizes infancy stage
   5. Child begins to walk, run, climb, and jump; newfound abilities present challenges for the family to adjust to.

B. Stages of Growth and Development
   1. Eighteen months
      a) Is able to climb stairs and onto furniture; can get into everything
      b) Has rapidly changing objects of attention; speaks about 10 words
      c) Is capable of drinking from a cup and holding and filling a spoon, although generally spilling contents of these utensils
      d) May desire potty
      e) May often stay awake after having been put to bed
      f) Should receive haemophilus influenzae (Hib) immunization
   2. Two years
      a) Height—33 inches
      b) Weight—26–28 pounds
      c) Teeth—16 baby teeth
      d) Vital signs
         (1) Pulse—90-120 per minute
         (2) Respiration—20-35 per minute
      e) Can talk in short sentences
      f) Indulges in imitative play
      g) Starts to postpone going to bed or may climb out of crib
      h) Although appetite may fluctuate, is now capable of self-feeding
      i) Needs constant supervision in outdoor play or must be kept in fenced-in area
   3. Two and one-half years
      a) Has all deciduous ("milk" or temporary) teeth
      b) In play, can throw a ball, play with blocks and construct towers with them, and jump and dance about the room
      c) May develop stuttering because of being unsure of him-/herself socially
      d) Will become overtired in active play
      e) Is easily distracted at table and dawdles
      f) May awaken during night

C. Guidance of the Toddler
   1. Emotional behavior fluctuates enormously, and parents must learn to deal with this wisely.
   2. Toddler must learn how to conduct him-/herself, but activities should not be totally directed by parents.
   3. Toddler must be disciplined, but this does not mean constant punishment.
   4. Toddler seeks approval of his/her actions; such approval tends to instill self-confidence.

D. Daily Care of the Toddler
   1. Consistent routine—essential

2. Clothing—simple so that toddler can help dress and undress him-/herself; clothes should be fairly loose so as not to impede movements

3. Shoes—should fit shape of foot and should have firm soles

4. Good posture—ensured by
   a) Plenty of exercise
   b) Plenty of fresh air
   c) Proper nutrition
   d) Sufficient rest and sleep

5. Slouching—may be evident in children who feel insecure or lack self-confidence

6. Meals
   a) Toddler is inconsistent in eating habits; mealtime can become a means of obtaining attention; toddler may also refuse to eat because he/she is tired or is not hungry
   b) Food must be chopped into fine pieces.
   c) Toddler should be given a nutritious variety of food, in colorful dishes, and should be encouraged to use his/her own set of small silverware

7. Play
   a) Method for toddler to exercise
   b) Means of obtaining relief from emotional tensions
   c) Educational value
   d) Adult supervision required
   e) No toys having small, removable parts—can be dangerous

8. Toilet training
   a) There is no set method for toilet-training toddler.
   b) Success of training is determined by person training toddler and by toddler's reaction to training.
   c) Usually mother will start training with training pants.
   d) Bowel training is generally first aspect of training attempted.
   e) Bladder training usually starts when child remains dry for 2 hours at a time.
   f) Either child's potty chair or attachment for adult toilet seat should be used.
   g) Toddler who has been toilet trained should continue to use potty if hospitalized to prevent regression of bladder and bowel training.

9. Preventing accidents in or near home
   a) Most accidents occur in or near home.
   b) Accidents are leading cause of childhood death.
   c) Practical nurse must teach and demonstrate adequate safety precautions to patients and families.
   d) Practical nurse should set good example in accident prevention.
   e) Preventing burns
      (1) Keep cigarettes and matches out of sight and out of reach.
      (2) Turn handles of cooking utensils toward rear of stove, away from edge.
      (3) Do not leave cups, especially those containing hot liquids, on tables and within child's reach.
      (4) Always test temperature of hot foods and liquids before giving to child.
      (5) Never leave bathroom when hot water is running or when tub has water in it.
      (6) Cover all unused electrical outlets with plugs made specifically for that purpose.
      (7) Screen all fireplaces whether or not fires are burning.
   f) Preventing automobile accidents
      (1) Watch toddler constantly when he/she is outside; enclose play area.
      (2) Hold toddler's hand when crossing street.
      (3) Teach child to look both ways and to honor red, yellow, and green lights when crossing streets.
      (4) Teach child not to jaywalk, and to follow instructions of school crossing guards.

(5) Do not leave child alone in car for any reason whatsoever.
(6) Do not allow child to play inside car.
(7) Use seat belts in car; obtain and use child seats.
(8) Do not permit child to ride in the back of an open truck.
(9) Do not back out of a driveway if you cannot see child, i.e., if you cannot ascertain his/her whereabouts

g) Preventing falls
(1) Make sure that crib sides are fastened securely; keep them up whenever child is in crib.
(2) Use side rails on a large bed, especially immediately after changing child from crib to bed.
(3) Teach child how to climb staircase as soon as he/she is ready.
(4) Lock door leading to stairs to cellar or attic; use gates to prevent access to other staircases.
(5) Secure toddler to Bathinette or changing table when in use.
(6) Wipe up spills immediately.
(7) Do not wax floors when toddler is learning how to walk.
(8) Place screens in all open windows and all windows that can be opened.

h) Preventing suffocation and choking
(1) Be aware of goal—to keep small objects away from child and, therefore, out of his/her mouth.
(2) Remove all small objects from toddler's reach.
(3) Do not feed child popcorn, nuts, or small candies.
(4) Remove all bones from fish and any small bones from chicken.
(5) Keep all plastic bags away from child; do not use plastic bags to line cribs.
(6) Do not allow child to play with deflated balloons.
(7) Do not permit child to play with strings, such as those on venetian blinds.
(8) Do not use bedclothes with drawstrings around neckline.
(9) If toddler vomits while lying down, elevate hips slightly and turn to side to allow fluid to drain from mouth.

i) Preventing poisoning
(1) Keep medicines locked in sturdy medicine cabinet.
    (a) Do not allow child to handle medications
    (b) Make sure all medicines are clearly and accurately labeled, and follow dosage instructions
    (c) Discard old medicines promptly by flushing them down toilet.
(2) Keep all household cleaning supplies out of child's reach, preferably locked away.
(3) Use paint labeled "for indoor use" on any surfaces that child might chew on.
(4) If child or adult has taken poison, call a doctor at once.
(5) If you must go to the hospital or emergency room, take container that held poison—antidote may be found on container's label.

j) Preventing drowing
(1) Remain with toddler when he/she is in bathtub; never leave toddler alone.
(2) Never leave basins full if they are accessible to child.
(3) Keep constant watch on child at beach or pool.
(4) Teach child to swim, and show him/her safety techniques pertaining to water activities.
(5) Always empty wading pools after use.

E. Immunizations If Not Given in Infancy   See Table 3 of the Appendix.

II. Hospitalization of the Toddler

A. Traumatic Experience for Toddler and Parents
1. Child is suffering and cannot understand why he/she has been separated from parents.
2. Toddler who is kept away from family for a long period of time may begin to appear uninterested in seeing them; important for parents to realize that this is a natural defense reaction and is not a genuine expression of child's real feelings toward them.

B. Return Home from Hospital
1. Toddler or child may change his/her behavior upon discharge from hospital and subsequent return home.
2. Parents must regain child's trust by giving him/her extra attention and reassurance.

III. Disorders of the Toddler

A. Fractures
1. Definition of **fracture:** Break in a bone, most frequently caused by accidents
2. Types
   a) Greenstick fracture—occurs in children whose bones are still soft and likely to splinter; one side of bone is broken, other side is bent but not broken
   b) Simple fracture—bone is broken but overlying skin is not
   c) Compound fracture—bone punctures tissue and overlying skin; this may lead to infection
   d) Complete fracture—bone is broken into two pieces
3. Assessment
   a) Pain and tenderness on moving bone
   b) Swelling
   c) Skin discoloration
   d) Numbness
   e) Skin—may or may not be broken
4. First aid
   a) Do not move injured part.
   b) Keep child warm.
   c) In case of compound fracture, cover wound with sterile dressing.
   d) If it is necessary to move victim, immobilize adjacent joints by applying a splint.
   e) Call doctor at once.
5. Fracture common in children
   a) Skull
   b) Femur
   c) Humerus
   d) Wrist
   e) Fingers
6. Nursing treatment
   a) If there is the possibility of skull fracture, or if skull fracture has been determined:
      (1) Observe child for signs of increasing intracranial pressure or
         (a) Vomiting
         (b) Irritability
         (c) Changes in pupillary signs
         (d) Clear fluid from nose or ears
         (e) Coma
      (2) Measure vital signs frequently.
      (3) Report all symptoms immediately.

    b) If femur is fractured:
        (1) Make sure child is in good anatomical position.
        (2) Make sure circulation to toes is adequate.
        (3) Check for cyanosis and numbness or irritation from cast or traction attachments.
        (4) Bathe child daily.
        (5) Give back rubs to prevent ulceration.
        (6) Change soiled clothing and bed linen immediately.
        (7) Encourage child to drink plenty of fluids.
        (8) Give balanced diet high in roughage.
        (9) Provide child with interesting diversions.
    c) Cast (body spica) has been applied to hospitalized child:
        (1) Explain procedure of application to child.
        (2) Aid physician with drying and molding.
            (a) Use firm mattress with bed board under it.
            b) Have child's head and shoulders flat with no pillow underneath.
            (c) Support body curves by pillows.
            (d) Handle cast with palms of hands.
            (e) Turn child every 2 hours.
        (3) Observe for complications
            (a) Poor circulation
            (b) Complaints of pain or pressure
        (4) Give daily skin care to avoid breakdowns.
        (5) Closely watch skin around edge of cast.
        (6) Prevent soiling of cast by urine and feces.
        (7) Give periods of muscle exercises daily.
        (8) Encourage deep breathing to aerate lungs.
        (9) Note bladder and bowel function.
        (10) Be sure child remains in correct position.
        (11) As much as possible, provide normal environment for child.
        (12) Work with social service to evaluate home situation.
        (13) At time of cast removal, work with physician.
        (14) After cast is removed, assist family to have child's situation return to normal.

B. Cerebral Palsy
  1. Definition of **cerebral palsy:** Loss or deficiency of muscle control caused by permanent, nonprogressive brain damage
  2. Causes
    a) Gestational damage
    b) Birth injuries
    c) Infections such as encephalitis or meningitis
    d) Intracranial hemorrhage
    e) Anoxia
  3. Assessment
    a) Symptoms depend on size and location of brain lesion.
    b) There is spasticity of voluntary muscles.
        (1) Jerking movements
        (2) Difficulty in coordination
    c) Speech is indistinct and halting.
    d) Mental retardation may be indicated.
    e) Athetosis may be indicated.
  4. Treatment and nursing care
    a) Goal of treatment and care of child is to help him/her to use remaining resources and to adjust to his/her handicap.

      b) Good skin care is mandatory to prevent pressure sores.

      c) Child should be encouraged to do as much for him-/herself as is possible.

      d) Passive exercise, changing positions, use of splints, and maintenance of good posture are all necessary to prevent deformities and/or contractures.

      e) When braces are used, they must be checked regularly for fit and general condition.

      f) Child must be protected against injury; use safety precautions.

C. Croup (Acute Laryngotracheo bronchitis)

  1. Definition of **croup:** Acute viral infection of upper and lower respiratory tracts, sometimes referred to as *spasmodic laryngitis*

  2. Assessment

      a) Hoarse metallic cough

      b) Dyspnea

      c) Difficult inspiration occurring suddenly during night

      d) Stridor

      e) Fever

  3. Treatment

      a) Purpose is to reduce laryngeal spasms.

      b) Emetic is sometimes given to induce vomiting.

      c) Sedative is given.

      d) Patient is placed in area of high humidity; steam inhalators are used.

      e) Croup tent may be used.

  4. Nursing care upon hospitalization

      a) Prepare croup tent.

      b) Acquaint child with croup tent.

      c) Reassure parents.

      d) When administering an emetic, remain with child until vomiting has subsided; then wash child's hands and face and change bed linen if necessary; give sips of water to rinse mouth.

      e) Observe respirations, color, restlessness, and anxiety; watch for diminishing respiratory distress.

      f) Record temperature, pulse, respiration, and blood pressure.

      g) Keep tracheotomy set nearby; if tracheotomy is performed, give appropriate nursing care.

      h) Administer oxygen if necessary.

      i) Encourage oral intake.

      j) Supply fluid replacement if dehydrated.

      k) Provide for rest.

D. Pneumonia

  1. Definition of **pneumonia:** Inflammation of lungs in which air sacs fill with exudate

  2. Causes

      a) Bacteria

      b) Virus

      c) Aspiration of lipid substances

  3. Types

      a) Lipid pneumonia—occurs chiefly during infancy and is caused by inhalation of an oily substance, e.g., nose drops, into air passages

      b) Hypostatic pneumonia—occurs in patients who have poor circulation in lungs or remain in one position for too long a period of time

      c) Primary pneumonia—occurs as initial disease

      d) Secondary pneumonia—occurs as complication of another illness

4. Assessment
   a) Dry cough
   b) High fever
   c) Increase in respiration rate
   d) Shallow respirations
   e) Listlessness, poor appetite
5. Treatment
   a) Antibiotics or sulfonamide administration
   b) Isolation
   c) Oxygen if necessary
   d) Intravenous fluids if necessary
6. Nursing care
   a) Provide for necessary rest.
   b) Check and record vital signs at regular intervals.
   c) Suction if necessary (nasal-oral).
   d) Give sponge baths to help reduce fever.
   e) Administer fluids and antibiotics.
   f) Turn patient regularly.
   g) Observe patient for weak and rapid pulse, distension, constipation, cyanosis, and disorientation.
   h) Monitor liter flow of oxygen.
   i) Check humidifier.
   j) Provide restful environment.

E. Nephrosis
   1. Definition of **nephrosis:** Kidney disease characterized by degeneration of epithelial cells of renal tubules
   2. Cause—unknown
   3. Assessment
      a) Edema—occurs around eyes and ankles before becoming generalized
      b) Weight gain caused by accumulation of fluids
      c) Appearance of striae on abdomen
      d) Paleness, irritability, listlessness
      e) Poor appetite
      f) Albuminuria
      g) Hypoproteinemia
      h) Increased cholesterol content in blood
      i) Vomiting and diarrhea
   4. Treatment
      a) Diuretics to increase urine output
      b) Antibiotics to treat possible infection
      c) Normal diet
      d) Abdominal paracentesis to relieve ascites when present (abnormal accumulation of fluid in the peritoneal cavity, seen in advanced cases of nephrosis)
      e) Hospitalization only for special therapy
   5. Nursing care
      a) Give long-term care throughout periodic hospitalizations.
      b) Provide good skin care.
      c) Turn patient frequently to prevent sores.
      d) Elevate head to reduce edema of eyelids.
      e) Bathe eyes with normal saline.
      f) Encourage patient to eat; increase protein calories; decrease sodium.
      g) Record fluid intake.
      h) Measure and record urinary output.

     i)   Protect against infection.
     j)   Maintain bedrest until edema decreases.
     k)   Determine specific gravity and albumin content of urine.
     l)   Weigh patient to determine changes in edema.
     m) Protect against infection and drafts.
     n)   Record vital signs.
     o)   Provide for play and rest periods.

F. Deafness
   1. Definition of **deafness:** Loss of hearing in one or both ears
   2. Causes
     a)   Maternal viral infections during pregnancy
     b)   Childhood infections
     c)   Allergic reactions
     d)   Trauma
     e)   Toxic result (could be from medications)
     f)   Neoplasm
   3. Assessment
     a)   Failure to react to noises
     b)   Failure to talk
     c)   Apparent mental retardation
   4. Treatment
     a)   Early detection
     b)   Evaluation at an approved speech and hearing center
     c)   Early training
        (1) Lip reading
        (2) Sign language
        (3) Speaking
     d)   Hearing aids as prescribed at speech and hearing center
   5. Role of practical nurse
     a)   Teach proper ear hygiene.
     b)   Teach importance of immunizations.
     c)   Do not treat child as invalid—meet needs related to his/her stage of growth and development.

UNIT 5: THE PRESCHOOL CHILD

VOCABULARY

antibiotic	tending to destroy life; organisms isolated from bacteria, molds, and fungi that destroy other organisms and thus are useful in medicine
communicable disease	disease that may be carried directly or indirectly from one individual to another
discipline	instruction or training that guides one's behavior or moral character
hemoptysis	expectoration of pure blood, usually as a result of lung hemorrhage
environment	internal or external conditions by which one is surrounded and with which one interacts
responsible	to be held accountable for one's actions
ulceration	suppuration occurring on the skin or on a mucous membrane

I. Introduction

   A. General Characteristics
     1. Preschool child is between 3 and 6 years old.

    2. Child's growth has slowed down since toddler stage; grows taller and becomes less chubby.

    3. Pulse rate is 90-110 per minute.

    4. Respiration rate is 20 per minute (relaxed).

    5. Blood pressures are as follows:

       a) Systolic—85-90 mm hg

       b) Diastolic—60 mm hg

    6. Muscle control is increasing—walking, swinging, jumping.

    7. Child becomes more confident in him-/herself and in ability to perform tasks.

B. Stages of Growth and Development

    1. The three-year-old

       a) Is able to assist with simple chores

       b) Can speak in longer sentences than toddler

       c) Can verbalize thoughts and ask questions about what is going on

       d) Begins to change in relationship with parents

          (1) Becomes less attached to mother

          (2) Becomes more interested in father

          (3) Begins to identify with parent of same sex

       e) Develops fears due to increasing intelligence and awareness of potential dangers

       f) Is sensitive, becomes possessive, and may react unpleasantly in presence of others

    2. The four-year-old

       a) Begins to play with other children, preferably of same sex

       b) Is more aggressive; likes to exert superiority feelings and show off

       c) Enjoys playing with simple toys such as those with which to build things

       d) Has an increasing curiosity about sex

       e) Begins to contemplate death and phenomenon of dying

    3. The five-year-old

       a) Is able to take on more responsibilities

       b) Is able to distinguish between what he/she can and cannot do

       c) Is curious about environment around him/her

       d) Talks constantly and asks questions to which he/she expects to receive answers

       e) Should be encouraged to develop more motor skills

       f) Can understand what is happening on television for longer periods of time

       g) May begin to lose deciduous teeth

C. Discipline

    1. Discipline must be administered promptly.

    2. It is helpful to reward child for good deeds.

    3. When disciplining child, penalty must deal with act performed, not child.

    4. One must be consistent in discipline.

    5. It is natural for child to imitate what he/she sees and hears; therefore, it is not unnatural for child to use bad language he/she has heard.

    6. It is natural for child to feel jealous toward new family member or of attention parents direct toward each other; child should be helped to overcome this jealousy by proper education.

D. Daily Care

    1. Daily bath and weekly shampoo; hair should be styled simply

    2. Simply styled clothing that permits child to dress and undress without assistance

    3. Both indoor and outdoor play periods

    4. Accident prevention

       a) Automobile accident prevention
       b) Burn prevention
       c) Poison prevention
   5. Regular sleep and elimination patterns

E. Other Needs
   1. Regular visits to the dentist
   2. Annual complete physical examination
   3. Booster injections for polio, DTP, MMR at 4–6 years*

II. Hospitalization of the Preschool Child

A. Emotional Needs of Child and Parents
   1. Preschool child is able to understand what is happening.
   2. Child will endure considerable stress because of fear of bodily harm.
   3. Child should not be made to feel he/she is being punished by being in the hospital.
   4. Parents will endure considerable stress because child is in the hospital.

*As of September 1990, kindergarten children in New York State are required to demonstrate receipt of TWO doses of measles vaccine. Thereafter, children born on or after January 1, 1985, will be required to have two doses for school attendance. Measles (two doses), mumps, and rubella vaccines are required for college attendance as of August 1, 1990.

B. Nursing Care
   1. Many diseases of preschool child are communicable.
   2. Medical aseptic techniques, including isolation, are required.

III. Noncommunicable Disorders of the Preschool Child

A. Leukemia
   1. Definition of **leukemia:** malignant neoplasm of blood-forming tissues
   2. Characteristics
       a) Uncontrolled increase in white blood cells
       b) Principal cancer in children
   3. Cause—unknown
   4. Peak incidence—from 3 to 5 years
   5. Assessment
       a) Listlessness, low-grade fever, pallor
       b) Tendency to bruise; pain in legs and joints
       c) Enlargement of lymph nodes
       d) Enlargement of liver and spleen in later stages of development
       e) Vomiting, weight loss, dyspnea, anorexia
       f) Infections
       g) Ulcerations of mucous membranes of mouth and anal region
       h) Anemia
   6. Diagnosis
       a) Blood smear
       b) Bone-marrow examination
   7. Treatment over 2½- to 3-year period
       a) Intensive multiple antimetabolite drug therapy
       b) Maintenance therapy for suppression of leukemic cells
   8. Nursing care
       a) Express genuine interest and concern for child and family.

  b) Be supportive.
  c) Handle child gently.
  d) Give daily baths, frequent changes of position.
  e) Give daily grooming and care of nails.
  f) Give special mouth care.
  g) Keep room neat, clean, cheerful, and free from infection.
  h) Provide interesting diversions suitable to child's condition.
  i) Encourage child to eat.
    (1) Provide adequate nutrition.
    (2) Increase proteins.
    (3) Increase calories.
    (4) Give small meals and fluids by mouth.
  j) Provide frequent rest periods.
  k) Assess for bleeding: gums, cuts, etc.
9. Prognosis—cure

B. Tonsillitis
  1. Tonsils
    a) Are part of body's defense against infection
    b) Consist of two masses of lymphoid tissue at back of mouth
  2. Assessment
    a) Persistent or recurrent sore throat
    b) Obstruction to breathing and swallowing
    c) Enlargement of tonsils
  3. Treatment
    a) Antibiotics
    b) Tonsillectomy—removal of tonsils
  4. Preoperative care for tonsillectomy
    a) Observe child for signs of upper respiratory infection.
    b) Observe child for any loose teeth.
    c) Withhold food and fluid before surgery.
    d) Administer preoperative medicines.
    e) Properly label bed and identify patient.
    f) Encourage child to void before leaving ward.
  5. Postoperative care for tonsillectomy
    a) Observe child carefully for signs of bleeding and hemorrhaging: rapid pulse, restless-ness, hemoptysis, pallor, frequent swallowing.
    b) Assure airway before total recovery from anesthesia.
    c) Place child in semisitting position upon regaining consciousness.
    d) Place child in prone position with head turned to side to allow drainage from the throat (usually most comfortable).
    e) Apply ice collar to relieve discomfort.
  6. Written instructions after discharge
    a) Diet of fluids and soft foods
    b) Frequent rest periods to stimulate recovery
    c) Tylenol for discomfort
    d) Protection from infections
    e) Encouragement of regular elimination
    f) Followup appointment with physician

C. Strabismus (Cross Eye)
  1. Definition of **strabismus:** Condition in which child cannot direct both eyes toward same object
  2. Treatment

        a) Eye exercises
        b) Corrective lenses (glasses)
        c) Surgery, if necessary
    3. Postoperative nursing care
        a) Allow child to be up and about on ward.
        b) Use elbow restraints to prevent child from touching eye dressings.
        c) Reassure restrained child.
        d) Give regular diet.
        e) Take precautions against startling child whose eyes are covered.

D. Reye's Syndrome
    1. Definition of **Reye's syndrome:** Poorly understood syndrome involving abnormal brain function and fatty infiltration of internal organs
    2. Characteristics
        a) Acute encephalopathy
        b) Fatty degeneration of viscera
    3. Occurrence—in children under age of 18 years after an acute viral infection
    4. Assessment
        a) Viral infection (may be common cold)
        b) Pernicious nausea and vomiting after sixth day
        c) Sudden change in mental status
        d) Fluid and electrolyte disturbances
        e) Cardiac arrhythmias
        f) Aspiration pneumonia
    5. Diagnosis
        a) Liver biopsy—definitive
        b) Increased pressure in CSF
    6. Stages
        a) I: Vomiting, lethargy, liver dysfunction
        b) II: Disorientation, combativeness, hyperventilation, hyperactive reflexes, liver dysfunction
        c) III: Decorticate positioning, coma, hyperventilation, pupillary light reaction, liver dysfunction
        d) IV: Deepening coma, fixed and dilated pupils, improvement of liver dysfunction
        e) V: Seizures, loss of reflexes, respiratory arrest, correction of liver dysfunction
    7. Treatment—symptomatic
    8. Nursing care
        a) Closely monitor vital signs.
        b) Do hourly neurologic assessment for increased intracranial pressure.
        c) Watch for seizure activity.
        d) Monitor intake and output of urine.
        e) Pay constant attention to respiratory status and necessary procedures.
        f) Be aware that patient may need intensive nursing care.
    9. Prognosis
        a) Prognosis is related to severity.
        b) Early diagnosis critical; disease is rapidly fatal.

E. Side Effects of Aspirin Intake
    1. Allergic reactions
    2. Gastric ulceration
    3. Hemorrhagic tendencies
    4. Liver damage
    5. Deafness (tinnitus)
    6. Reye's syndrome in children (see Section III.D above)

IV. **Communicable Diseases of the Preschool Child**

A. General Principles
1. Nursing adult patient and preschool child with communicable diseases entails use of same medical aseptic techniques.
2. Work with child is more challenging because child is less able to accept and to deal successfully with situation.
3. Preschool child with communicable disease is generally hospitalized only if complications arise.

B. Review of Medical Asepsis
1. All articles that come in contact with patient must be disinfected following their use.
2. It is nurse's responsibility to protect her-/himself and others from infection.
3. Isolation techniques and procedures used depend upon hospital.
4. Hand washing is of vital importance.
5. Gown and mask techniques must be utilized.
6. Special precautions must be taken to prevent transmission of infection from discharges from eyes, ears, throat, open wounds, and genitalia.
7. Patient's toys must be washable (books cannot be satisfactorily disinfected; therefore, their use is inadvisable).
8. Visitors must take adequate precautions to prevent transmission of infection; this includes wearing a gown and mask while in patient's room.

C. Isolation at Home
1. Child must be kept away from other family members.
2. Patient's room should not be near center of activities.
3. Doctor's orders are carried out either in patient's room or in a private bathroom.
4. Patient's bath water and all other fluid wastes are flushed down the toilet.
5. Toilet seat is washed and disinfected following use.
6. Patient's dishes must not be mixed together with those of other family members.
7. Nursing care is same as that used in hospital.

D. Chickenpox
1. Assessment
   a) Mild fever for 24 hours
   b) Small, red pimples or blisters, vesicles to crusts
   c) Pruritus
2. Treatment
   a) Isolation until all lesions have crusted
   b) Light diet
   c) Calamine lotion to relieve itching
3. Complications
   a) Reye's syndrome (see Section III.D)
   b) Encephalitis
   c) Pneumonia

E. Measles
1. Assessment
   a) Fever
   b) Dry cough
   c) Running nose and red eyes (coryza)
   d) Rash that spreads in blotches from hairline
   e) Peeling of skin
   f) Koplik's spots

2. Treatment
   a) Adherence to doctor's orders
   b) Isolation
   c) Bedrest until fever disappears
   d) Nasal-oral hygiene
   e) Antibiotics against secondary infections
3. Complications
   a) Otitis media
   b) Pneumonia
   c) Laryngitis
   d) Occasionally, encephalitis
   e) Croup

F. Mumps
   1. Assessment
      a) Fever and headache
      b) Vomiting
      c) Swelling of parotid glands
   2. Treatment
      a) Bedrest
      b) Fluids
      c) Bland diet
   3. Complications
      a) Meningitis
      b) Arthritis
      c) Nephritis
      d) Deafness
      e) Sterility in male

G. German Measles (Rubella)
   1. Assessment
      a) Mild fever
      b) Sore throat or cold symptoms
      c) Rash
      d) Enlarged glands of neck and ears
   2. Treatment—none required; disease is mild and self-limiting

H. Strep Throat
   1. Assessment
      a) Sore throat (usually white patches on throat)
      b) Fever
      c) Vomiting
   2. Treatment
      a) Antibiotics
      b) Isolation
      c) Rest
      d) Analgesics
      e) Ice collar
      f) Throat irrigation
   3. Complications
      a) Sinusitis
      b) Ear infection
      c) Rheumatic fever if inadequately treated

I. Whooping Cough (Pertussis)
    1. Assessment
        a) Cold symptoms
        b) Low fever
        c) Paroxysmal cough that changes to "whooping" sound at end of second week
    2. Treatment
        a) Careful medical supervision by doctor
        b) Isolation
        c) Nutritious diet
        d) Sedative cough mixtures
        e) Antibiotics
        f) Steam inhalation

J. Other Infectious Disease
    1. Polio (poliomyelitis or infantile paralysis)
    2. Rocky Mountain spotted fever
    3. Infectious hepatitis
    4. Meningitis
    5. Encephalitis
    6. Impetigo
    7. Rheumatic fever
    8. Ringworm

V. **Common Parasitic Infestations of the Preschool Child**

A. Pinworm (Enterobiasis)
    1. Causes
        a) Eggs of pinworm are transported from perianal area to mouth via fomites.
        b) Airborne eggs are inhaled and then swallowed.
    2. Assessment
        a) Perianal itching and excoriations
        b) Abdominal pain
        c) Insomnia
        d) Convulsions
        e) Gastrointestinal symptoms
    3. Diagnosis—by microscopic identification of female worms
    4. Treatment
        a) Pyrantel pamoate
        b) Antipruritic ointments

B. Roundworms
    1. Causes
        a) Fecal contamination of soil
        b) Eating of contaminated vegetables
    2. Assessment
        a) Colicky abdominal pains
        b) Bronchial symptoms
        c) Eosinophilia
    3. Diagnosis
        a) Microscopic identification of eggs
        b) Visual identification of worms in stool
    4. Treatment—Pyrantel pamoate

C. Hookworms
   1. Causes
      a) Eggs in stool—then to soil
      b) Infection of human skin by larvae
      c) Penetration of lungs via blood and lymphatics
   2. Assessment
      a) Pulmonary symptoms
      b) Maculopapular rash
      c) Gastrointestinal symptoms
      d) Growth retardation
   3. Treatment
      a) Supportive measures
      b) Pyrantel pamoate

UNIT 6: THE SCHOOL-AGE CHILD

VOCABULARY

disoriented	confused; having lost one's sense of time, place, and/or identity
hereditary	genetically transmitted from parent to child
preadolescence	period immediately preceding adolescence
shock	disturbance of all body functions due to circulatory disruption

I. **Introduction**

   A. Characteristics
      1. Age is from 6 to 12 years old.
      2. There is increasing interest and participation in activities with others of same age group.
      3. Child shows preference for friends of same sex.
      4. Child tends to identify with parent of same sex.
      5. There is a decrease in growth rate, extending until just before puberty.
      6. Muscular coordination improves.
      7. Permanent teeth appear
      8. Vital signs are nearly the same as those of adult.
         a) Temperature—average is 98.6° F
         b) Pulse—85-100 per minute
         c) Respiration rate—18-20 per minute
         d) Blood pressures
            (1) Systolic—90-108 mm hg
            (2) Diastolic—60-68 mm hg

   B. Stages of Growth and Development
      1. The six-year-old
         a) Has a lot of energy, which comes in bursts that in turn, cause overtiring
         b) Has short attention span
         c) Is very sensitive to criticism
         d) Loses temporary teeth
         e) Requires about 12 hours of sleep nightly
         f) Must receive preschool immunizations and yearly physical examination
      2. The seven-year old

    a) Has progressed from stage of not knowing when to rest to having an appreciation of rest periods to offset active periods

    b) Needs to have interesting toys with bit of realism

    c) Is making progress in school

        (1) Can count in multiples (such as by 2's)

        (2) Can recite days, months, and seasons

    d) Is more fun and less of a problem than 6-year-old

3. The eight-year-old

    a) Is capable of doing creative work

    b) Can work and play alone for periods of time

    c) Likes to be considered important

    d) Enjoys and participates in competitive sports

    e) Actively participates in group activities, fads, clubs, etc.

4. The nine-year-old

    a) Shows interest in family activities

    b) Is dependable and can assume responsibility for personal belongings

    c) Resists adult authority

    d) Is more able to accept criticism

    e) Requires about 10 hours of sleep nightly

5. The ten-year-old

    a) Wants to act independently of authoritative figures

    b) Pays much attention to the group

    c) If girl, has matured more physically than have boys

    d) Takes interest in personal appearance

    e) Is entering the preadolescent stage of growth

6. The preadolescent (10–12 years)

    a) Growth is influenced by body hormones.

    b) The preadolescent has 24-26 permanent teeth.

    c) The preadolescent has limitless energy.

    d) The preadolescent appears disoriented.

        (1) Intense

        (2) Argumentative

        (3) Preoccupied

        (4) Emotional

    e) The preadolescent needs freedom to develop, yet is still in need of adult guidance.

C. Physical Care

  1. Good eating habits must be encouraged.

    a) Good breakfast is necessary.

    b) Nutritious, balanced meals are necessary for growth.

  2. Good health must be promoted.

    a) Yearly physical examination

    b) Booster shots (see Tables 4 and 5 of the Appendix)

    c) Dental checkups

  3. Active school-age child needs plenty of rest.

    a) For 6–8 year old—11–13 hours sleep

    b) For 9–12 year old—about 10 hours of sleep

  4. Child can accept major responsibility for dressing and personal hygiene.

    a) Brushing teeth

    b) Combing hair

    c) Washing face and hands

  5. Clothing should be durable and simple in design; shoes should fit properly and be sturdy.

II. Guidance of the School-Age Child

A. General Principles
1. Child must learn not to be overly self-critical; he/she must learn self-acceptance.
2. Child should be encouraged to participate in group activities.
3. Child must learn to accept responsibility for personal tasks and assignments.
4. Child must be taught value and management of money.
   a) Child can earn an allowance or have a task or job.
   b) Child can make visits to store.
5. Child must be taught about bodily changes that occur at puberty.

III. Hospitalization of the School-Age Child

A. Child's Attitude
1. School-age child is able to accept hospitalization when he/she becomes ill.
2. Even though school-age child may appear to be very brave under stressful situation of being hospitalized, he/she may be upset and frightened.
3. School-age child must continue education throughout illness.

B. Nurse's Responsibilities
1. In addition to children with acute illnesses, nurse will encounter school-age children who are long-term patients or who have handicaps; it is very likely that these patients will be difficult to handle.
2. Nurse must find out as much as possible about children on pediatric wards in order to be most effective in caring for them.

IV. Disorders of the School-Age Child

A. Burns
1. Description
   a) First degree—burn is superficial, skin is reddened
   b) Second degree—skin blisters
   c) Third degree—skin is charred, tissues are injured
      (1) Second- and third-degree burns are treated as open wounds.
      (2) Death from severe burns usually occurs within 48 hours, the result of shock and toxic conditions stemming from it.
2. Treatment
   a) Treatment for shock—given by physician
   b) Local treatment of wound
      (1) Open technique—no covering is placed on wound
      (2) Closed technique (pressure bandage)—wound is bandaged to prevent loss of body fluids
   c) Prevention of infection
      (1) Administration of antibiotics
      (2) Aseptic techniques
   d) Maintenance of body fluids
   e) Medications to relieve pain

B. Appendicitis
1. Definition of **appendicitis:** Inflammation of appendix
2. Occurrence–generally between ages of 5 and 20; rare before fifth year
3. Cause—obstruction of opening of appendix into cecum by infection, allergy, or fecal matter
4. Assessment

a) Nausea and vomiting
b) Abdominal tenderness localized generally over McBurney's point (lower right quadrant)
c) Constipation
d) Fever
e) Increased white blood cell count
5. Treatment
a) Appendectomy—requires surgery
b) Penicillin, streptomycin, or sulfonamides to minimize danger of infection
6. Postoperative nursing care
a) Monitor and record vital signs immediately upon return to room.
b) Observe kind, amount, and rate of IV.
c) Record observations, time of patient's arrival on ward, state of consciousness of patient.
d) Observe for symptoms of complications: hemorrhage, peritonitis, shock.
e) Change patient's position frequently.
f) Keep record of input and output.
g) Change sterile dressings or assist doctor in changing them if called upon to do so.
h) Encourage early ambulation
i) Monitor, assess, and medicate postoperative pain.

C. Diabetes Mellitus
1. Definition of **diabetes mellitus:** Complex and chronic disorder of metabolism that results from deficiency of insulin
2. Cause—unknown, possibly hereditary
3. Cure—none known
4. Occurrence
a) Is rare in children
b) If occurs, generally develops at age 3, 6, or 12 (juvenile diabetes)
5. Assessment
a) Polydipsia—excessive thirst; skin becomes dry; boils develop
b) Polyphagia—constant hunger; weight loss, irritability
c) Polyuria—frequent large volumes of urine
d) Diabetic acidosis
(1) Acetoacetic acids accumulate in body fluids more rapidly than they can be oxidized by tissue cells.
(2) Condition results from contraction of secondary infection or failure to take proper care of child.
(3) Symptoms of diabetic acidosis are as follows:
(a) Flushed appearance of face
(b) Dehydration of the body; dry skin
(c) Thirst
(d) Restlessness
(e) Pain throughout body
(f) Fruity odor of breath
(g) Weakness and drowsiness
(h) Coma
6. Treatment—subcutaneous insulin administration
a) Insulin enables body to utilize carbohydrates.
b) Dosage is measured in units and injected with special syringes.
c) Child must be taught why he/she must take insulin.
d) Child over 7 years of age must be taught to take insulin.

7. Diet
    a) Free diet
        (1) Exact intake is not adhered to.
        (2) Snacking and high-carbohydrate intake are discouraged.
        (3) Regular, consistent meals are encouraged.
    b) Measured diet
        (1) Physician prescribes caloric intake.
        (2) Physician prescribes food types to be eaten and in what amounts.
    c) Role of nurse
        (1) Prepare patient for meals.
        (2) Make certain correct meal tray is served to correct patient on time.
        (3) Assist patient in eating if necessary.
        (4) Report any observations about patient's food likes and dislikes, as well as failure to finish meals, to head nurse.
8. Exercise
    a) Exercise causes utilization of sugar by body.
    b) Exercise promotes blood circulation.
    c) Patient must guard against insulin reactions following vigorous exercise.
9. Education of child and parents
    a) Importance of proper diet and exercise
    b) Administration of insulin
    c) Symptoms of insulin shock and diabetic coma
10. Urine tests
    a) Three types are used:
        (1) Clinitest for sugar in urine
        (2) Benedict's test for sugar in urine
        (3) Acetone test for ketone bodies in urine
    b) These tests are very important in management of diabetes and should be taken regularly.
    c) Practical nurse may be called upon to do these tests and should be familiar with them.
11. Insulin shock
    a) Occurrence
        (1) Insulin shock occurs when blood sugar level is extremely low.
        (2) Diabetes is more unstable in children than in adults; therefore, children are more likely to suffer from an insulin reaction.
    b) Causes
        (1) Poor planning of exercise
        (2) Reduction or omission of food intake
        (3) Incorrect insulin dosage
        (4) Severe vomiting
    c) Assessment
        (1) Paleness, hunger, and weakness
        (2) Profuse sweating
        (3) Disorders of nervous and muscular systems due to absence of glucose in body
        (4) Coma and convulsions
    d) Treatment
        (1) Administer sugar, or orange juice with 2 tablespoons sugar.
        (2) Contact physician if rapid response is not obtained.
        (3) Keep unconscious patient warm.
    e) Nursing management
        (1) Recognize signs of diabetic acidosis.

    (2)   Administer treatment as ordered.

    (3)   Monitor symptoms.

    (4)   Assess gastrointestinal disturbances—abdominal distention.

    (5)   Monitor urine output exactly, and test each specimen.

    (6)   Provide nutritional diet, and encourage child to eat.

    (7)   Administer insulin as ordered.

    (8)   Be knowledgeable about hypoglycemic reactions.

        (a)   Causes—overdose of insulin, reduction in diet

        (b)   Symptoms—trembling, sweating, tachycardia, hunger, odd behavior, seizures, coma

        (c)   Treatment—orange juice or other readily available source of sugar

    (9)   Evaluate diabetic control by monitoring child's blood glucose.

  (10)   Adjust insulin and diet.

  (11)   Prevent infection.

  (12)   Provide emotional support for child and parents.

V. Child Abuse (Battered Child Syndrome)

A. Definition of **child abuse:** Maltreatment, either physical or mental, of child under 18 years by a parent or other person responsible for the child's welfare

B. Causes
1. Isolation of family—lack of support system
2. Parental personality or educational defects
3. Factors related to child—very young, hyperactive, irritable
4. Situational stress—poverty, parental conflicts, unemployment, etc.
5. Parental abuse of mother or father when she/he was a child

C. Types
1. Overt—e.g., child is severely beaten
2. Covert—e.g., child is deprived of affection

D. Assessment of Abuse
1. Inconsistent history of apparent injury
2. Skin lesions, e.g., cigarette or scald burns
3. Bony injuries shown by X ray in various stages of healing
4. Repeated injuries
5. Depression and withdrawal

E. Assessment of Sexual Abuse
1. Difficulty in walking or sitting
2. Sexually transmitted infections
3. Vaginal discharge
4. Insomnia
5. Behavioral problems

F. Assessment of Neglect
1. Inadequate provision of basic needs
2. Retardation of emotional growth
3. Delay in seeking care for illnesses

G. Role of the Practical Nurse
1. Carefully observe child with above symptoms.

2. Report observations to nursing supervisor.
3. Try to identify certain at-risk families through observation and history of familial setting.
4. Assess parent-child relationship
   a) Encourage parents to accept guidance.
   b) Work with mother's strengths.
   c) Provide psychological support for mother.
   d) Be aware that treatment of parents helps to ensure physical and emotional safety of child.

UNIT 7: THE ADOLESCENT

VOCABULARY

adolescent	individual in the period of life from puberty to maturity
chemotherapy	use of chemical agents to treat disease
cryosurgery	surgery done after freezing the part
dermabrasion	removal of top layer of skin by abrasive process; generally performed to remove acneiform scarring
infestation	harboring of microscopic parasites
intradermal	between layers of skin
menarche	onset of menses, occurring between 10th and 17 years
menstruation	monthly discharge of blood, secretions, and tissue debris from uterus of non-pregnant female
nocturnal emissions	involuntary discharge of semen during sleep
puberty	time at which sexual maturity occurs and reproduction becomes possible
secondary infection	infection occurring as the result of infection already present
social	relating to one's interactions with other individuals or groups

I. Introduction

   A. General Characteristics
      1. The adolescent desires to be independent.
      2. Period is marked by rapidly changing body growth.
      3. The adolescent is generally described as irritable, aggressive, and unstable.

   B. Physical Characteristics
      1. Preadolescence—period immediately before adolescence ending with onset of puberty
         a) Height and weight gains
         b) Excessively active sweat glands
         c) Development of acne
      2. Female characteristics
         a) Onset of menstruation
         b) Body changes
            (1) Fat deposited on breasts, hips, and thighs
            (2) Growth of external genitalia
            (3) Growth of hair under arms and in pubic area
            (4) End of bone growth
      3. Male characteristics
         a) No one significant event (such as menstruation)
         b) Body changes
            (1) Increase in size of pectoral muscles and depth of shoulders
            (2) Growth of hair on face, chest, underarms, and pubic area

        (3)   Enlargement of genitals
        (4)   Production of sperm, erections, and nocturnal emissions

C.   Guiding the Adolescent through Physical Development
    1.   Preadolescents must be taught what bodily changes to expect in next few years.
    2.   "Early" and "late" developers must be assured that they are developing normally.
    3.   Periodic medical and dental examinations should be made and kept by child.
    4.   Adolescents need 8–9 hours of sleep each night.
    5.   Adolescents need to eat three well-balanced meals daily.
       a)   Nutrition plays important role in physical and mental health.
       b)   Food habits developed now will remain with them the rest of their lives.

D.   Guiding Adolescent through Mental and Social Development
    1.   Adolescents need to have a certain amount of independence.
    2.   Adolescents need to gain self-confidence and be able to accept responsibilities.
    3.   Adolescents need guidance in selecting a suitable career objective.
       a)   They should be encouraged to take advantage of their talents.
       b)   Active search for information is important.
       c)   School guidance counselors can be important sources of encouragement and information.
    4.   Adolescents must learn how to deal with today's social problems, which they will encounter.
       a)   Drugs and alcohol
       b)   Premarital sex and sexually transmitted diseases
    5.   It is natural for adolescents to worry and daydream.

E.   Parent's Role in Guiding the Adolescent
    1.   Parents must adjust their attitudes to accommodate changing world and sometimes new values.
    2.   Parents must not be afraid to exert authority over their children; however, they must exert neither too much nor too little.
    3.   Parents must not hinder their children from growing up and achieving independence.
    4.   Parents should instill a set of values in their children so that they will be prepared to go out into world on their own.
    5.   Adolescents need to learn how to earn money and how to spend it wisely.
    6.   Parents play a decisive role in adolescent's ability to get along with members of opposite sex.
       a)   Difficulties in social life are very likely to arise.
       b)   Dating and group activities help adolescent to become comfortable around and familiar with members of the opposite sex.
    7.   Parents should continue to emphasize accident prevention.
       a)   Automobile accidents
       b)   Swimming, diving, and boating accidents
    8.   Parents should stress relationships between alcohol use and accidents.
    9.   If adolescent is sexually active, or is likely to be, parents should educate regarding condoms and other contraceptives

II. Disorders of the Adolescent

A.   Introduction
    1.   Generally adolescents tend to be healthy.
    2.   When hospitalization becomes necessary, homesickness is not as prevalent.
    3.   Because of major changes that adolescent experiences, emotions may play large part in illnesses.

4. Adolescent who is handicapped or who has been ill since childhood may experience emotional difficulties at this stage in life.

B. Rheumatic Fever
   1. Etiology
      a) Is collagen disease characterized by destruction of connective tissues of body
      b) Is extremely destructive to heart
      c) Occurs most frequently between ages 7 and 10
      d) Is caused primarily by infection of throat by allergic reaction to hemolytic streptococci
   2. Assessment
      a) Polyarthritis—wandering (migratory) joint pains, mainly of larger joints
      b) Skin eruptions—body rash of small, red circles and wavy lines on trunk and abdomen
      c) Chorea or St. Vitus's dance—involuntary, puposeless movements of muscles
      d) Abdominal pain
      e) Fever
      f) Pallor, fatigue, anorexia, unexplained nosebleeds, poor appetite, dyspnea upon exertion
      g) Uncoordinated vital signs (pulse and respirations versus temperature)
      h) Carditis
   3. Treatment
      a) Rest
      b) Medication (one or all of following may be ordered)
         (1) Salicylates—aspirin
         (2) Steroids—cortisone, ACTH, or prednisone
         (3) Digitalis
         (4) Phenobarbital
         (5) Penicillin or erythromycin
   4. Nursing care
      a) Administer medication.
         (1) Observe carefully for side effects and excessive dosages (particularly steroid reactions).
         (2) Always count patient's pulse rate before administering digitalis; hold if more than 120 or less than 60; notify R.N.
      b) Be aware that joints should be rested (if acutely inflamed) by application of sandbags, splints, bivalved casts, or an mechanical device that will maintain them in functional positions.
      c) Provide for systematic range-of-motion exercises.
      d) If patient is on strict bedrest, maintain bedrest precautions.
      e) Carry out nursing procedures so as not to pain or tire patient.
      f) Provide good skin and mouth care.
      g) Count pulse for a full minute.
      h) Protect patient from all persons with infections.
      i) Prepare child for tutoring sessions; after acute phase he/she should be permitted to continue schoolwork.
      j) Maintain bland, high-protein, high-carbohydrate diet.

C. Pediculosis Capitis
   1. Definition of **pediculosis capitis:** Infestation of hair and scalp with head lice; nits (eggs of lice) are attached to hair and hatch in 3–4 days, producing more lice
   2. Occurrence
      a) Head lice are more common in girls, because of their long hair, than in boys.
      b) Head lice are easily transferred from one person to another.

3. Assessment
   a) Severe itching and scratching of scalp
   b) Pustules and excoriations about face
   c) Matting of hair
4. Treatment
   a) Kill lice with pesticides prescribed by physician.
   b) Remove nits by combing hair with comb and hot vinegar, followed by washing.
   c) Treat facial and scalp infections.
   d) Cut hair.
   e) Remove lice and nits in bedding and clothing.
   f) Prevent infestation.
      (1) Cleanse hair and head gear properly.
      (2) Do not wear apparel belonging to people with lice.

D. Tuberculosis
   1. Definition of **tuberculosis:** Infectious disease caused by tubercle bacillus; it usually affects the lungs but may also affect other organs
   2. Occurrence—more frequent in adolescent girls than boys
   3. Two types
      a) Bovine strain
         (1) Is transmitted through cow's milk
         (2) Attacks other parts of body besides lungs
      b) Human strain
         (1) Is transferred from person to person
         (2) Primarily affects lungs—referred to as *pulmonary tuberculosis*
   4. Etiology
      a) Can live outside body for long periods of time
      b) Can live inside body in dormant form for long periods of time
      c) Enters body through respiratory or digestive tract
   5. Assessment
      a) Primary lesion
         (1) Malaise, fatigue
         (2) Weight loss, anorexia
         (3) Irritability
      b) Secondary infection from reinfection or activation of healed lesion
         (1) Cough and expectoration
         (2) Fever in late afternoon, night sweats
         (3) Bloody sputum
         (4) Weight loss
   6. Diagnosis
      a) Tuberculin tests
         (1) Intradermal test (Mantoux)
         (2) Patch test (Vollmer)
      b) Chest X ray
      c) Examination of sputum (microscopic dark-field)
      d) Examination of stomach contents
   7. Treatment
      a) Early diagnosis and treatment are essential.
      b) Treatment is by chemotherapy.
         (1) Commonly used drugs
            (a) Isoniazid
            (b) Rifampin
            (c) Pyrazinamide

     (d) Ethambutol
    (2) Less commonly used drugs
     (a) Capreomycin
     (b) Kanamycin
     (c) Ethionamide
     (d) Para-aminosalicylic acid
     (e) Cycloserine
  8. Nursing management
    a) Isolate infectious patient in a well-ventilated room until no longer infectious.
     (1) Patient to cough and sneeze into tissues.
     (2) Used tissues to be placed in nearby covered receptacle.
     (3) Patient to wear mask when outside room.
     (4) Hospital personnel and visitors to wear masks when in patient's room.
    b) Encourage patient to get plenty of rest.
    c) Urge patient to eat small meals throughout day; weigh patient weekly.
    d) Watch for drug side effects.
     (1) Isoniazid sometimes leads to hepatitis or peripheral neuritis.
     (2) Ethambutol sometimes leads to optic neuritis.
     (3) Rifampin can lead to hepatitis or purpura.
    e) Before discharge, teach patient about potential side effects of medication(s).
    f) Emphasize importance of regular follow-up exams.
    g) Stress importance of following long-term care as ordered.
    h) Advise prophylaxsis for exposed persons.

 E. Obesity
  1. Definition of **obesity:** Presence of excess fat (20% over that in standard weight tables) on body; differs from overweight only in degree of severity
  2. Cause—overeating
    a) Parents may overfeed the adolescent.
    b) Adolescent may use eating to escape from or compensate for problems.
  3. Effects during adolescence
    a) Adolescent will be subject to ridicule.
    b) Adolescent will not conform to standards of his/her peers.
    c) Adolescent may be unable to participate in sports or other physical activities.
    d) Personal appearance may be less than desirable.
  4. Treatment
    a) Adolescent should be placed on carefully prescribed diet, controlled by medical or nursing regimen.
    b) Adolescent's psychological and emotional needs must be met.

 F. Acne Vulgaris
  1. Definition of **acne:** Inflammatory disease of the sebaceous glands of the skin
  2. Sequence of events
    a) Adolescence is marked by increased hormonal and glandular activity.
    b) Folliolo openings in skin become clogged.
    c) Blackheads form when dirt enters already enlarged and overactive pores.
    d) Pimples form.
    e) Pustules (pus-filled pimples) form.
    f) Acne occurs on cheeks, chin, forehead, shoulders, and back.
  3. Treatment
    a) Proper cleansing of skin
    b) Proper nutrition—avoidance of chocolate, peanuts, soft drinks, and fried food
    c) Adequate rest

       d) Adequate exercise and elimination
       e) Topical and local antibiotics, e.g., tetracycline—but not before permanent dentition
       f) X-ray therapy in severe cases
       g) Dermabrasion
       h) Cryosurgery

G. Lyme Disease (may occur at any age)
  1. Definition of **Lyme disease:** Tick-transmitted, spirochetal, inflammatory disease that affects one or more joints
  2. Assessment
       a) An expanding maculopapular rash (most important clue to diagnosis)
       b) Flulike symptoms: chills, fever, headache, dizziness, fatigue, stiff neck
       c) Swelling and pains in joints, especially knees
       d) Lymphadenopathy
       e) Splenomegaly
       f) Cardiac arrhythmias
       g) Facial paralysis
       h) Weakness in legs
  3. Diagnosis (difficult, but early diagnosis is important)
       a) Sometimes antispirochetal antibodies in high titre
       b) Negative findings important
          (1) Absence of morning stiffness in knees
          (2) Absence of rheumatoid factor
          (3) Absence of antinuclear antibodies
          (4) Absence of previous streptococcal infection
  4. Treatment
       a) Tetracycline for 10–20 days (first choice)
       b) Penicillin for 10–20 days (second choice; used for pregnant women and for children)
       c) Erythromycin (third choice)
       d) Aspirin or other nonsteroidal, anti-inflammatory drugs
       e) Aspiration of fluid from knee joints
       f) Use of crutches
       g) Synovectomy, if necessary
       h) For resistant cases; ceftriaxone (can penetrate blood-brain barrier and enter CNS)

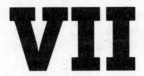

VII

Nursing Care of the Older (Geriatric) Patient

UNIT 1: THE AGING PROCESS

VOCABULARY

aphasia	inability to express oneself through speech
atrophy	wasting of a part
benign	not malignant
cataract	opacity of lens of eye
chronic disease	long, drawn-out disease; not acute
geriatrics	study and treatment of diseases and disabilities of old age
gerontology	study distinguishing normal aging from disease effects
hemorrhoids	anal blood tumors due to dilated anal veins
keratosis	horny growth
pain threshold	point at which a stimulus produces a feeling of pain
personality	that which makes up the distinctive character of a person
presbycusis	difficulty in hearing due to old age
senility	mental and physical infirmity due to old age
spermatogenesis	formation of spermatozoa
tactile	pertaining to touch

I. **General Principles**

    A. Importance of Geriatrics
        1. Population of aged is expanding.
        2. Increase in need for care of elderly will be greater.
        3. After age 45 individuals tend to suffer more chronic conditions—arthritis, rheumatism, heart disease, hypertension, diabetes, visual and hearing impairments
            a) Treatment of chronic diseases is costly.
            b) There is higher utilization of medical services by elderly because of Medicare and Medicaid.

    B. Gradual Physiological Changes Extending over 20–35 Years (onset between 40 and 90 years)
        1. Skin and subcutaneous tissues
            a) Skin
                (1) Skin becomes wrinkled, atrophic, dry; discolorations (yellow and brown) occur.

335

      (2) Ecchymoses frequently appear from trivial trauma because of increased fragility of subcutaneous vessels

      (3) Angiomas and keratoses are common.

      (4) Fissures often occur around mouth.

  b) Hair—graying, whitening, and thinning are generally universal

  c) Sweating—aged persons sweat less than younger persons

2. Musculoskeletal system

  a) Height—decrease noted

  b) Posture—some bending of joints noted

  c) Muscle power—some loss evident

      (1) Makes carrying out of ordinary tasks difficult

      (2) Impairs efficiency of respiration

      (3) Causes problems in defecation and urination

      (4) Causes loss of reserve sugar needed for energy

3. Nervous system

  a) Tactile discrimination is diminished.

  b) Pain threshold may be raised.

  c) Reflexes are generally slower and less efficient.

  d) Balance is affected.

  e) Vulnerability to shock increases.

  f) Short-term memory is impaired, but long-term memory preserved; there is increase in factual knowledge from experience.

4. Personality changes

  a) May be reluctant to accept new ideas and may have narrower interests.

  b) Are often pessimistic and melancholy.

  c) May suffer loss of adaptability and lessening of emotional response

  d) May exhibit abnormal possessiveness

  e) Often show increasing mental confusion with advanced age

5. Special senses

  a) Vision

      (1) Presbyopia (farsightedness)—near vision decreases because of increasing rigidity of lens and loss of accommodations

      (2) Cataract—may or may not be handicapping; visual efficiency can be reduced

      (3) Glaucoma—more common in elderly people; leads to destruction of optic nerve tissue

      (4) Accomodation to light and dark—slower because of sclerosis of pupillary sphincter

  b) Hearing

      (1) Presbycusis begins at about age 30 and progresses to lower.

      (2) It starts in higher frequencies.

      (3) Leads to limitations in social relationships and thus causes withdrawal and changes in personality.

  c) Smell and taste—progressive loss common; may be hazardous as detection of noxious gases may be faulty

  d) Touch

      (1) Ability to detect heat, cold, and touch decreases.

      (2) There is some vibration sense loss.

6. Speech

  a) Changes in voice, pronunciation, and language usage

  b) Aphasia as result of cerebral lesions

7. Cardiovascular system

  a) Tendency toward increase in systolic blood pressure

  b) Decline in cardiac output at rest

    c) Sometimes, degenerative changes
    d) Loss in vessel elasticity
    e) Increased rigidity of heart valves

8. Respiratory system
    a) Reduction in vital capacity
    b) Increase in residual volume
    c) Increase in pulmonary arteriosclerosis, although slower than systemic arteriosclerosis
    d) Some increase in emphysema

9. Gastrointestinal system
    a) Anorexia due to decline in senses of smell and taste
    b) Poor dental health
    c) Reduction in gastric volume common
    d) Tendency toward loss of gastric juice
    e) Constipation due to decrease in peristalsis (weakening of muscular activity)
    f) Hemorrhoids—may lead to anemia from bleeding
    g) Lessening in nutritional needs
    h) Gallstones—frequency increases with age

10. Urinary system
    a) Filtration rate, renal blood flow, and tubular function decrease.
    b) Nocturia and polyuria are common.
       (1) Due to enlargement of prostate in male, which can lead to urinary stasis and thus cystitis
       (2) Due to infections of urethra with resultant cystitis in female
    c) Bladder capacity decreases.

11. Reproductive system
    a) Female
       (1) Menopause occurs; may present discomfort.
       (2) Low-grade estrogenic activity continues for some years as the result of adrenal and pituitary activity.
       (3) Vaginal dryness and thinning of mucosa occur.
    b) Male
       (1) Cessation of spermatogenesis in later life
       (2) Some atrophy of genitals in later life

12. Endocrine system
    a) Few endocrine deficits are recognized except menopause (diminution of estrogen secretion).
    b) Secretion of adrenal 17-ketosteroids and anabolic steroids is reduced.
    c) There is a gap in our knowledge of utilization of some hormones.
    d) In resting state, hormone activity may be normal, but under stress, abnormalities are detected.

13. Blood
    a) Poor nutritional state may affect level of hemoglobin.
    b) Improvement of anemia may decrease because of hemorrhage.
    c) Response of leukocytes to infection may decrease.

14. Nutrition—generally poor
    a) Many elderly have a preference for sugars.
    b) Reduced water intake is the rule.
    c) Motivation for preparing adequate meals is lacking.
    d) Taste buds are lost, and sense of smell reduced.
    e) Loss of teeth and presence of ill-fitting dentures make eating difficult.
    f) There is a reduction in gastric juice and gastric enzymes.
    g) Basal metabolic rate decreases.

II. **Symptoms, Signs, and Disorders Common in the Elderly**

  A. Accidental Hypothermia
    1. Definition of **hypothermia:** Condition in which the body temperature is below 35°C (95°F)
    2. Characteristics—decreased function and disease of organ systems
    3. Causes
      a) Inadequate heating of living quarters
      b) Prescribed medications

  B. Urinary Incontinence
      a) Cause is decreased bladder capacity.
      b) There is also incompetence of urinary sphincter.

  C. Degenerative Osteoarthritis
    1. Cause is unknown.
    2. Condition becomes universal by age 70.

  D. Hip Fracture and Repair (more often in female)

  E. Stroke
    1. Cerebral ischemia
    2. Cerebral hemorrhage
    3. Cerebral infarction due to embolism or thrombosis

  F. Metabolic Bone Disease (e.g., Osteomalacia)

  G. Prostatic Carcinoma
    1. Cause is unknown but may be due to excessive testosterone.
    2. Disease is slowly progressive.

  H. Basal Cell Carcinoma
    I. Herpes Zoster (Shingles)

  J. Chronic Lymphatic Leukemia
    1. Cause is unknown.
    2. Disease is commoner in males.

  K. Parkinsonism (Parkinson's Disease)
    1. Definition of **Parkinsonism:** Slowly progressive, degenerative disorder of central nervous system
    2. Four characteristic features—slowness, muscular rigidity, resting tremor, postural instability
    3. Etiology
      a) Cause is unknown, but viruses are suspected.
      b) There may be genetic susceptibility.
    4. Assessment
      a) Tremor
      b) Loss of spontaneous movement
      c) Rigidity
      d) Weakness affecting eating, swallowing, talking, writing
      e) Depression
      f) Dementia

     5. Nursing interventions
        a) Encourage patient to function at highest capacity.
        b) Assess and improve nutrition of patient.
        c) Refer patient to speech pathologist for therapy.
        d) Encourage independence in activities of daily living.
        e) Help patient and family to participate actively in therapy.
        f) Educate patient regarding the following:
            (1) Equipment that can help condition
            (2) Planned programs of activity
            (3) Regular physical routines
            (4) Well-balanced diet

L. Decubitus Ulcers
    Occurrence
    1. Patients with decreased sensation
    2. Generally patients who have been bedridden for long periods

M. Alzheimer's Disease
    1. Etiology
        a) Cause is unknown.
        b) Some change in brain cells is suspected.
    2. Assessment
        a) Loss of memory, gradually worsening
        b) Inappropriate behavior
        c) In many instances, good physical health

UNIT 2: SPECIAL PROBLEMS AND NEEDS OF THE ELDERLY AND AGED

I. **Financial and Social Implications of Aging**

    A. Financial Problems
        1. Retirement may create financial hardship.
        2. Many individuals have no pension plans, and Social Security without supplementation may be inadequate for needs.
        3. Problems are exacerbated if chronic illness occurs.
            a) Many persons are covered by Medicare, but benefits may not be adequate for long-term care.
            b) Many aged are not eligible for Medicaid coverage, and lack funds for expensive drugs and other medical costs.

    B. Housing
        1. High rents, especially in large cities, may absorb much of retiree's income.
        2. In cases of long-term disability, special housing may be needed.
            a) For skilled nursing care
            b) For intermediate nursing care
            c) For custodial care

    C. Emotional Needs
        1. Feeling of independence
        2. Feeling of being needed

3. Feeling of making valued contributions to community and to family
4. Recreation and socialization

II. Role of the Practical Nurse

General Principles
1. Is important member of medical team in institutional care of aged
2. Is important member of medical team in home care of aged
3. Must understand physical, mental, and psychological aspects of aging
4. Must be familiar with chronic manifestations of disease in elderly
5. Must understand need for protective devices
6. Must be sympathetic to aged persons

III. Duties of the Practical Nurse

A. General
1. Appreciate patient's desires in light of his/her ethnic, cultural, and religious background.
2. Protect patient from inappropriate behavior that would threaten his/her feelings of self-worth or interfere with interaction with other patients.
3. Urge patient to take part in recreational activities.
4. Try to understand patient's actions in light of past economic and social problems.

B. Specific
1. Assist R.N. in developing and implementing a nursing care plan for patient.
2. Give treatments, medications, and diet as ordered by physician.
3. Assist with restorative nursing care.
4. Accurately observe and record the following:
   a) Physical and mental condition of patient
   b) Changes in patient's condition
5. Apprise supervisors and/or physician of changes in patient's condition.
6. Give care to prevent decubitus ulcers and deformities.
7. Keep patient comfortable, clean, and well groomed.
8. Protect patient from accidents as much as possible.
9. Keep patient active and out of bed as much as possible.
10. Help patient to understand necessity for an adequate diet.
    a) High protein
    b) Roughage to keep bowels regular (check bowel patterns and chart)
11. Encourage and assist in helping patient in activities of daily living.
12. Allow patient to do as much as he/she can for self.
13. Respect dignity and rights of patient.
14. Maintain Foley catheter when needed.
15. Supervise range-of-motion exercises.

VIII

Nursing Care of the Oncology Patient

VOCABULARY

oncology	study of tumors
benign tumor	noncancerous growth that does not spread to other parts of the body; recovery is favorable with treatment
biopsy	removal and microscopic examination of tissue from the living body for purposes of diagnosis
cancer	general term for more than 100 diseases characterized by abnormal and uncontrolled growth of cells. The resulting mass, or tumor, can invade and destroy surrounding normal tissues. Cancer cells from the tumor can spread through the blood or lymph to start new cancers in other part of the body.
chemotherapy	treatment with anticancer drugs.
combination therapy	use of two or three methods to treat an individual cancer patient
immune system	body's system of defenses against disease, composed of white cells and antibodies, i.e., protein substances that react against bacteria and other harmful material
immunotherapy	experimental method of treating cancer that used substances that stimulate the body's immune system
malignant tumor	tumor having properties of invasion and metastasis
mammography	technique for X-raying the breast
Pap test	microscopic examination of material taken from the cervix to determine whether cancer cells are present
proctoscopic examination	examination made with a proctoscope, i.e., a lighted tube through which a doctor can see the interior of the rectum and lower colon; the proctoscope is inserted through the anus
radiation therapy	treatment using high-energy radiation from X-ray machines, cobalt, radium, or other sources
radioactive isotopes	substances that emit radiation while disintegrating; used in small, harmless amounts in cancer diagnosis and treatment
stoma	opening in the abdominal wall created as a new outlet for urine or feces
X rays	high-energy radiation used in high doses to treat cancer or in low doses to diagnose the disease
ultrasonography	process by which sound waves are reflected off points of variation to develop an image of a structure
computed tomography (CT)	process by which density differences are revealed by passing a very narrow X-ray beam over tiny cubes of tissue; a computer reconstructs a transverse section of the body and displays the image on a television monitor
magnetic resonance imaging (MRI)	technique that combines advantages of CT scan with ultrasound in using nonionizing radiation and providing tomography in any desired plane

NURSING CARE OF THE ONCOLOGY PATIENT

I. General Principles

A. Introduction
1. Definition of **cancer**: An abnormal and uncontrolled growth of cells
2. Characteristics
   a) Cancer is not one disease; word is general term for more than 100 diseases.
   b) Cancer is easily spread to other parts of body.
   c) Cancer nourishes itself by consuming normal cells.
   d) Cancer can strike any organ.

B. Incidence
1. Annual death toll from cancer is high in the United States, where it ranks second as cause of death.
2. Cancer can strike at any age.
3. Incidence increases as age advances.

C. Assessment: Seven Warning Signs and Symptoms
1. Change in bowel or bladder habits
2. A sore that does not heal
3. Unusual bleeding or discharge
4. Thickening or lump in breast or elsewhere
5. Indigestion or difficulty in swallowing
6. Obvious change in wart or mole
7. Nagging cough or hoarseness

D. Characteristics of Tumors
1. Malignant
   a) Multiply rapidly
   b) Are not encapsulated; are invasive and infiltrative
   c) Are composed of undifferentiated cells
   d) Can detach themselves from tumor site, travel through blood and lymph system, and establish new tumors in distant regions of body
2. Benign
   a) Grow slowly
   b) Are often encapsulated, so tumor cannot spread and invade surrounding tissue
   c) Do not form secondary tumors in other regions of the body

II. Treatment

A. Kinds of Treatment
1. Surgery
2. Radiotherapy (radiation treatment)
3. Radioisotopes
4. Drugs (chemotherapy)
5. Immunotherapy

B. Method of Treatment—depends on
1. Type of cancer
2. Extent of spread
3. Condition of patient
4. Decision of oncologist

III. **Role of Nutrition**

A. National Cancer Institute Nutritional Guidelines
   1. Avoid obesity.
   2. Decrease total fat intake.
   3. Increase intake of high-fiber foods.
   4. Increase intake of cruceriferous vegetables, e.g., broccoli, brussels sprouts, cabbage, cauliflower.
   5. Include foods high in vitamins A and C.
   6. Decrease use of smoked, nitrite-cured, and salt-cured foods.
   7. Drink alcoholic beverages very sparingly.

B. No evidence that any special diet will prevent cancer

IV. **Nursing Interventions in Cancer Treatment**

A. Maintaining Nutritional and Fluid Balance
   1. Obtain comprehensive dietary history of patient.
   2. Confer with dietician to plan diet.
   3. Encourage patient's family to bring home-cooked foods.
   4. Make mealtime relaxed and pleasant.
   5. If patient can't eat, give protein formulas and semiliquid foods through tube.
      a) Flush tube well after each use.
      b) Give 4–6 ounces of water or fluid between feedings.
   6. Be aware that hyperalimentation is very important in cancer cases.

B. Controlling Pain
   1. Pain is caused by inflammation, pressure, and tumor infiltration into adjoining tissues.
   2. Narcotic analgesics and narcotic analgesics with phenothiazines are effective.
   3. Radiation helps at times.

C. Monitoring and Alleviating Chemotherapy Side Effects
   1. Report signs of infection immediately.
   2. Force fluids to 2–3 liters daily.
   3. Warn of possibility of hair loss.
      a) Suggest wig.
      b) Reassure patient that hair will grow back after therapy ends.
   4. Check skin for rashes, petechiae, and cellulitis during certain treatments.
   5. Maintain a properly running I.V.
   6. Notify the physician immediately if extravasation occurs.
   7. Emphasize beneficial results of chemotherapy to patient.
   8. Provide antiemetic if necessary.
   9. Provide support and encouragement during treatment.

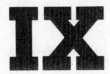

Public Health

VOCABULARY

demography	study of distribution of people
morbidity	illness or disease
mortality	death
natality	birth
pollute	to make impure
quarantine	isolation because of suspected contagion
reticuloendothelial system	cell group found in bone marrow, liver, spleen, and lymph nodes; aid in making new blood cells and in disintegrating old ones
sewage	matter found in sewers, e.g., garbage, human and animal excretions
sewerage	system of pipes arranged for carrying off sewage of house or town
vital statistics	branch of biostatistics which deals with data of human mortality, morbidity, natality, and demography

I. **Introduction**

    A. Definition of **Public Health**: Combination of sanitary science and medical science to improve physical, social, and mental well-being of community as a whole

    B. Characteristics
       1. Involves more than individual doctor-patient relationship
       2. Is generally controlled by legislation and/or government policy
       3. Has strong local community input today

II. **Health Agencies**

    A. Governmental
       1. United States Public Health Service
          a) Was originally formed to provide public health care to the merchant marine
          b) Presently involves the following:
             (1) International and interstate quarantine
             (2) Research and demonstration health projects
          c) Gives technical advice
          d) Gives financial support to health programs of states and local health agencies
          e) Provides public information and education
          f) Has several units, including the following:
             (1) National Institutes of Health
             (2) National Institutes of Mental Health
             (3) Consumer Protection and Environmental Health Service

2. Department of Health and Human Services
   a) Is umbrella organization
   b) Is composed of major federal agencies involved in health and human services
3. Food and Drug Administration
   a) Evaluates drugs before they are released for public use
   b) Monitors side effects of all drugs on market
   c) Monitors rules and laws relative to food processing
4. Children's Bureau
   a) Helps states improve maternal and child health services
   b) Provides funds for state Bureaus of Handicapped Children
5. State and local departments of health
   a) Functions legislated
      (1) Control of communicable disease
      (2) Control of environmental sanitation
      (3) Recording of vital statistics and other health statistics
      (4) Maternal and child health services
      (5) Rehabilitation services for patients with certain groups of diseases
      (6) Mental health care
      (7) Financial and advisory aid to local health districts
   b) Local health departments
      (1) Provide direct services in environmental control
      (2) Provide some diagnostic and therapeutic clinical services
      (3) Provide preventive medicine clinics, well-baby clinics, immunization clinics

B. Voluntary
   1. Professional societies
      a) American Medical Association
         (1) Sets standards for medical profession
         (2) Encourages public and professional education
         (3) Supports some health legislation if it conforms to views of association
      b) American Nurses' Association
         (1) Is official organization for registered nurses
         (2) Sets standards for professional practice and nursing education
      c) National Association of Practical Nurse Education and Services
         (1) Was formed to improve standards of practical nurse education
         (2) Accepts as members M.D.'s, R.N.'s, L.P.N.'s, and lay persons
         (3) Seeks to raise quality of care rendered by practical nurses
         (4) Accredits schools of practical nursing
      d) National Federation of Licensed Practical Nurses
         (1) Was formed to improve working conditions of licensed practical nurse
         (2) Seeks to promote better understanding of practical nursing
         (3) Is official organization for L.P.N.'s and R.N.'s
      e) National League of Nursing
         (1) Was formed to improve nursing education and nursing services at all levels
         (2) Includes professional nurses, practical nurses, allied professionals, and other interested persons
   2. Agencies concerned with specific diseases and research
      a) American Cancer Society
      b) American Diabetic Association
      c) American Association for Help of Retarded Children
   3. Large funding organizations
      a) Community Chest
      b) Red Cross

c) Rockefeller Foundation
d) United Fund

III. Communicable Disease Control

A. Environmental Control
1. Milk sanitation
   a) Milk is effective transmitter of diseases such as typhoid, dysentery, tuberculosis, streptococcal infections, diphtheria, poliomyelitis, infectious hepatitis.
   b) Milk must be protected at three levels.
      (1) Production—healthy cows
      (2) Processing—pasteurization
      (3) Distribution—correct refrigeration, adequate and sterilized containers
2. Control of water supplies
   a) Water supplies are derived from the following:
      (1) Rain and snow
      (2) Surface water—rivers, ponds, lakes, etc.
      (3) Groundwater—wells and springs
   b) Water-borne diseases include infectious hepatitis, bacillary and amebic dysentery, typhoid and paratyphoid fevers, cholera, and diseases resulting from chemical pollution.
   c) Water is purified by
      (1) Evaporation and condensation
      (2) Storage in ponds and lakes
      (3) Self-purification of running streams
      (4) Filtering action of soil
   d) Protection of water supplies is necessary in national emergencies.
      (1) Danger of intentional contamination by saboteurs.
      (2) Disruption of supplies necessary for drinking, fire fighting, etc.
3. Improvement in methods of sewage disposal to avoid
   a) Pollution of water
   b) Danger to water supplies
   c) Danger to livestock
   d) Poisoning and contamination of fish and shellfish
   e) Objectionable floating matter
   f) Decreased oxygen in water, leading to death of aqueous plants, etc.
4. Proper food handling
   a) Proper handling of food is effective in reducing prevalence of intestinal diseases.
   b) Improperly handled or cooked food is a good transmitter of the following:
      (1) Animal parasites such as tapeworms
      (2) Bacteria
      (3) Bacterial toxins such as botulinus and salmonellosis
   c) Poisons are sometimes used as pesticides or preservatives.
   d) Health department programs include the following:
      (1) Restaurant inspections
      (2) Meat and fish inspections
      (3) Examinations of food handlers
5. Control of arthropod vectors
   a) Drainage of swampy areas
   b) Ratproofing of buildings
   c) Use of insecticides
   d) Use of screens
   e) Use of insect repellents

B. Isolation and Quarantine of Infected Persons
  1. This measure is not entirely effective because healthy carriers spread disease.
  2. Also, the incubation period of disease is symptom-free.

C. Immunization (most important measure in preventing infectious disease)
  1. Smallpox
  2. Diphtheria
  3. Whooping cough
  4. Tetanus
  5. Measles
  6. German measles
  7. Mumps
  8. Poliomyelitis
  9. Pneumococcal pneumonia

D. Antibiotics and Chemotherapeutics (often important, especially in treating infections)

IV. **Chronic Disease Control**

Early Detection Advantageous
  1. Necessitates periodic physical examination
  2. Necessitates periodic screening tests for diseases common after middle age
     a) Cervical cytology (Pap smear) in all women yearly during childbearing years
     b) Periodic breast examination, including mammography, for older and high-risk women
     c) EKG yearly after age 35
     d) Tonometry yearly after age 35 (2% of persons tested over age 40 years found to have glaucoma)
     e) Blood chemistry especially for glucose (1% of persons over age 25 years found to be diabetic)
     f) TB screening

V. **Immunity and Immunization**

A. Types of Immunity
  1. Natural
     a) Is resistance of body to invasion of bacteria, viruses, or other infectious agents or toxins
     b) Results from
        (1) White blood cells and reticuloendothelial system
        (2) Presence of nonspecific antibodies in blood
  2. Acquired
     a) Development of immunity to many destructive agents
        (1) Proteins of toxins stimulate production of specific antibodies.
        (2) These immune bodies (antibodies) can destroy specific organisms.
     b) Types of acquired immunity
        (1) Active—established by having the disease or by artificial means (vaccines, toxoids, etc.)
        (2) Passive—established by administration of immune serum

B. Active Immunization Procedures in Pediatrics (schedule recommended by New York State Department of Health)
  1. Oral polio vaccine—2 months, 4 months, 15 months, 4–6 years

2. Diphtheria-tetanus-pertussis—2 months, 4 months, 6 months, 15 months, 4–6 years
3. Measles, mumps, rubella—15 months, 4–6 years
4. Haemophilus influenza (Type B): 18 months (as of 1/1/90, required for children 18 months to 5 years in daycare or any preschool program)

C. Other Immunization Procedures
   1. BCG—recommended for tuberculin-negative persons who will live or travel in a high-tuberculous area
   2. Immunization against rabies, which is fatal if not treated properly and immediately
      a) Immunity before exposure is limited to persons living in areas where rabies is prevalent.
      b) Immunity is generally given after exposure.
   3. Immunization before foreign travel
      a) Certain immunizations are given, depending upon need and country or countries to be visited
         (1) Cholera
         (2) Yellow fever (given by USPHS)
         (3) Typhoid fever
         (4) Typhus
         (5) Plague
      b) Complete physical examination is essential in conjunction with screening tests.
   4. Difficulties in maintaining effective program in the United States
      a) Continual rise in costs of diagnostic examinations and tests
      b) Unequal distribution of manpower and facilities for health care

VI. Current Major Health Problems

A. Congenital Heart Disease   See also Chapter VI, Unit 3.
   1. Of live births, 0.3% are affected.
   2. Many die in neonatal period.
   3. Prevention includes the following:
      a) Avoidance of rubella infection by pregnant women
      b) Adequate immunization against rubella during childhood
      c) Early case history and treatment

B. Arteriosclerosis, Hypertension, and Coronary Artery Disease   See also Chapter IV, Unit 4.
   1. Early diagnosis is imperative.
   2. Proper management includes the following:
      a) Dietary management
      b) Occupational adaptation
      c) Therapeutic procedures, e.g., use of drugs, salt restriction
      d) Emotional support

C. Cancer   See also Chapter VIII.
   1. Primary prevention is generally improbable.
   2. Elimination of smoking is desirable.
   3. Removal of industrial carcinogens is important.
   4. Removal of precancerous lesions—skin lesions, cervical lesions—is important.
   5. Early detection is important.
   6. Vigorous treatment is essential.
   7. Population should be educated regarding abnormal signs.
   8. Rehabilitation after diagnosis and treatment is very important.

D. Chronic Respiratory Disease   See also Chapter IV, Unit 5.
1. Extent of problem
   a) Deaths from pneumonia and tuberculosis have declined in past 50 years.
   b) Incidence of emphysema and bronchitis has risen.
2. Causes
   a) Degree of poverty has correlation with incidence.
   b) Atmospheric pollution and cigarette smoking are important factors.
3. Prevention and/or amelioration
   a) Early diagnosis
   b) Vigorous treatment
   c) Rehabilitation

E. Diabetes Mellitus See also Chapter IV, Unit 8.
1. Etiology
   a) Hereditary influence is important.
   b) Obesity is a factor.
   c) Insulin only controls, but does not cure, this disease.
2. Prevention and/or control
   a) Early detection and case finding
   b) Proper management
      (1) Dietary control
      (2) Reducing obesity
      (3) Avoidance of infections
      (4) Use of insulin where indicated
   c) Avoidance of marriage between diabetics

F. Arthritis   See also Chapter IV, Unit 2.
1. Extent of problem
   a) Causes great disability and discomfort but rarely death
   b) Disables possibly over 3.2 million persons in the United States
2. Types of arthritis
   a) Osteoarthritis
      (1) Is degenerative joint disease
      (2) Obesity and resultant faulty posture may be factors.
   b) Rheumatoid arthritis
      (1) Leads to deformity and disability
      (2) Is more frequent in females
      (3) Familial tendency is present.
   c) Gout
      (1) Is more frequent in men
      (2) Dietary and alcoholic factors are important
   d) Infectious arthritis
      (1) May be caused by many organisms
      (2) Usually affects a single joint

G. Deafness   See also Chapter IV, Unit 3.
1. Causes
   a) Congenital
   b) Infections
   c) Brain disorders
   d) Environmental factors (noise)
   e) Drugs, e.g., quinine, streptomycin
2. Prevention

    a) Case history
    b) Removal of environmental hazards
    c) Adequate treatment of infections

  H. Blindness   See also Chapter IV, Unit 3.
    1. Causes
       a) Cataract
       b) Diabetes
       c) Glaucoma
       d) Infections
       e) Trauma
    2. Extent of problem
       a) Persons with corrected visual acuity of 20/200 or less are classified as legally
          blind.
       b) Of persons in the United States, 0.2% are legally blind.
       c) There are about 0.5 million blind persons in the United States.
    3. Prevention
       a) Control of opthalmia neonatorum by use of silver nitrate or antibiotic in eyes at
          birth
       b) Treatment and control of syphilis in pregnant women
       c) Control of oxygen given to premature infants, thereby preventing retrolental fibro-
          plasia
       d) Periodic visual screening of schoolchildren
       e) Early diagnosis of glaucoma
    4. Rehabilitation
       a) Special classes for blind children
       b) Vocational rehabilitation

VII. Maternal, Child, and Other Health Programs

  A. Purpose
    1. To provide complete and continuous health supervision, integrated with other health
       department programs for effectiveness, from conception to adulthood
       a) Maternal supervision and care
       b) Well-baby care
       c) Preschool screening
       d) School screening
    2. To serve as measures for population control by providing birth control education.
  B. School Health Programs
    1. Goals
       a) Educate child and family in good health habits
       b) Stimulate child and family to use this knowledge
       c) Lead to early discovery of physical and mental abnormalities
       d) Provide adequate immunization programs
       e) Prevent communicable disease
    2. School health team
       a) Teacher—sees child daily
          (1) Does daily screening
          (2) Notes abnormalities of vision, hearing, actions, nutrition
          (3) Teaches health studies
       b) Public health nurse
          (1) Sees child referred by teacher
          (2) Has conferences with teacher concerning child

        (3)   Refers child for further followup
    c) School physician
        (1)   Provides periodic examinations
        (2)   Provides necessary immunizations if requested by parent
    d) Dental and audiometric screening in some schools
  3. Special programs in schools for disabled children

VIII. Nutrition Programs

A. Extent of Problem
1. Problem in the United States is to maintain good nutrition in all people.
2. Malnourishment is common in certain areas because of inadequate or poor food.
3. Ethnic culture and age are factors.

B. Examples of Programs
1. Many health departments sponsor nutrition programs.
2. School lunch programs are funded by federal government.
3. There are federally funded programs for elderly, such as "Meals on Wheels."

IX. Mental Health   See also Chapter XII.

A. Mental Retardation
1. Of general population, 3% are affected.
2. Numbers of mentally retarded are growing.
    a) There is an increase in general population itself.
    b) Physical health of retarded is improving, and longer life results.
3. Early diagnosis (tests are done at birth) and treatment of certain metabolic disorders, e.g., phenylpyruvic acid oligophrenia and galactosemia, can prevent retardation.

B. Psychosis, Alcoholism, and Organic Mental Syndrome (Senile Psychosis)
1. Many state and federal programs support treatment of psychosis.
2. There are federally funded programs for treatment of alcoholism in local communities.
3. Many senile psychotics are in nursing homes (mental hospitals tend not to admit patients for whom there is no rehabilitation).

Institutional, Community, and Rehabilitation Nursing

UNIT 1: INSTITUTIONAL NURSING

I. **Kinds and Levels of Institutional Care**

   A. Kinds of Institutional Care as Defined by Federal and State Legislation
      1. Acute hospital care
      2. Skilled nursing care
      3. Intermediate nursing care
      4. Intermediate supervised personal care
      5. Institutional room and board

   B. Levels of Institutional Care Defined
      1. By approved medical care practices
      2. By approved health care concepts
      3. By current legislation
         a) Medicare
         b) Medicaid
         c) State health codes
         d) Local health codes
      4. By current health programs

   C. Levels of Care Not All-Inclusive or Rigid
      1. Many patients' needs overlap, depending upon diagnosis and level of functioning
      2. There may be periodic changes upward or downward in patient's condition
      3. Standards of quality and quantity of care depend upon the judgment and skill of health professionals

II. **Medical and Nursing Care in Acute General or Specialty Hospitals**

   A. Medical Care
      1. Medical care is under direction of patient's attending physician.
      2. Quantity and quality are governed by official agencies and standards of the hospital uitlization review committee.

   B. Nursing Care and Services
      1. Patient usually stays for only a short time.

2. Nursing care is provided under direction of R.N., who serves as director of nursing services.
   a) Practical nurses, attendants, aides, and orderlies assist R.N. and work directly under her/his supervision.
   b) Nurses collaborate with and carry out physician's orders.
   c) Individual patient's needs are met according to nursing care plan.
   d) Close observation is provided.
3. Social services is under direction of social work department.

III. Medical and Nursing Care in Nursing Homes and Chronic Care Hospitals

A. Medical Care
   1. Medical care is under direction of attending physician.
   2. Current legislation requires physician to see patient every 30 days, but visits may be more frequent if medically necessary.
   3. Medicare (Title XIX) requires documentation for acute visits.
   4. Utilization review committee monitors necessity for care

B. Nursing Care
   1. Nursing care is under direction of R.N.
   2. Adequate number of licensed nurses must be on duty throughout each 24-hour period as specified by federal and state statutes.
   3. Nursing care is provided by L.P.N. or R.N.
   4. Average stay of patient is long term, but stay may be short term.
   5. Basic social services are under direction of social service department.

C. Needs Met in This Type of Care (depend upon other needs)
   1. Skilled observations of patients with chronic conditions
   2. Administration of intravenous or subcutaneous fluids by an R.N. upon physician's order
   3. Daily nasopharyngeal aspiration
   4. Daily administration of oxygen and/or positive pressure treatments by licensed nursing personnel
   5. Comprehensive dressings, required on daily basis by order of physician, performed by R.N. or L.P.N.
   6. Tube feeding or gastrostomy feeding given by licensed nurses on physician's order
   7. Continuous supervision by licensed nurse because of unpredictable behavior of patient
   8. Administration of potent injectible medications daily
   9. Bowel and bladder training
   10. Gait training (short-term) and other restorative procedures

D. Nursing Service
   1. Characteristics
      a) Must be in accordance with established nursing care plan
      b) Develops and maintains nursing care plan to complement attending physician's plan of medical care
      c) Reviews and updates plan as necessary
   2. Goals
      a) Provide skilled care to prevent decubiti and contractures
      b) Keep patient comfortable, clean, and protected from injury
      c) Encourage patient to take part in group activities
      d) Rehabilitate patient in activities of daily living

e) Supervise patient's nutrition
f) Administer medications according to physician's orders
g) Help meet patient's psychological needs

IV. Intermediate Medical and Nursing Care in Nursing Homes

A. Medical Care
   1. Medical care is under direction of attending physician.
   2. Physician attendance for each resident is required at least every 60 days by federal and state statute, but may be more frequent if patient's condition requires it.
   3. Documentation is required by Medicare for frequent visits.

B. Nursing Care
   1. Nursing care is under direction of R.N.
   2. L.P.N., as charge nurse, works under supervision of R.N.

C. Average Length of Stay—varies according to patient's needs but may be long term

D. Services Provided
   1. Assisting bed patients and patients who need wheelchair and/or other ambulatory aids
   2. Supervision of activities of daily living, e.g., bathing, personal hygiene, dressing, eating.
   3. Prevention and treatment of skin irritation and of uncomplicated decubiti
      a) Severe irritations and ulcers may mandate skilled care.
      b) Proper documentation in patient's record is necessary.
   4. Assistance and training in self-care
   5. Assistance and training in patient transfer techniques, e.g., bed to chair, wheelchair to toilet
   6. Range-of-motion exercises as part of routine maintenance nursing care
   7. Administration of medications—all medications should be administered by licensed personnel
   8. Administration of oxygen on a less-than-daily basis
   9. Use of nebulizers and intermittent positive pressure breathing equipment on less-than-daily basis
   10. Basic social services under direction of social work department

V. Intermediate Supervised Personal Care in Old-Age Homes and Similar Facilities

A. Characteristics
   1. Care and services emphasize protection and supervison; nursing care is not given.
   2. Routine medical care is ambulatory and on outpatient basis.
   3. Physician services are provided on emergency basis only and are arranged by individual patient.
   4. Daily care and services are directed by trained nonprofessional persons.
   5. Average stay is long term, but length is determined on individual basis.

B. Services Provided
   1. Supervision and protection from hazards
   2. Regular and therapeutic diets
   3. Supervision and assistance with personal care
   4. Assistance with physical exercise according to individual needs
   5. Recreation activities

6. Basic social services
7. Help with securing medical care when necessary

VI. Institutional Room and Board in Domiciliary Facilities

Characteristics
1. Services are limited to room and board for otherwise independent persons.
2. This level of care is required mostly for social and economic reasons.
3. Medical services are the responsibility of individual.

UNIT 2: COMMUNITY NURSING

1. Nursing in the Community

A. Nature of Home Care—may be sporadic or organized, according to plan

B. Types of Organized Home Care
   1. Hospital-based
   2. Community-based

C. Advantages of Home Care (see Data Summary 18)
   1. Allows ill patient to receive needed nursing care at home
   2. Keeps family group intact
      a) Ill mother remains home with family.
      b) Ill child does not have feeling of abandonment by family.
   3. Allows patient to continue as much as possible in culture and life-style to which he/she is accustomed
      a) Ethnic foods may not be readily available in an institution.
      b) Visiting is easier for family and friends.
      c) Sounds of family activity are important.
   4. Frees hospital bed for more acutely ill patients
   5. Is less expensive than hospital nursing

II. Hospital-Based Home Care

A. Advantages
   1. Home care frees expensive hospital bed for a more acutely ill patient.
   2. Hospitals are generally depressing to long-term patients.
   3. Patients are made more dependent in hospitals.
   4. Patients are exposed to fewer infections at home.
   5. Continuity of hospital care is assured although patient is at home.

B. Standards
   1. Home care department should be separate unit of hospital.
   2. Full-time professional personnel and competent nonprofessionals should be assigned with full-time physician director.
      a) Professional personnel
         (1) Administrator
         (2) Chief of professional services (physician)
         (3) Staff physicians
         (4) Public health nurse coordinator
         (5) Staff nurses

           (6)   Social worker
           (7)   Physical therapist
           (8)   Occupational therapist
           (9)   Vocational rehabilitation specialist
           (10) Recreational therapist
           (11) Professional consultants

      b) Nonprofessional personnel
           (1)   Administrative medical secretary and necessary clerical staff
           (2)   Workshop staff

   3. Total needs of patient should be considered in determining eligibility for admission to program.
      a) Complete medical evaluation
      b) Complete nursing evaluation
      c) Complete social evaluation to determine whether
           (1)   Facilities in patient's home are adaptive to care.
           (2)   Family is willing to have patient home.

C. Coordination of Services
   1. Team evaluation conference, in which all information—medical, nursing, and social—is considered in developing a treatment plan for patient
   2. Interagency referral form to help coordinate information and thus assure continuity of services
   3. Adequate discharge planning
      a) Good physician services must be available.
      b) Plans must be made to maintain patient gains.
      c) Other necessary services must be available to patient.

D. Financing
   1. Third-party insurance carriers, e.g., Blue Shield-Blue Cross
   2. Public programs such as Medicaid (Title XIX)
   3. Other prepayment and third-party programs

E. Criteria for Selection of Patients
   1. This type of program must fit patient's needs; program is not a substitute for inpatient care.
   2. Criteria must include medical, nursing, and social factors.
   3. Patients must be unable to afford to pay individually for services received under home care.
   4. Nearness of patient to hospital facilities must be considered.
   5. Staff travel time must be considered.

III. Community-Based Home Care

A. Advantages
   1. Home care is available to patients not eligible for hospital-based programs.
   2. This type of care offers the advantages listed in Section I.C.

B. Disadvantages
   1. This type of care serves primarily as coordinating agent.
   2. Standards are more difficult to set and maintain than in hospital-based program.
   3. Supervision of physicians is more difficult.
   4. It is more difficult to get physicians to attend conferences.
   5. It is difficult to get physicians to submit reports.

C. Standards
1. Program must have adequate professional staff.
   a) Physician (generally attending physician of patient)
   b) Public health nurse (may be L.P.N. under supervision of R.N.)
   c) Caseworker
2. Attending physican must make referral on appropriate form.
   a) May be his letterhead
   b) Must contain necessary information as to condition of patient
   c) Must include orders for medical and nursing care
   d) If rehabilitation or physiotherapy necessary, must include these orders (see Data Summary 19)
3. Attending physician must arrange for necessary consultations by other medical specialists; referrals to outpatient department of local hospital or to other agencies may be included.

D. Financing
1. Private insurers, e.g., Blue Shield-Blue Cross, Travelers.
2. Public funds such as Medicaid (Title XIX)
3. Patient's own funds, although this care is very costly

E. Criteria for Selection of Patients
1. Physician's request
2. Evaluation of necessary nursing care, made by nursing agency

F. Coordination
1. Interagency referral form necessary
2. Physicians encouraged to attend conferences

IV. **Role of Practical Nurse in Organized Home-Care Programs**

A. Important Member of Health Team
1. Is supervised by professional public health nurse
2. Has major responsibility of caring for patient; carries out nursing care plan developed by public health nurse

B. Duties and Responsibilities
1. Must be very knowledgeable regarding all bedside nursing procedures
2. Must be able to improvise with facilities available in patient's home
3. Must keep adequate and accurate records of patient's condition
4. Must report changes in patient's condition to supervising nurse
5. Must educate patient's family
   a) Assist family to understand care needs in patient's disease
   b) Assist family to help in care of patient
6. Must provide psychological assistance to patient
   a) Must be able to empathize with patient
   b) Must help patient to accept his/her illness
   c) Must not identify with patient to excessive degree
7. Must be able to cope with emergency conditions
   a) Must be able to recognize emergent conditions
   b) Must be able to intervene in such conditions by seeking necessary help

---

DATA SUMMARY 18
Services Offered under Community Home-Care Programs

1. Physician services
2. Home nursing sevices including home health aide
3. Social services
4. Homemaker or housekeeper services
5. Transportation services for medical services
6. Physical therapy
7. Speech therapy
8. Home-delivered food services
9. Medical laboratory services

DATA SUMMARY 19
Rehabilitation Services Offered under
Home-Care Programs, Both Community- and Hospital-Based

1. Routine evaluation of patients for rehabilitation
2. Physical therapy services
3. Speech and hearing therapy services

UNIT 3: REHABILITATION NURSING

I. Introduction

A. Definition of **rehabilitation:** Restoration of patient's function to as nearly normal as possible
   1. Includes care by specialists in fields of physical therapy, occupational therapy, speech therapy, eye therapy, hearing therapy, etc.
   2. Seeks maximum reduction of physical or mental disability

B. Objectives of Rehabilitation
   1. Patient is taught to be as independent as possible.
   2. Patient is taught to stress his/her assets rather than handicaps.

II. Handicapping Disorders

A. Neurological Conditions
   1. Stroke
      a) Paralysis
      b) Aphasia
   2. Paralysis or loss of limb(s) as a result of accident or pathological condition
      a) Hemiplegia
      b) Quadriplegia
      c) Paraplegia
      d) Amputation
   3. Multiple sclerosis
   4. Parkinsonism (Parkinson's Disease)
   5. Poliomyelitis

6. Cerebral palsy
7. Brain injury

B. Heart Disease

C. Psychosis

D. Loss of Vision

E. Deafness

III. Immediate Goals of Rehabilitation and Factors Affecting Results

A. Immediate goals
   1. Restore function as much as possible
   2. Maintain function
   3. Help patient adjust to conditions in which function cannot be restored, as in sensory loss (blindness, deafness)
   4. Aid patient to move from an intensive level of care (hospital) to a lesser level of care and ultimately to community

B. Considerations Affecting Results of Rehabilitation
   1. Age of patient
   2. Physical condition of patient
   3. Duration of disability
   4. Nature of disability
   5. Psychological reaction of patient to disability
   6. Intelligence and understanding of patient
   7. Attitude of patient's family
   8. Community resources convenient to patient
   9. Professional help and facilities available to patient

IV. The Rehabilitation Team

A. Medical
   1. Attending physician
   2. Medical consultants

B. Nursing

C. Ancillary
   1. Speech therapist
   2. Occupational therapist

V. Facilities for Rehabilitation

Types
   1. Rehabilitation centers connected with large medical centers and teaching hospitals
   2. Specialized nursing homes with physiotherapy departments and staff
   3. Home care organized by voluntary agencies
   4. Special public schools for brain-injured, cerebral palsy, cardiac, and orthopedic-handicap patients
   5. Private specialized schools for the handicapped

INSTITUTIONAL, COMMUNITY, AND REHABILITATION NURSING

6. Halfway houses for psychiatric rehabilitation
7. Foster homes

VI. Rehabilitation Therapies

A. Educational Therapy
1. Patient must be assisted in understanding his/her limitations and in using whatever functions he/she has.
2. Patient's family must be encouraged to accept patient's limitations.
3. Family must be trained to help patient.

B. Surgical Therapy
1. Surgical correction when feasible
2. Fitting of artificial limbs and other aids

C. Physical Therapy
1. Positioning
2. Bracing
3. Splinting
4. Exercise
5. Practice with artificial aids
   a) Prostheses
   b) Walkers
   c) Wheelchairs
   d) Low-vision lenses
   e) Hearing aids

D. Occupational Therapy—medically prescribed
1. Training in activities of daily living
2. Recreational therapy, useful in restoring function of small muscles of hand and fingers (weaving, woodcarving, needlework)
3. Prevocational activites, e.g., typing

E. Speech Therapy
1. Importance—patients become frustrated when they cannot communicate
2. Speech disorders
   a) Congenital conditions—cleft palate and lip
   b) Acquired aphasia after CVA
   c) Special need after laryngectomy
   d) Stammering and stuttering
   e) Articulative dysfunctions

VII. Rehabilitation Nursing

A. Goals
1. Maintain skin intact in immoble patient
2. Keep posture as normal as possible to avoid contractures and relieve dependent edema
3. Keep functional range of joint motion
4. Restore or maintain bladder function
5. Restore or maintain bowel function
6. Aid patient in activities of daily living toward independence
7. Aid patient in transfer

B. Role of the Practical Nurse
    1. Help patient become as independent as possible in
        a) Activities of daily living
        b) Transfer from bed to wheelchair
        c) Ambulation
        d) Use of artificial limbs
        e) Use of aids for eating and walking
    2. Develop occupational and recreational interests.
    3. Gain cooperation of family in aiding patient.
    4. See that physician's orders are carried out.
    5. Help to maintain emotional balance of patient (more favorable if patient knows that
        medical plan includes feasible restorative plans).

C. Specific Nursing Needs and Procedures
    1. Complications affecting bedridden patient
        a) Decubitus
        b) Disturbances leading to constipation, indigestion, abdominal distension, etc.
        c) Urinary infection from stasis
        d) Thrombophlebitis due to blood stagnation
        e) Stagnation of respiratory secretions leading to pneumonia, etc.
        f) Contractures, osteoporosis, and diminution in muscle tone
    2. Prevention of contractures
        a) Frequently move and turn patient
        b) Use various types of supports to maintain position.
        c) Provide gentle passive exercise of spastic or contracted joints.
    3. Bowel-bladder training program
        a) Be aware that program is useful except in patients with spinal cord injuries.
        b) Follow procedures outlined in textbook or regimen outlined by particular institu-
            tion.
    4. Range-of-motion function—follow procedures initiated by physiotherapy department
    5. Activities of daily living
        a) Cooperate in team effort with physician and therapists.
        b) Set realistic objectives
        c) Have available devices necessary to aid patient
    6. Other functions
        a) Maintain effective respiratory function.
        b) Maintain excellent skin care; reduce threat of pressure sores.
        c) Monitor for neurologic deficit.
        d) Monitor nutrition; provide adequate diet according to diagnosis.
        e) Promote patient's comfort.
        f) Help patient cope with psychological disturbances.

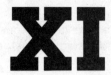

Disaster and Emergency Nursing

VOCABULARY

abrasion	spot rubbed bare of skin or mucous membrane
accident	unforeseen occurrence, especially one involving injury
artificial respiration	procedure for causing air to flow from and into lungs by mechanical means when natural breathing ceases
disaster	event that causes great misfortune, e.g., flood, fire, earthquake
dislocation	displacement of bone end from joint
emergency	occasion of urgency; situation that arises suddenly and requires immediate action
first aid	immediate and temporary care given victim of sudden illness or accident until skilled medical care can be obtained
fracture	break or rupture in bone
hemorrhage	bleeding; escape of blood from vessels
laceration	wound made by tearing of the skin
poison	any substance applied to body, ingested, inhaled, or developed within body that may cause damage or disturbance of function
rabies	specific infectious disease of certain animals, e.g., dogs and wolves, transmitted to humans by bite of infected animal
shock	condition of acute peripheral circulatory failure due to loss of circulating fluid after injury
sprain	injury to soft tissue surrounding joints
strain	injury to muscles due to overexertion
wound	break in skin or mucous membrane that extends into underlying tissue

I. **Introduction**

    A. General Principles
        1. During major disaster, practical nurse does not function in usual role.
        2. Nurse administers first aid.
        3. Nurse directs care of people.

    B. Functions of Rescuers
        1. Save lives
        2. Give comfort
        3. Preserve function
        4. Preserve cosmetic appearance

II. **Disaster**

    A. Characteristics

    1. Emergency situation has arisen.
    2. Large number of people are involved
    3. Nursing care may be either first aid or emergency care.

B. Types
    1. Natural
        a) Flood
        b) Tornado
        c) Earthquake
        d) Hurricane
    2. Man-made
        a) Airplane crash
        b) Train crash
        c) Multiple automobile crash
        d) War
        e) Violent civil disturbance, e.g., riot

C. Major Problems
    1. Psychologic reaction to disaster may be panic.
    2. Integrity of water and food supplies may be threatened.
    3. Proper organization of treatment needs to be determined.
        a) Follow disaster drills as previously practiced.
        b) Apply triage procedure, which establishes priorities of treatment.
            (1) First priority—immediate treatment
            (2) Second priority—delayed treatment
            (3) Third priority—expectant treatment

D. General Nursing Principles
    1. Proper identification—uniforms of medical personnel
    2. Proper reporting to designated treatment area
    3. Proper tagging of patients for identification and treatment
        a) Ambulatory patients to be given tasks
        b) Self-care disabled persons to be moved
    4. Close observation of patients for
        a) Psychologic reaction
        b) Medical emergencies

III. **Emergency**

A. General Characteristics
    1. Any number of persons may be involved.
    2. Care can be given only in hospital or doctor's office.

B. Types
    1. Hemorrhage
        a) Pressure bandage or tourniquet
        b) Administration of blood or fluids to combat shock
        c) Administration of necessary drugs
    2. Respiratory disorders (asphyxiation, acute bronchial asthma, etc.)
        a) Administration of oxygen
        b) Administration of necessary drugs
        c) Tracheotomy

DISASTER AND EMERGENCY NURSING

    3. Burns
      a) First degree—skin reddened
      b) Second degree—skin blistered
      c) Third degree—tissues charred
    4. Fractures
      a) Simple—bone broken
      b) Compound—bone broken and external wound
      c) Comminuted—bone broken or splintered into pieces
      d) Greenstick—bone partially broken and bent
    5. Shock
      a) Traumatic
      b) Electric
      c) Insulin
      d) Toxic
      e) Vasovagal
      f) Cardiogenic
    6. Anaphylactic shock
      a) Hypersensitivity to injected or ingested substance, e.g., penicillin, shellfish
      b) Insect stings
    7. Coma
      a) Diabetic
      b) Hypoglycemic
      c) Uremic
      d) Alcoholic
      e) Apoplectic
    8. Poisoning—may be accidental or deliberate
    9. Wounds
      a) Incision
      b) Abrasion
      c) Laceration
      d) Puncture
   10. Special wounds (see Data Summary 20)
      a) Animal bites
      b) Infected wounds
      c) Wounds with danger of tetanus (see Table 6 of the Appendix)

  C. General Rules for Emergency Treatment
    1. Plan course of action.
    2. Examine victim.
    3. Give necessary first-aid treatment.
    4. Make victim comfortable.
    5. Keep victim warm.
    6. Keep crowd away.
    7. Provide for safe followup care.
    8. Report treatment given.

IV. First Aid

  A. Basic Principles
    1. Give immediate and temporary care to victim until skilled medical care is available.
    2. Evaluate situation and perform all life-saving procedures first.
      a) Be sure that breathing has been restored or maintained.

b) Control any hemorrhaging if possible.
c) Administer appropriate antidotes in cases of poisoning.

B. Procedures
1. Place victim in supine position—lying on back with face upward.
    a) Avoid excessive handling.
    b) Prevent exposure to cold or heat; maintain normal body temperature.
2. Examine victim to detect single or multiple injuries, particularly in cases involving traffic accidents or falls.
    a) Find injuries.
    b) Obtain information about accident.
3. Plan and execute specific course of action.
    a) Call for ambulance or physician.
    b) Continue administering first aid.
    c) Clearly instruct any helpers.
    d) Prevent shock that may occur whenever there is loss of blood, crushing injury, major injury, or large bone fracture.
    e) Reassure victim.
    f) Work carefully instead of rushing (the few emergencies that require rapid movement to medical facility are cases of respiratory difficulty, uncontrolled bleeding, and imminent delivery).
4. Care for unconscious patients.
    a) Be sure that breathing is maintained or, if needed, restored.
        (1) Maintain jaw and head in position to assure clear airway.
        (2) Only if necessary and compatible with other injuries, place patient on side in order to permit drainage of regurgitated material or secretions.
    b) Check for Medic-Alert bracelet or necklace and for contact lenses.
        (1) Be aware that Medic-Alert tags indicate special emergency treatments; they are worn by cardiacs, diabetics, epileptics, hemophiliacs, patients on special drugs or with specific allergies, and the like.
    c) Remove contact lenses carefully, in order to prevent injury to cornea.

V. Emergency Childbirth

A. General Principles
1. During a disaster, abortions, premature births, and full-term births will be precipitated.
2. The goal is to provide best chance of survival and safety for baby and mother.

B. Procedure
1. Place victim on back.
2. Keep vaginal area as free from contamination as possible.
3. Remain calm so that mother does not become panic stricken.
4. Deliver baby slowly, guiding his/her passage carefully.
5. Do not push or pull infant through birth canal.
6. Wipe mucus from infant's mouth and nose with clean cloth.
7. Place baby across mother's abdomen in a postural drainage position; this allows for drainage of mucus.
8. Tie cord securely in two places and cut between ties.
9. Put baby to breast if placenta is not expelled shortly; never pull out placenta.
10. Wrap baby in clean cloth or blanket to keep warm.
11. Massage fundus after placenta is expelled.
12. Get medical help at once.

VI. **Disaster Nursing, Emergency Nursing, and First Aid**

A. Roles of the Practical Nurse
   1. Roles are similar in all cases.
   2. Nursing functions are essentially the same
   3. Differences result from numbers of persons involved and conditions under which care must be given.

B. Procedures
   1. Basic nursing procedures
   2. Administration of antibiotics
   3. Administration of analgesic drugs for pain
   4. Catheterization
   5. Lavage
   6. Injection of tetanus toxoids
   7. Administration of antidotes for poisoning
   8. Administration of oxygen
   9. Assisting doctor in applying plaster cast
   10. Assisting doctor with major surgical procedures
   11. Proper identification of victims
   12. Proper record of drugs and procedures given

VII. **Cardiopulmonary Resuscitation Techniques**

A. Artificial Ventilation
   1. Mouth-to-mouth or mouth-to-nose ventilation with expired air
      a) Remove foreign bodies that obstruct air passages.
      b) Tilt head back and lower jaw into projected position; move tongue away from base of throat.
      c) Pinch nostrils closed
      d) Blow air into victim's mouth at rate of 12 times per minute; for small children, blow air into nose and mouth simultaneously at rate of 2 times per minute.
   2. Use of S tube; requires special training
   3. Use of bag and mask

B. Artificial Circulation
   1. External cardiac compression is necessary to circulate blood; give 60–80 compressions per minute at 80–100 pounds of pressure
   2. Effective circulation is indicated by constriction of pupils and presence of palpable carotid pulse.

C. Drugs Used
   1. Epinephrine
      a) Is both cardiotonic and vasoconstrictor
      b) Is given directly into heart or intravenously
   2. Sodium bicarbonate
      a) Corrects metabolic acidosis
      b) Restores pH to normal

D. Equipment
   1. Electrocardiographic monitor
   2. Defibrillator

DATA SUMMARY 20
Special Wounds

Note: In all of the following cases, medical attention should be obtained as soon as possible.

Type	Symptoms	Treatment
Animal bites	Teeth marks Saliva in wound If untreated: Headache, malaise, fever, muscle spasms in mouth and throat, partial paralysis	Cleanse wound by washing thoroughly with soap and water. Do not let animal escape. Contact police, physician, and veterinarian immediately. Consider possibility of rabies or tetanus.
Insects	Localized pain Slight swelling In some cases, allergic response	Apply ice packs or ice water. Relieve itching with baking soda paste, ammonia water compresses, or calamine lotion.
Jellyfish (marine animal)	Weakness Nausea In occasional cases, shock	Immerse part in hot water. Liberally apply mixture of equal parts of ammonia and water or hot magnesium sulfate soaks.
Plant poisoning	Itching Small blisters Local swelling Fever	Wash part with soap and running water. Cleanse with alcohol. Apply calamine lotion to help relieve itching.
Snake bites (Poisonous)	Fang marks evident Pain at site of bite Swelling Tissue discoloration Shortness of breath Rapid pulse Nausea and vomiting Dimming vision or unconsciousness	Immobilize victim. Keep injured part higher than other body parts. Make cross cuts ¼ inch long at fang marks and where venom was deposited. If bite is on extremity, apply tourniquet, but allow slight blood oozing from wound. Remove venom from tissues by suction. Apply ice to bite.
Scorpion	Skin discoloration Local swelling Pain for approx. 1 hour In some cases, (allergic response) Burning sensations Headache, nausea, vomiting when poison is introduced	Use tight tourniquet for 5 minutes if sting is on extremities. Pack part in ice for 2 hours.
Spider	Redness at site Slight swelling Generalized pain Painful breathing Excessive perspiration	Apply tight tourniquet for 5 minutes. Apply hot packs to relieve muscle pain.
Stingray (marine animal)	Painful swelling Later, oozing blood from tissues	Irrigate wound with cold salt water. Apply tourniquet. If feasible, immerse leg or other part in hot water.
Ticks	Evidence of tick's body or head	Cover tick with heavy oil in order to close its breathing pores. Wait for it to remove its head. After 30 minutes, remove tick immediately; (1) Rocky Mountain spotted fever or (2) Lyme disease may have been introduced into system.

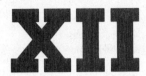

Nursing Care of the Mentally Ill, the Alcoholic, and the Drug-Addicted Patient

UNIT 1: BASIC PSYCHIATRIC NURSING

VOCABULARY

abnormal behavior	any single act or pattern of behavior considered to be outside social limits set for given chronologic age, time, place, and culture
amnesia	loss of memory or recall
compensation	mechanism by which an approved character trait is put forward to conceal from the ego the existence of an opposite trait
displacement	transfer of hostility or other strong feelings from original cause to another object or person
fabrication	lying without direct intent to deceive
fantasy	imagined scenes or occurrences
frustration	prevention of satisfaction and attainment
habit	constant pattern of behavior more or less automatically fixated and determined
hostility	unfriendliness; feeling and/or acting as an enemy does
hydrotherapy	treatment of disease by various types of baths
identification	assuming, for oneself, the mannerisms, attitudes, and achievements of someone else
illusion	mistaken impression resulting from actual stimulus
overactivity	frantic physical activity, usually without direction
regression	reverting to childish behavior that was successful in one's past
sadism	sexual perversion in which satisfaction is derived from infliction of cruelty upon another
underactivity	extreme apathy, depression, and lack of response to any stimulus

I. Introduction

    A. Characteristics of Mentally Healthy Behavior
        1. Independent personality
        2. Flexible personality
        3. Toleration of stress and frustrations
        4. Adjustability to change
        5. Acceptance and knowledge of self
        6. Sincere concern for others
        7. Ability to love others

369

       8.   Ability to be directed by inner values
       9.   Ability to find outlets for basic needs
     10.   Ability to appraise reality objectively

  B.   Characteristics of Psychotic/Neurotic Behavior
       1.   Agitation
       2.   Suspicion
       3.   Worry
       4.   Guilt
       5.   Loneliness
       6.   Illusion
       7.   Insomnia
       8.   Repression
       9.   Compulsive manner
     10.   Somatic complaints
     11.   Delusions of grandeur
     12.   Hallucinations

II. The Psychiatric Team

  A.   Members
       1.   Psychiatrist
       2.   Psychologist
       3.   Psychiatric social worker
       4.   Psychiatric nurse (R.N.)
       5.   Licensed practical nurse
       6.   Psychiatric aide
       7.   Occupational therapist

  B.   Qualities Psychiatric Nurse Needs to Establish Rapport with Patient
       1.   Poise
       2.   Interest
       3.   Skill
       4.   Tact
       5.   Politeness
       6.   Truthfulness
       7.   Friendliness
       8.   Even temperament
       9.   Ability to assume role of counselor or teacher (offering understanding and tolerance)

III. Principles of Nursing Care for Various Types of Psychiatric Patients

  A.   Patients Requiring Constant Observation
       1.   All new patients
       2.   Depressed patients
       3.   Drug-addicted patients
       4.   Alcoholic patients
       5.   Suicidal patients
       6.   Patients who talk about suicide
       7.   Patients receiving special treatments
       8.   Patients with sudden impulses
       9.   Patients with persecution complexes
     10.   Hypochondriacal patients

B. Patients with Personality Disorders
  1. Establish basis of therapeutic nurse-patient relationship.
     a) Negative behavior will not receive approval.
     b) Positive behavior will receive approval.
  2. Deal with anxiety and frustration.
     a) Must be identified
     b) Must be allowed expression
  3. Deal with aggression and hostility.
     a) Accepted
     b) Channeled into appropriate outlet
  4. Give appropriate praise and encouragement.

C. Hyperactive Patients
  1. Provide safe environment.
  2. Provide outlet for excessive energy.
  3. Maintain nonjudgmental attitude.
  4. Anticipate destructive behavior.

D. Underactive Patients
  1. Maintain patient's physical appearance.
  2. Provide appropriate and reasonable activity.
  3. Provide undemanding tasks.
  4. Observe for rigors of acidosis and dehydration.
  5. Maintain good nutrition.
  6. Regularly check bowel movements.
  7. Prevent suicide.

E. Schizophrenic Patients
  1. Establish therapeutic relationship; maintain nonthreatening environment.
  2. Assist patient in maintaining good personal hygiene.
  3. Provide stimulation of social activities.
     a) Development of feeling of trust by patient
     b) Development of sense of self
  4. Help patient to reestablish effective contact with reality.

F. Patients with Chronic Brain Disorders
  1. Provide reassurance and security.
  2. Provide carefully regulated daily routine.
  3. Provide well-balanced, easily digested diet.
  4. Recognize intellectual and emotional limitations.
  5. Protect patient from emotional upsets.
  6. Protect patient from judgmental defects.
  7. Assist patient in maintaining good personal hygiene (including bowel and bladder hygiene).
  8. Keep patient comfortable.
  9. Help patient to use his/her intellectual capacity.
  10. Extend sympathy and kindness to patient.
  11. Help maintain patient's individuality.

IV. **Organic Behavioral Disorders**

A. Causes
  1. Traumatic experiences
  2. Nervous system injury

B. Forms
  1. Acute
     a) Cause—presence of toxins in body
     b) Treatment
        (1) Removal of toxins
        (2) Prevention of complications
  2. Chronic
     a) Other designations
        (1) Senile dementia
        (2) Dementia paralytica
        (3) Arteriosclerotic dementia
        (4) Alzheimer's disease
     b) Treatment—objective is to help patient function to best of his/her ability

C. Nursing Care
  1. Follow physician's orders.
  2. Avoid excessive stimulation of patient.
  3. Observe patient closely.
  4. Help reestablish feeling of worth.
  5. Provide companionship.
  6. Provide social acceptance.
  7. Help develop self-respect.
  8. Provide safety.

V. **Deviation from Normal Behavior**

A. Aggressive Patterns
  1. Traits
     a) Open expression of hostility
     b) Extreme mood changes
  2. Nursing care
     a) Provide quiet environment.
     b) Provide adequate rest.
     c) Avoid outside stimulants.
     d) Allow patient to express hostility.
     e) Answer patient's questions directly.
     f) Do not criticize or condone inappropriate actions.

B. Underactivity
  1. Traits
     a) General state of depression
     b) Extreme apathy
  2. Nursing care
     a) Provide for regular exercise.
     b) Pay special attention to personal hygiene.
     c) Administer good skin care.
     d) Avoid circulatory complication.
     e) Avoid musculoskeletal disorder.
     f) Prevent patient from standing or sitting in one position for long **period**.
     g) Be direct in conversation.

C. Overactivity

1. Traits—excessive, undirected, frantic physical activity
2. Nursing care
    a) Handle patient calmly.
    b) Provide quiet, nonstimulating environment.
    c) Provide physical outlets.
    d) Provide outdoor recreational activities.
    e) Provide opportunities for patient to develop talents.
    f) Provide opportunities to pursue hobbies.
    g) Keep patient from injuring self.

D. Withdrawal Patterns
    1. Traits
        a) Seriously withdrawn attitude and behavior
        b) Lack of self-respect
        c) Sense of unworthiness
        d) Isolation from others
        e) Fear of not being accepted
    2. Nursing care
        a) Show interest in patient.
        b) Provide objective, friendly attitude.
        c) Exert a firm attitude.
        d) Do not condone unacceptable actions.

E. Suicidal Patient
    1. Traits
        a) Patient threatens to take his/her life.
        b) Cause stems from extreme feelings of unworthiness, depression, and despair.
    2. Warning signs
        a) Earlier attempts with instruments, drugs, poisons, etc.
        b) Statements that provide a warning
            (1) "I want to end my life."
            (2) "Life isn't worth living."
            (3) "I no longer want to live."
            (4) "I'm just a burden to everyone."
        c) Actions that provide a warning, e.g., giving away possessions
        d) Moods
            (1) Depression
            (2) Defiance
            (3) Dissatisfaction with dependency on others
            (4) Disorientation
        e) Changes in eating and sleeping patterns
    3. Nurse's role
        a) Listen to patient.
        b) Show consideration for patient.
        c) Try to convince the patient that he/she is worthy of respect and attention.
        d) Report any attempt at suicide or early warnings.
        e) Observe patient closely.
        f) Win patient's confidence.
        g) Anticipate patient's behavior.
        h) Never leave patient alone.
        i) Remove any articles that can be used for self-destruction.
        j) Help patient gain a motive for living.

VI. Preventive Measures

    A. Early Detection of Symptoms
        1. Special training for teachers
        2. Public education in early recognition of symptoms

    B. Establishment of Healthful Living Patterns

    C. Expanded Mental Health Research

    D. Stable Home Life

VII. Role of the Nurse in Caring for Psychiatric Patients

    A. General Principles
        1. Focus nursing care on patient as person.
        2. Avoid physical and verbal force.
        3. Communicate on level of patient's understanding.
        4. Be consistent in attitude for patient's security.
        5. Extend yourself to patient.
        6. Anticipate patient's needs.
        7. Reassure patient.
        8. Recognize patient's needs.
        9. Know patient.
      10. Understand patient's behavior.
      11. Plan for patient's care.
      12. Implement plan.
      13. Evaluate results of care.
      14. Share your observations with other members of health care team.

VIII. Drug Therapy—the Nurse's Responsibilities

    A. Goals
        1. Relieve anxiety of patient in regard to administration of medication and its effect on illness.
        2. Relieve symptoms and signs of illness.
        3. Administer drug correctly—correct patient, drug, dose, route, and time.
        4. Assemble proper equipment for administration of ordered medication.

    B. Procedures
        1. Medications are given only on physician's order.
        2. All orders should be complete as to name of drug, dose, route, and interval (if route not specified, oral administration is inferred).
        3. Medications must be prepared and administered with utmost care.
           a) See Chapter 1, Unit 3, Section iv.
           b) Exercise accuracy when converting from apothecaries' system to metric and vice versa.

    C. Responsibilities
        1. Observe reaction of drug on patient.
        2. Record all signs and symptoms.
        3. Immediately report any untoward signs after administration of drug.
        4. Make certain patient swallows medication during oral administration.

5. Chart medication when given.
6. Chart omission of scheduled dose.
7. Educate patient.
   a) Instruct patient as to name of drug, how to take it, and what reactions to expect.
   b) Inform patient of names of drugs causing allergic responses.

IX. Treatment and Rehabilitation of the Mentally Ill Patient

A. Drugs (tranquilizers, sedatives, etc.)

B. Hydrotherapy

C. Occupational Therapy

D. Electroshock Therapy

E. Psychotherapy

F. Psychoanalysis

X. Public Mental Health

A. Role of the Community
   1. Develop programs to enlighten and educate public concerning needs of mental health field.
   2. Establish institutional facilities for mental health.
   3. Establish recreational facilities for all age groups.
   4. Establish day and night care for all age groups—halfway houses, foster homes, after care (should be included in all community planning).
   5. Sex education should be taught in elementary and high schools in order to provide correct and intelligent information for children and to help prepare young people for marriage and parenthood.

UNIT 2: CLASSIFICATION OF MAJOR MENTAL ILLNESSES

VOCABULARY

affect	emotional tone or feeling
aggression	unprovoked attack or act of hostility
ambivalence	simultaneous existence of conflicting emotions, e.g., love and hate, in one person toward another person or thing
autistic thinking	extreme withdrawal; failure to relate to others
compulsion	irresistible impulse to perform, usually repeatedly, some irrational act or ritual
delusion	impression or idea inconsistent with reality
depression	unremitting feeling of sadness, discouragement, or hopelessness
hallucination	perception of sights or sounds that are not actually present
obsession	idea that persists in spite of one's efforts to ignore or avoid it
phobia	an unrealistic fear
projection	unconscious act of ascribing to others one's own ideas or impulses
rationalization	mental process by which a plausible explanation is concocted for ideas or actions that one wishes to hold or do
sublimation	direction of strong impulses into acceptable channels so that behavior is acceptable to society

I. Introduction

A. Importance of Mental Illness
1. Mental illnesses are major health problems in the United States.
2. Patient admissions to public mental hospitals have increases 75% in past 25 years.

B. Necessary Measures
1. Educational programs to change public's attitudes toward mental illness
2. Larger community role in providing good mental health for all
3. More research in prevention of mental illness and care for mentally ill

II. Classifications

A. Neurosis
1. definition of **neurosis:** Mild personality disorder in which contact with reality is maintained; there is no organic condition
2. Types
   a) Anxiety neurosis
   b) Hypochondriacal neurosis
      (1) Preoccupation with body
      (2) Fear of presumed diseases
   c) Hysterical neurosis
   d) Depressive neurosis—excessive reaction of depression
   e) Neurasthenia neurosis
   f) Phallic neurosis
   g) Other types—phobias, obsessions, compulsions
3. Symptoms
   a) Anxiety
   b) Fear
   c) Depressed feelings
   d) Agitation
   e) Guilt feelings
   f) Loneliness
   g) Insomnia
   h) Repression
   i) Compulsive manner
   j) Somatic complaints
   k) Worry

B. Psychosis
1. Definition of **psychosis:** Severe personality disorder in which contact with reality is lost; patient is unable to care for self and may be danger to others
2. Types
   a) Postpartum psychosis
   b) Functional psychosis
      (1) No determinable etiology
      (2) Examples—mania, melancholia, paranoia, schizophrenia
   c) Organic psychosis
      (1) Significant pathological changes in body, especially in central nervous system
      (2) Characteristics—dementia and impaired effective control
      (3) Examples—vitamin deficiency, chronic alcoholism, cerebral tumor, syphilis, endocrine disorder, infectious disease, poison

    d) Involutional psychosis
      (1) Occurs in involutional periods
      (2) Varies widely in etiology
  3. Symptoms
    a) Delusions
    b) Erratic train of thought
    c) Hallucinations
    d) Delusions of grandeur
    e) Suspicion
    f) Distortion of reality
    g) Anxiety
  4. Definitions of some common psychoses
    a) Schizophrenia
      (1) Definition of **schizophrenia:** Group of disorders manifested by disturbances of thinking, mood, and behavior
      (2) Forms—simple, hebephrenic, catatonic, paranoid
    b) Manic-depressive psychosis—characterized by varying degrees of elation and depression
    c) Paranoia—characterized by delusions of persecution based on false premises but logical and consistent
    d) Alzheimer's disease
      (1) Cause—exact cause unknown
      (2) Characteristics—progressive loss of memory, inappropriate behavior, personality changes
    e) Senile psychosis
      (1) Cause—senile degenerative or arteriosclerotic brain changes
      (2) Characteristics—progressive dementia, habit deterioration, and regression to childhood dependence
    f) Suicidal behavior

C. Mental Retardation
  1. Definition of **mental retardation:** subnormal intellectual functioning, manifested during developmental period and associated with impairment of learning and social adjustment
  2. Degrees
    a) Relatively mild—IQ between 50 and 70
    b) Moderate—IQ between 20 and 49
    c) Severe—IQ under 20

D. Psychosexual Disorders
  1. Homosexuality
    a) Homosexuality is no longer regarded as a mental disorder.
    b) Cause of this condition is not known.
    c) Sexually transmitted diseases are relatively frequent among homosexuals.
    d) AIDS is predominant among male homosexuals.
    e) Psychiatric illnesses are less common among lesbians than among male homosexuals.
    f) Treatment is not indicated without strong motivation to change sexual orientation.
  2. Gender identity disorders
    a) Etiology of transsexualism is not known.
    b) Condition dates from early childhood.
  3. Paraphilia
    a) Sadism

        b) Exhibitionism
        c) Masochism
        d) Transvestism
        e) Voyeurism
        f) Fetishism
        g) Pedophilia
           (1) This disorder manifests itself in child molestation.
           (2) Pedophilia accounts for a significant proportion of sexual criminal acts.
           (3) Acts are repeated in high percentage of cases.

III. **Factors Contributing to Mental Disorders**

    A. Heredity

    B. Environment

    C. Physical Diseases

    D. Psychological Factors

    E. Trauma

    F. Toxic Influences
       1. Drugs
       2. Alcohol

UNIT 3: DRUG ADDICTION AND ALCOHOLISM

I. **Drug Addiction**

    A. Introduction
       1. Definition of **drug addiction:** Physical and psychological dependence on a drug or drugs
       2. Causes
          a) Dependency on drugs in order to adjust to conflict
          b) Excessive misuse of drugs
       3. Characteristics
          a) Continuing compulsive use to prevent discomfort of withdrawal
          b) Risk of harm implied

    B. Commonly Misused Drugs
       1. Opiates
       2. Cocaine; crack-cocaine
       3. Demerol sodium
       4. Methadone
       5. Barbiturates
       6. Hallucinogenic drugs
          a) LSD (lysergic acid diethylamide)
          b) Phencyclidine (PCP); street term is *angel dust*
          c) Peyote
       7. Alcohol

        8.   Amphetamines
        9.   Cannabis (marijuana)
     10.   Volatile solvents
     11.   Volatile nitrites
     12.   Nicotine (tobacco) (This is so widely used that its use is not considered a misuse.)

C. Assessment
   1. Signs of addiction
      a) Poor personal hygiene
      b) Needle marks (tracks) on body along veins
      c) Red eyes
      d) Constant, clear nasal discharge
      e) Unreactive pupils; may be dilated or constricted
      f) Drowsiness or hyperactivity
      g) Poor ocular focus—constant oscillations of eyes
      h) Speech blurred, not fluent
   2. Symptoms of addiction
      a) Abdominal cramping
      b) Constipation
      c) Anorexia
      d) Apparent nutritional deficiences
      e) Nausea and vomiting
      f) Poor work or school history

D. Nursing Care
   1. Monitor vital functions.
   2. Monitor neurologic status.
   3. Seizure precautions.
   4. Provide quiet environment.
   5. Assure adequate airway and ventilation.
   6. Administer oxygen if needed.

E. Symptoms upon Withdrawal
   1. Muscle cramps
   2. High blood pressure
   3. Diarrhea
   4. Prostration
   5. Nausea
   6. Less severe symptoms—weakness, insomnia, and anorexia

F. Treatment and Rehabilitation
   1. Long-term rehabilitation
   2. Chemotherapy
   3. Psychotherapy
   4. Therapeutic communities
   5. Hypnotherapy
   6. Yoga

II. **Alcoholism**

A. Causes and Development
   1. There is no one specific cause.

2. Genetic and biochemical, as well as cultural and psychosocial, factors are believed to be important.
3. Alcohol provides a temporary "escape" from emotional problems (depression).
4. As a result, psychological dependency on alcohol develops.

B. Assessment
   1. Impaired motor activity
   2. Disturbed motor coordination
   3. Depressant effect on brain and nervous system
   4. Physical effects of toxicity
   5. Delirium tremens in alcoholism that has persisted for 5–10 years
      a) Perspiring; shaking
      b) Delusions
      c) Excitement
      d) Hallucinations
      e) Disorientation

C. Nursing Care
   1. Watch patient closely in order to prevent self-injury or injury to others.
   2. Avoid physical strain and/or exhaustion.
   3. Administer medications prescribed by physician (medications often include tranquilizers).
   4. Prevent respiratory infections.
   5. Maintain sound nutritional program for patient.
   6. Provide calm, quiet atmosphere; avoid criticism.
   7. Prevent additional toxic complications.
   8. Inform patient of the value of support groups such as Alcoholics Anonymous
   9. Encourage family members to join support groups such as Al-Anon and Al-Ateen.

D. Role of the Community
   1. The dangers of drug addiction and alcoholism should be taught in elementary and high schools.
   2. Alcohol and drug-abuse programs should be coordinated for maximum benefit to community.

Mastery Test

Set aside a day to take the mastery test. Allow 2 consecutive hours in the morning for Part I, have your lunch and a break, and then take Part II in 2 consecutive hours in the afternoon. Take the examination in a quiet room, without interruption, and do not use aids such as notes or textbooks.

This mastery test, unlike the actual NCLEX-PN, uses an answer sheet and designates answer choices by letters—A, B, C, D. This is necessary in order to provide an answer key.

As you take the test, remember to:

1. Read each question and the four answer choices carefully.
2. Answer first the questions you are sure of, and then go back to the others.
3. Using a #2 pencil, indicate each answer by blackening completely the circle that corresponds to your choice:
   Ⓐ ● Ⓒ Ⓓ, not Ⓐ Ⓑ̸ Ⓒ Ⓓ or Ⓐ ⓧ Ⓒ Ⓓ.
4. Answer every question. Eliminate one or two choices if you can, and then select from the remaining answers.

MASTERY TEST

ANSWER SHEET FOR MASTERY TEST

Part I

1 Ⓐ Ⓑ Ⓒ Ⓓ	26 Ⓐ Ⓑ Ⓒ Ⓓ	51 Ⓐ Ⓑ Ⓒ Ⓓ	76 Ⓐ Ⓑ Ⓒ Ⓓ	101 Ⓐ Ⓑ Ⓒ Ⓓ
2 Ⓐ Ⓑ Ⓒ Ⓓ	27 Ⓐ Ⓑ Ⓒ Ⓓ	52 Ⓐ Ⓑ Ⓒ Ⓓ	77 Ⓐ Ⓑ Ⓒ Ⓓ	102 Ⓐ Ⓑ Ⓒ Ⓓ
3 Ⓐ Ⓑ Ⓒ Ⓓ	28 Ⓐ Ⓑ Ⓒ Ⓓ	53 Ⓐ Ⓑ Ⓒ Ⓓ	78 Ⓐ Ⓑ Ⓒ Ⓓ	103 Ⓐ Ⓑ Ⓒ Ⓓ
4 Ⓐ Ⓑ Ⓒ Ⓓ	29 Ⓐ Ⓑ Ⓒ Ⓓ	54 Ⓐ Ⓑ Ⓒ Ⓓ	79 Ⓐ Ⓑ Ⓒ Ⓓ	104 Ⓐ Ⓑ Ⓒ Ⓓ
5 Ⓐ Ⓑ Ⓒ Ⓓ	30 Ⓐ Ⓑ Ⓒ Ⓓ	55 Ⓐ Ⓑ Ⓒ Ⓓ	80 Ⓐ Ⓑ Ⓒ Ⓓ	105 Ⓐ Ⓑ Ⓒ Ⓓ
6 Ⓐ Ⓑ Ⓒ Ⓓ	31 Ⓐ Ⓑ Ⓒ Ⓓ	56 Ⓐ Ⓑ Ⓒ Ⓓ	81 Ⓐ Ⓑ Ⓒ Ⓓ	106 Ⓐ Ⓑ Ⓒ Ⓓ
7 Ⓐ Ⓑ Ⓒ Ⓓ	32 Ⓐ Ⓑ Ⓒ Ⓓ	57 Ⓐ Ⓑ Ⓒ Ⓓ	82 Ⓐ Ⓑ Ⓒ Ⓓ	107 Ⓐ Ⓑ Ⓒ Ⓓ
8 Ⓐ Ⓑ Ⓒ Ⓓ	33 Ⓐ Ⓑ Ⓒ Ⓓ	58 Ⓐ Ⓑ Ⓒ Ⓓ	83 Ⓐ Ⓑ Ⓒ Ⓓ	108 Ⓐ Ⓑ Ⓒ Ⓓ
9 Ⓐ Ⓑ Ⓒ Ⓓ	34 Ⓐ Ⓑ Ⓒ Ⓓ	59 Ⓐ Ⓑ Ⓒ Ⓓ	84 Ⓐ Ⓑ Ⓒ Ⓓ	109 Ⓐ Ⓑ Ⓒ Ⓓ
10 Ⓐ Ⓑ Ⓒ Ⓓ	35 Ⓐ Ⓑ Ⓒ Ⓓ	60 Ⓐ Ⓑ Ⓒ Ⓓ	85 Ⓐ Ⓑ Ⓒ Ⓓ	110 Ⓐ Ⓑ Ⓒ Ⓓ
11 Ⓐ Ⓑ Ⓒ Ⓓ	36 Ⓐ Ⓑ Ⓒ Ⓓ	61 Ⓐ Ⓑ Ⓒ Ⓓ	86 Ⓐ Ⓑ Ⓒ Ⓓ	111 Ⓐ Ⓑ Ⓒ Ⓓ
12 Ⓐ Ⓑ Ⓒ Ⓓ	37 Ⓐ Ⓑ Ⓒ Ⓓ	62 Ⓐ Ⓑ Ⓒ Ⓓ	87 Ⓐ Ⓑ Ⓒ Ⓓ	112 Ⓐ Ⓑ Ⓒ Ⓓ
13 Ⓐ Ⓑ Ⓒ Ⓓ	38 Ⓐ Ⓑ Ⓒ Ⓓ	63 Ⓐ Ⓑ Ⓒ Ⓓ	88 Ⓐ Ⓑ Ⓒ Ⓓ	113 Ⓐ Ⓑ Ⓒ Ⓓ
14 Ⓐ Ⓑ Ⓒ Ⓓ	39 Ⓐ Ⓑ Ⓒ Ⓓ	64 Ⓐ Ⓑ Ⓒ Ⓓ	89 Ⓐ Ⓑ Ⓒ Ⓓ	114 Ⓐ Ⓑ Ⓒ Ⓓ
15 Ⓐ Ⓑ Ⓒ Ⓓ	40 Ⓐ Ⓑ Ⓒ Ⓓ	65 Ⓐ Ⓑ Ⓒ Ⓓ	90 Ⓐ Ⓑ Ⓒ Ⓓ	115 Ⓐ Ⓑ Ⓒ Ⓓ
16 Ⓐ Ⓑ Ⓒ Ⓓ	41 Ⓐ Ⓑ Ⓒ Ⓓ	66 Ⓐ Ⓑ Ⓒ Ⓓ	91 Ⓐ Ⓑ Ⓒ Ⓓ	116 Ⓐ Ⓑ Ⓒ Ⓓ
17 Ⓐ Ⓑ Ⓒ Ⓓ	42 Ⓐ Ⓑ Ⓒ Ⓓ	67 Ⓐ Ⓑ Ⓒ Ⓓ	92 Ⓐ Ⓑ Ⓒ Ⓓ	117 Ⓐ Ⓑ Ⓒ Ⓓ
18 Ⓐ Ⓑ Ⓒ Ⓓ	43 Ⓐ Ⓑ Ⓒ Ⓓ	68 Ⓐ Ⓑ Ⓒ Ⓓ	93 Ⓐ Ⓑ Ⓒ Ⓓ	118 Ⓐ Ⓑ Ⓒ Ⓓ
19 Ⓐ Ⓑ Ⓒ Ⓓ	44 Ⓐ Ⓑ Ⓒ Ⓓ	69 Ⓐ Ⓑ Ⓒ Ⓓ	94 Ⓐ Ⓑ Ⓒ Ⓓ	119 Ⓐ Ⓑ Ⓒ Ⓓ
20 Ⓐ Ⓑ Ⓒ Ⓓ	45 Ⓐ Ⓑ Ⓒ Ⓓ	70 Ⓐ Ⓑ Ⓒ Ⓓ	95 Ⓐ Ⓑ Ⓒ Ⓓ	120 Ⓐ Ⓑ Ⓒ Ⓓ
21 Ⓐ Ⓑ Ⓒ Ⓓ	46 Ⓐ Ⓑ Ⓒ Ⓓ	71 Ⓐ Ⓑ Ⓒ Ⓓ	96 Ⓐ Ⓑ Ⓒ Ⓓ	121 Ⓐ Ⓑ Ⓒ Ⓓ
22 Ⓐ Ⓑ Ⓒ Ⓓ	47 Ⓐ Ⓑ Ⓒ Ⓓ	72 Ⓐ Ⓑ Ⓒ Ⓓ	97 Ⓐ Ⓑ Ⓒ Ⓓ	122 Ⓐ Ⓑ Ⓒ Ⓓ
23 Ⓐ Ⓑ Ⓒ Ⓓ	48 Ⓐ Ⓑ Ⓒ Ⓓ	73 Ⓐ Ⓑ Ⓒ Ⓓ	98 Ⓐ Ⓑ Ⓒ Ⓓ	123 Ⓐ Ⓑ Ⓒ Ⓓ
24 Ⓐ Ⓑ Ⓒ Ⓓ	49 Ⓐ Ⓑ Ⓒ Ⓓ	74 Ⓐ Ⓑ Ⓒ Ⓓ	99 Ⓐ Ⓑ Ⓒ Ⓓ	124 Ⓐ Ⓑ Ⓒ Ⓓ
25 Ⓐ Ⓑ Ⓒ Ⓓ	50 Ⓐ Ⓑ Ⓒ Ⓓ	75 Ⓐ Ⓑ Ⓒ Ⓓ	100 Ⓐ Ⓑ Ⓒ Ⓓ	125 Ⓐ Ⓑ Ⓒ Ⓓ

MASTERY TEST

Part II

1 Ⓐ Ⓑ Ⓒ Ⓓ	26 Ⓐ Ⓑ Ⓒ Ⓓ	51 Ⓐ Ⓑ Ⓒ Ⓓ	76 Ⓐ Ⓑ Ⓒ Ⓓ	101 Ⓐ Ⓑ Ⓒ Ⓓ
2 Ⓐ Ⓑ Ⓒ Ⓓ	27 Ⓐ Ⓑ Ⓒ Ⓓ	52 Ⓐ Ⓑ Ⓒ Ⓓ	77 Ⓐ Ⓑ Ⓒ Ⓓ	102 Ⓐ Ⓑ Ⓒ Ⓓ
3 Ⓐ Ⓑ Ⓒ Ⓓ	28 Ⓐ Ⓑ Ⓒ Ⓓ	53 Ⓐ Ⓑ Ⓒ Ⓓ	78 Ⓐ Ⓑ Ⓒ Ⓓ	103 Ⓐ Ⓑ Ⓒ Ⓓ
4 Ⓐ Ⓑ Ⓒ Ⓓ	29 Ⓐ Ⓑ Ⓒ Ⓓ	54 Ⓐ Ⓑ Ⓒ Ⓓ	79 Ⓐ Ⓑ Ⓒ Ⓓ	104 Ⓐ Ⓑ Ⓒ Ⓓ
5 Ⓐ Ⓑ Ⓒ Ⓓ	30 Ⓐ Ⓑ Ⓒ Ⓓ	55 Ⓐ Ⓑ Ⓒ Ⓓ	80 Ⓐ Ⓑ Ⓒ Ⓓ	105 Ⓐ Ⓑ Ⓒ Ⓓ
6 Ⓐ Ⓑ Ⓒ Ⓓ	31 Ⓐ Ⓑ Ⓒ Ⓓ	56 Ⓐ Ⓑ Ⓒ Ⓓ	81 Ⓐ Ⓑ Ⓒ Ⓓ	106 Ⓐ Ⓑ Ⓒ Ⓓ
7 Ⓐ Ⓑ Ⓒ Ⓓ	32 Ⓐ Ⓑ Ⓒ Ⓓ	57 Ⓐ Ⓑ Ⓒ Ⓓ	82 Ⓐ Ⓑ Ⓒ Ⓓ	107 Ⓐ Ⓑ Ⓒ Ⓓ
8 Ⓐ Ⓑ Ⓒ Ⓓ	33 Ⓐ Ⓑ Ⓒ Ⓓ	58 Ⓐ Ⓑ Ⓒ Ⓓ	83 Ⓐ Ⓑ Ⓒ Ⓓ	108 Ⓐ Ⓑ Ⓒ Ⓓ
9 Ⓐ Ⓑ Ⓒ Ⓓ	34 Ⓐ Ⓑ Ⓒ Ⓓ	59 Ⓐ Ⓑ Ⓒ Ⓓ	84 Ⓐ Ⓑ Ⓒ Ⓓ	109 Ⓐ Ⓑ Ⓒ Ⓓ
10 Ⓐ Ⓑ Ⓒ Ⓓ	35 Ⓐ Ⓑ Ⓒ Ⓓ	60 Ⓐ Ⓑ Ⓒ Ⓓ	85 Ⓐ Ⓑ Ⓒ Ⓓ	110 Ⓐ Ⓑ Ⓒ Ⓓ
11 Ⓐ Ⓑ Ⓒ Ⓓ	36 Ⓐ Ⓑ Ⓒ Ⓓ	61 Ⓐ Ⓑ Ⓒ Ⓓ	86 Ⓐ Ⓑ Ⓒ Ⓓ	111 Ⓐ Ⓑ Ⓒ Ⓓ
12 Ⓐ Ⓑ Ⓒ Ⓓ	37 Ⓐ Ⓑ Ⓒ Ⓓ	62 Ⓐ Ⓑ Ⓒ Ⓓ	87 Ⓐ Ⓑ Ⓒ Ⓓ	112 Ⓐ Ⓑ Ⓒ Ⓓ
13 Ⓐ Ⓑ Ⓒ Ⓓ	38 Ⓐ Ⓑ Ⓒ Ⓓ	63 Ⓐ Ⓑ Ⓒ Ⓓ	88 Ⓐ Ⓑ Ⓒ Ⓓ	113 Ⓐ Ⓑ Ⓒ Ⓓ
14 Ⓐ Ⓑ Ⓒ Ⓓ	39 Ⓐ Ⓑ Ⓒ Ⓓ	64 Ⓐ Ⓑ Ⓒ Ⓓ	89 Ⓐ Ⓑ Ⓒ Ⓓ	114 Ⓐ Ⓑ Ⓒ Ⓓ
15 Ⓐ Ⓑ Ⓒ Ⓓ	40 Ⓐ Ⓑ Ⓒ Ⓓ	65 Ⓐ Ⓑ Ⓒ Ⓓ	90 Ⓐ Ⓑ Ⓒ Ⓓ	115 Ⓐ Ⓑ Ⓒ Ⓓ
16 Ⓐ Ⓑ Ⓒ Ⓓ	41 Ⓐ Ⓑ Ⓒ Ⓓ	66 Ⓐ Ⓑ Ⓒ Ⓓ	91 Ⓐ Ⓑ Ⓒ Ⓓ	116 Ⓐ Ⓑ Ⓒ Ⓓ
17 Ⓐ Ⓑ Ⓒ Ⓓ	42 Ⓐ Ⓑ Ⓒ Ⓓ	67 Ⓐ Ⓑ Ⓒ Ⓓ	92 Ⓐ Ⓑ Ⓒ Ⓓ	117 Ⓐ Ⓑ Ⓒ Ⓓ
18 Ⓐ Ⓑ Ⓒ Ⓓ	43 Ⓐ Ⓑ Ⓒ Ⓓ	68 Ⓐ Ⓑ Ⓒ Ⓓ	93 Ⓐ Ⓑ Ⓒ Ⓓ	118 Ⓐ Ⓑ Ⓒ Ⓓ
19 Ⓐ Ⓑ Ⓒ Ⓓ	44 Ⓐ Ⓑ Ⓒ Ⓓ	69 Ⓐ Ⓑ Ⓒ Ⓓ	94 Ⓐ Ⓑ Ⓒ Ⓓ	119 Ⓐ Ⓑ Ⓒ Ⓓ
20 Ⓐ Ⓑ Ⓒ Ⓓ	45 Ⓐ Ⓑ Ⓒ Ⓓ	70 Ⓐ Ⓑ Ⓒ Ⓓ	95 Ⓐ Ⓑ Ⓒ Ⓓ	120 Ⓐ Ⓑ Ⓒ Ⓓ
21 Ⓐ Ⓑ Ⓒ Ⓓ	46 Ⓐ Ⓑ Ⓒ Ⓓ	71 Ⓐ Ⓑ Ⓒ Ⓓ	96 Ⓐ Ⓑ Ⓒ Ⓓ	121 Ⓐ Ⓑ Ⓒ Ⓓ
22 Ⓐ Ⓑ Ⓒ Ⓓ	47 Ⓐ Ⓑ Ⓒ Ⓓ	72 Ⓐ Ⓑ Ⓒ Ⓓ	97 Ⓐ Ⓑ Ⓒ Ⓓ	122 Ⓐ Ⓑ Ⓒ Ⓓ
23 Ⓐ Ⓑ Ⓒ Ⓓ	48 Ⓐ Ⓑ Ⓒ Ⓓ	73 Ⓐ Ⓑ Ⓒ Ⓓ	98 Ⓐ Ⓑ Ⓒ Ⓓ	123 Ⓐ Ⓑ Ⓒ Ⓓ
24 Ⓐ Ⓑ Ⓒ Ⓓ	49 Ⓐ Ⓑ Ⓒ Ⓓ	74 Ⓐ Ⓑ Ⓒ Ⓓ	99 Ⓐ Ⓑ Ⓒ Ⓓ	124 Ⓐ Ⓑ Ⓒ Ⓓ
25 Ⓐ Ⓑ Ⓒ Ⓓ	50 Ⓐ Ⓑ Ⓒ Ⓓ	75 Ⓐ Ⓑ Ⓒ Ⓓ	100 Ⓐ Ⓑ Ⓒ Ⓓ	125 Ⓐ Ⓑ Ⓒ Ⓓ

MASTERY TEST, PART I

Mr. White, a 51-year-old cabinet maker, has been suffering from shortness of breath, increased fatigability, dizziness, and headaches. His physician has admitted him to the hospital for diagnostic tests and treatment. His diagnosis on admission is anemia.

---

1. Laboratory tests ordered for Mr. White include a hemoglobin test. Hemoglobin is BEST defined as the
   A. material in the plasma that aids in the formation of red blood cells.
   B. pigment in the erythrocytes that combines with oxygen.
   C. chief component of platelets.
   D. material in leukocytes that destroys bacteria.

2. One of the most important qualities of hemoglobin is its ability to
   A. aid in the formation of antibodies.
   B. aid in the formation of platelets.
   C. combine with oxygen.
   D. produce red blood cells.

3. The laboratory report shows that Mr. White's hemoglobin is 6 gm per 100 ml, which is
   A. within normal limits for a man of his age.
   B. lower than normal for males.
   C. markedly above the normal range for males.
   D. slightly above the normal range for males.

4. In addition to the other laboratory tests, Mr. White is also scheduled for a sternal puncture. The sternum is the
   A. hipbone.
   B. shoulder blade.
   C. collarbone.
   D. breastbone.

5. The purpose of doing a sternal puncture is to
   A. suction fluid from the chest.
   B. obtain a sample of breast tissue.
   C. aspirate blood cells from the bone marrow.
   D. allow for drainage of purulent material in the bone.

6. Mr. White has experienced an increasing loss of appetite for several months. The medical term for this condition is
   A. anoxia.
   B. anorexia.
   C. cachexia.
   D. dyspnea.

7. Frequent dizzy spells or fainting are not uncommon in anemic patients like Mr. White, primarily because
   A. these patients often receive a large amount of narcotic drugs for relief of their headaches.
   B. these patients generally do not eat an adequate diet.
   C. a decrease in the number of red cells in these patients leads to a deficiency in oxygen supply to the brain.
   D. most of these patients have mental deterioration brought about by loss of blood.

8. When Mr. White requests more heat in his room, the nurse should
   A. realize that he is mentally deranged and is trying to get attention.
   B. tell him that the room must be kept cool for others who are working in the area.
   C. ignore his complaint because he should be kept in a cool environment.
   D. realize that most anemic persons cannot tolerate cold as well as others.

9. The BEST way to provide additional warmth for Mr. White is to
   A. give him extra blankets and slightly increase the temperature in his room.
   B. apply several hot water bottles to his feet and legs.
   C. allow him to sleep in his robe.
   D. place a small electric heater near his bed.

10. While helping Mr. White brush his teeth, the nurse notices that his gums appear very sore and bleed easily. This is
    A. an indication of inadequate oral hygiene.
    B. an indication of decaying teeth.

C. a result of brushing the teeth too vigorously.

D. a common condition in patients with severe chronic anemia.

11. Special mouth care for Mr. White should include
    A. gentle cleansing of the mouth and teeth with cotton applicators dipped in a mild mouthwash or hydrogen peroxide.
    B. cleansing of the mouth several times a day, using alcohol to destroy bacteria.
    C. brushing the teeth several times a day, using a brush with very stiff bristles.
    D. using a highly astringent mouthwash to decrease bleeding and stimulate the gums.

12. Mr. White is scheduled to receive a blood transfusion during the day. In planning nursing care for him, it will be best to
    A. omit his bath and change of linens that day because the blood transfusion is more important.
    B. postpone the bath and bed making until several hours after the transfusion is completed.
    C. give the bath and morning care early before the transfusion is started, so Mr. White will be more comfortable during the procedure.
    D. wait until the transfusion is started and then give morning care to divert his attention from the procedure.

Mrs. Chavez, a 51-year-old former nurse, is seriously ill with chronic leukemia. You are assigned to care for her while she is in the hospital.

13. Leukemia is
    A. a malignant disease.
    B. a disorder characterized by an increase in the red blood cell count.
    C. a disease of the blood vessels.
    D. a disease that is always fatal within 6 months from the onset of symptoms.

14. The white blood cells of a leukemia patient do not function like normal white blood cells. Since this is true, you might expect Mrs. Chavez to have
    A. an abnormality of the bone marrow.

B. higher resistance to infections.
C. enlargement of the blood vessels.
D. a tendency to develop clots in the blood vessels.

15. Which of the following may be signs of internal bleeding and should be reported if you notice them while you are nursing Mrs. Chavez?
    1. Tarry stools.
    2. Smoky urine.
    3. Yellowing of the skin.
    4. Coffee-grounds-colored vomitus.

    A. 1, 2, 3 and 4.
    B. 1, 2, and 4.
    C. 1 and 4.
    D. 2 and 3.

16. At times Mrs. Chavez is very irritable and difficult to please. As a nurse you should consider this behavior to be
    A. usual for a person of her age and background.
    B. a sign that she is neurotic.
    C. a symptom of her illness that she may not be able to control.
    D. indicative of lack of spiritual depth that leaves her unable to accept her illness.

Mrs. Marino, aged 65, has varicose veins in both legs. She also has an ulceration on the anterior surface of the right leg.

17. Varicose veins are veins that have become
    A. enlarged and engorged with blood.
    B. hardened and their openings narrowed.
    C. infected by the invasion of bacteria.
    D. atrophied because of constriction of the surface blood vessels.

18. A condition that may have made Mrs. Marino more vulnerable to the development of varicose veins is
    A. accumulations of material along the walls of the veins.
    B. repeated bacterial infections in the veins.
    C. incorrect functioning of the valves that control the flow of blood through the veins.

D. congenital malformations of the lower extremities, resulting in improper circulation.

19. Predisposing causes in the development of varicose veins include
   1. obesity.
   2. prolonged sitting or standing.
   3. wearing circular garters or tight girdles.
   4. wearing shoes with high heels.
   A. 1, 2, 3, and 4.
   B. 1 and 2.
   C. 3 and 4.
   D. 1 and 3.

20. If Mrs. Marino's varicose veins cannot be treated successfully by medical means, surgical correction will be necessary. Tying off the affected vein is referred to as a
   A. venogram.
   B. venectomy.
   C. vein ligation.
   D. phlebectomy.

21. Surgical removal of a varicose vein is referred to as a
   A. venotomy.
   B. varicosity.
   C. vein ligation.
   D. vein stripping.

Mrs. Corey, aged 35, is in her 35th week of gestation. This is her third pregnancy, and she has received good prenatal care. She has just been admitted to the hospital because she has been experiencing labor pains for the past 2 hours. The pains are now occurring every 10 minutes and are lasting for approximately 1 minute.

---

22. Which of the following steps is NOT part of the admissions procedure for Mrs. Corey?
   A. Listening to the fetal heart sounds.
   B. Recording Mrs. Corey's blood pressure.
   C. Recording Mrs. Corey's temperature, pulse, and respiration.
   D. Obtaining Mrs. Corey's urine for a culture and sensitivity test.

23. The doctor orders a pubic shave for Mrs. Corey. Before the practical nurse performs this procedure, she will
   A. isolate the patient.
   B. explain what procedure is to be done.
   C. order the patient's diet for the labor room.
   D. take the patient's history.

24. When Mrs. Corey is in labor, the nurse should check her blood pressure every
   A. 2 hours.
   B. hour.
   C. 3 hours.
   D. half-hour.

25. The nurse should ascess the fetal heat sounds immediately
   A. after the membranes have ruptured.
   B. upon admission to the labor suite.
   C. if bradycardia is present.
   D. in all of the above circumstances.

26. A clean urine specimen should be collected from Mrs. Corey
   A. immediately before the perineal preparation.
   B. immediately after the rectal examination.
   C. immediately after she is admitted.
   D. immediately after cleansing and shaving the vulva.

27. To check Mrs. Corey's contractions, the nurse feels Mrs. Corey's abdomen and determines
   A. the character of the contractions.
   B. the strength of the contractions.
   C. the frequency of the contractions.
   D. all of the above.

28. Fetal heart sounds should be checked by the nurse in order to determine the
   A. sex of the fetus.
   B. heart rate of the fetus.
   C. position, rate, and regularity of the fetal heart.
   D. mother's condition.

Mrs. Celia Dunn, a 45-year-old legal secretary, tells her doctor that she feels a lump in her left breast. After an examination, she is admitted to the hospital for a biopsy. The growth proves malignant, and Mrs. Dunn is scheduled for a radical mastectomy.

---

29. Mrs. Dunn appears very nervous and asks the nurse, "Will I have a hole in my chest?" Which one of the following would be the BEST answer for the nurse to make in response to this preoperative question from an anxious patient?
  A. "Ask your doctor, Mrs. Dunn."
  B. "Don't worry. It's nice your husband visited you this afternoon."
  C. "No, Mrs. Dunn, you won't have a hole in your chest. You sound upset. Do you want to talk?
  D. "I'm busy now. I'll come back later to talk to you."

30. The anesthesiologist orders atropine sulfate preoperatively for Mrs. Dunn. The nurse knows that the primary reason for giving this drug is that it helps to
  A. maintain cardiac status.
  B. supplement the action of the anesthesia.
  C. decrease the reflexes.
  D. suppress oral and respiratory tract secretions.

31. Which one of the following assessments should be made FIRST by the nurse when Mrs. Dunn is taken to the recovery room after her surgery?
  A. Checking the patient's dressings for bleeding and drainage.
  B. Taking and recording the patient's vital signs.
  C. Noting that the airway is unobstructed.
  D. Noting that the drainage tubes are functioning.

32. Mrs. Dunn's nursing care plan indicates that the nurse will position her
  A. with her left arm across her chest wall.
  B. in semi-Fowler's position with her left arm at her side.
  C. in semi-Fowler's position with her left arm elevated.
  D. with her left arm at her side at the level of her body.

33. After discharge from the hospital, Mrs. Dunn is treated with radiation and chemotherapy as an outpatient. In instructing the patient about these measures, it is important to tell her

  A. that radiation can cause pneumonitis.
  B. that radiodermatitis can occur during therapy.
  C. that gastroenteritis may occur.
  D. all of the above.

34. During the teaching session, which of the following activities of daily living will the nurse tell Mrs. Dunn to avoid?
  A. Taking a daily shower.
  B. Brushing her poodle.
  C. Doing the family wash.
  D. Doing her gardening.

35. During a later visit to the clinic for radiation, the nurse notices that a large area of Mrs. Dunn's skin appears red, wet, and oozing. The proper intervention is to
  A. instruct Mrs. Dunn to use Bacitracin ointment on the area.
  B. discontinue the treatment and explain to Mrs. Dunn that when the oozing stops the treatment will be resumed.
  C. give the treatment and note the condition in Mrs. Dunn's record.
  D. discontinue the treatment and notify the supervising nurse.

36. Mrs. Dunn has some gastrointestinal symptoms. Which of the following foods should she avoid?
  A. Chicken, canned thin soups, and vegetables.
  B. Milk, boiled eggs, canned vegetables, and fish.
  C. Fried foods, cheese, nuts, and raw vegetables.
  D. Pork, veal, beef, bread, and potatoes.

Mr. Earl Tompkins, 65 years old and retired, goes to his physician complaining of alternating constipation and diarrhea, bloody stools, and weight loss. The following schedule is set up for Mr. Tompkins:
Low-residue, meat-free diet for 3 days
Sigmoidoscopy the following day
Barium enema

---

37. The office nurse explains the low-residue diet to Mr. Tompkins. Which of the foods in the following list will he be allowed to eat?
  A. Ground beef.
  B. Chicken cutlet.

C. Spaghetti with cheese sauce.
D. Spaghetti with meat sauce.

38. In preparation for the sigmoidoscopy, given as an office procedure, which of the following is appropriate?
A. Have the patient fast the evening before the examination.
B. Give the patient an enema 1 hour before the examination.
C. Advise a liquid diet the entire day before the examination.
D. Have the patient take two Dulcolax tablets the evening before the examination, eat a light breakfast, and take a Fleet enema 1 hour before the examination.

39. The nurse knows that, after completion of the barium enema, the radiologist will order
A. a cathartic.
B. an emetic.
C. a sedative.
D. a stimulant.

40. False positive results may occur when the stool is examined for blood if the patient
A. has eaten foods containing iron.
B. has eaten meat.
C. has eaten fatty foods.
D. is diabetic.

41. After the diagnostic examinations and work-up, Mr. Tompkins's surgeon tells him that he has colon cancer and that a colostomy will be necessary. This procedure is defined as
A. surgical removal of the stomach.
B. insertion of a tube into the stomach for the purposes of feeding a patient with an obstruction in the digestive tract.
C. surgical removal of the affected portion of the colon and creation of an artificial anus through the abdomen.
D. surgical removal of the entire lower part of the intestinal tract and creation of a permanent anus through the abdomen.

42. An important preoperative nursing responsibility for a patient who is going to have a colostomy is
A. refusing to discuss the surgical procedure with patient.

B. discouraging the patient from asking questions of his/her doctor.
C. giving the patient emotional support.
D. discussing the advantages of the surgery with the patient.

43. After the surgery Mr. Tompkins is removed to the recovery room, where the first nursing intervention is to
A. check and record his vital signs.
B. check his airway.
C. check his dressings.
D. attach the indwelling catheter.

44. After Mr. Tompkins has been moved to his room, a unit of whole blood is started. Shortly thereafter, Mr. Tompkins complains of chills and of tingling in his fingers. The practical nurse should immediately
A. notify the surgeon.
B. stop the infusion of blood and notify the supervising nurse.
C. put a blanket on the patient.
D. rub the patient's hands.

45. Mr. Tompkin's colostomy is functioning by the 3rd postoperative day. What sign indicates this function?
A. Drainage from the nasogastric tube changes color.
B. Gas is passed from the colostomy.
C. Peristaltic waves can be seen.
D. There are no bowel sounds.

46. After the nasogastric tube is removed, the nurse explains to Mr. Tompkins that the surgeon has ordered clear fluids for his diet. Which of the following is CONTRAINDICATED?
A. Chicken broth.
B. Cranberry juice.
C. Ice cream.
D. Lemon Jell-O.

47. The next nursing intervention is to prepare Mr. Tompkins for the sight of his colostomy. This is MOST effectively done by
A. showing him pictures of a colostomy.
B. explaining how normal body functions work.
C. asking someone from the local ostomy club to talk to him.
D. urging him to discuss the colostomy.

48. On the 6th postoperative day the nurse tells Mr. Tompkins that the surgeon has ordered colostomy irrigations. She explains that such irrigations are intended to do all of the following EXCEPT
   A. dilate the sphincter.
   B. cleanse the lower intestinal tract.
   C. empty the colon of its contents: feces, gas, mucus.
   D. stimulate peristalsis and thus establish a regular pattern of evacuation.

49. To prevent skin irritation from colostomy drainage, which of the following should be applied around the surgical site?
   A. Bacitracin ointment.
   B. Petrolatum.
   C. Zinc oxide ointment.
   D. Talcum powder.

50. After the drain is removed from Mr. Tompkins's perineal wound, the most effective way of promoting healing is to
   A. apply antiseptic ointment to the area.
   B. take sitz baths.
   C. expose the area to air.
   D. apply warm, moist dressings of witch hazel to the area.

51. As the time nears for Mr. Tompkins's discharge, the practical nurse plans a dietary regimen, which she discusses with him. Which of the following will not apply to Mr. Tompkins?
   A. A diet high in roughage will help peristalsis and keep the bowels regular.
   B. An individualized diet is important in preventing constipation.
   C. A daily diary should be effective in determining what foods cause difficulty and should be eliminated from the diet.
   D. Gas-forming foods should be eliminated.

Mr. Harold Steinfeld, 70 years old, complains to his ophthalmologist of blurred, hazy vision in his eyes. Examination reveals lenticular opacity, and he is scheduled for cataract extraction of his left eye.

52. As the nurse is taking his history in the ambulatory care center, Mr. Steinfeld asks her the cause of cataracts in the elderly.

Which of the following statements is the BEST answer?
   A. Cataracts result from the heavy use of toxic substances like tobacco.
   B. Chronic systemic diseases are the cause of cataracts.
   C. Cataracts in the elderly are a result of the aging process.
   D. Cataracts can be due to early childhood injuries.

53. In the ambulatory care center, one of the preoperative orders for Mr. Steinfeld is as follows: Neo-Synephrine 10% and Ocufen, 1 drop of each O.S. every 5 minutes for 3 times. According to this order, the preoperative medications are to be placed
   A. only in the right eye.
   B. only in the left eye.
   C. in both eyes.
   D. in the right and the left eye alternately.

54. After the extracapsular extraction of the lens, an intraocular lens is implanted. After the surgery, Mr. Steinfeld is taken to a recovery room to rest for 2 or 3 hours before going home. The practical nurse monitoring him has to be aware of postoperative complications. Which of the following represents an emergency?
   A. Lacrimation affecting the operated eye.
   B. Sudden onset of double vision.
   C. Irritation of conjunctiva.
   D. Palpitations.

55. The function of the lens of the eye is to
   A. regulate near vision.
   B. focus light rays onto the retina.
   C. monitor the rods and cones.
   D. produce vitreous humor.

56. When Mr. Steinfeld is discharged, the nurse impresses upon him that he must limit his activities for about
   A. 1 week.
   B. 1 to 2 weeks.
   C. 2 to 4 weeks.
   D. 6 to 12 weeks.

57. During the discharge interview the nurse further instructs Mr. Steinfeld that he should comply with all of the following EXCEPT
   A. he must patch his eye 12 hours daily.
   B. he must not rub his eye.

C. he must use his eyes normally.

D. he must not allow himself to become constipated.

Marty Cole, 7 years old, is admitted to the pediatric service with a diagnosis of juvenile diabetes mellitus. He has not been under treatment previously.

---

58. As a practical nurse, you would expect Marty to exhibit all of the following symptoms EXCEPT
   A. increased thirst.
   B. fatigue.
   C. increased appetite with weight gain.
   D. increased urination with enuresis.

59. Because Marty is so young and because his mother works, it is decided to start him on
   A. regular insulin.
   B. regular + semilente insulin.
   C. semilente insulin.
   D. protamine zinc insulin (PZI).

60. When counseling Marty about his diabetes and its treatment, you would advise against eating
   A. French fries.
   B. ice cream.
   C. a tuna fish sandwich.
   D. a peanut butter sandwich.

61. When teaching Marty about regulating his diabetes mellitus, you will include information on
   A. testing his blood with a glucometer before meals.
   B. increasing concentrated carbohydrates in his diet.
   C. increasing calorie intake.
   D. avoiding exercise.

62. In counseling sessions about Marty, you will advise all of the following EXCEPT
   A. that the child carry with him at all times an identifying card with his diagnosis; his name, telephone number, and address; and the name and telephone number of his physician.
   B. that the child carry with him at all times a lump of sugar in case he should start to experience the symptoms of hypoglycemia.
   C. that the child eat a lump of sugar each day at noon.

D. that the parents, with Marty, discuss the diagnosis with the school nurse and/or the child's teacher.

Timmie Block, 3 months old, has been diagnosed as mentally retarded. His parents have brought him to the clinic where you work as a practical nurse for further assessment.

---

63. As you assess Timmie, the observation that will help confirm the diagnosis of mental retardation is that he
   A. has spadelike hands with simian creases.
   B. can follow bright objects with his eyes.
   C. frequently puts his foot in his mouth.
   D. has a tight hand grasp.

64. In working with Timmie's parents, you should develop a plan that
   A. will help the parents make future plans for their retarded child.
   B. is based on an accurate assessment of the family at the present time.
   C. will describe the family's feelings concerning the retarded child.
   D. will list appropriate institutions for the retarded child's placement.

John Barrows, a 67-year-old carpenter, is admitted to the hospital with the diagnosis of severe emphysema. Upon his admission, the nurse notices that he is severely dyspneic.

---

65. To make Mr. Barrows more comfortable in bed, the nurse places him in
   A. the Trendelenburg position.
   B. the high Fowler's position.
   C. Sims's position.
   D. the dorso-recumbent position.

66. For 40 years, Mr. Barrows has been a very heavy smoker. He asks the nurse to lower his bed so that he can get out to go into the sitting room to smoke. Her BEST answer is
   A. "It is against the rules to smoke on this floor."

B. "Your condition is serious, and if you want the treatment to work, you must refrain from smoking."

C. "Your doctor did not leave an order for you to smoke."

D. "No; you are to stay in bed."

67. The nurse encourages Mr. Barrows to drink water frequently because
   A. the patient's kidneys need a good flushing out.
   B. water helps to loosen the lung secretions.
   C. copious amounts of water are good for everybody.
   D. water will keep the patient from becoming constipated.

68. After the lung secretions have loosened, the nurse has Mr. Barrows sit up, leaning forward. This position helps to do all the following EXCEPT
   A. lessen the cough.
   B. drain the secretions.
   C. reduce the chest pain.
   D. decrease respiratory infection.

Mr. Joseph Jaworski, a 45-year-old accountant, comes to the emergency room at 2 A.M. complaining of severe indigestion, nausea, and vomiting for several hours. After examination, he is admitted to the hospital with a diagnosis of suspected myocardial infarction.

---

69. The practical nurse in the ER who is preparing Mr. Jaworski for admission knows that myocardial infarction is due to
   A. indigestion.
   B. reduced blood flow through one of the coronary arteries, causing myocardial ischemia.
   C. a decrease in ventricular contractions.
   D. an increase in ventricular contractions.

70. During the admitting process, the nurse reports that Mr. Jaworski's pulse has become irregular and he is experiencing premature ventricular contractions. The drug that the nurse expects to be ordered for Mr. Jaworski IMMEDIATELY is
   A. lidocaine.

B. morphine sulfate.
C. quinidine.
D. digitoxin.

71. The physician orders oxygen for Mr. Jaworski. In these cases oxygen
   A. reduces the patient's irritability.
   B. dilates the affected coronary artery.
   C. increases myocardial oxygenation.
   D. increases cardiac output.

72. When oxygen is administered, the nurse must put up a warning sign because oxygen
   A. is explosive.
   B. is combustible.
   C. supports combustion.
   D. combines with other gases.

73. The pain continues, and morphine sulfate is ordered for Mr. Jaworski. The purpose of this drug is
   A. to dilate the coronary artery.
   B. to depress respirations.
   C. to relieve pain and restlessness.
   D. to decrease cardiac output.

74. Nitroglycerine is ordered for Mr. Jaworski. The nurse knows that this drug
   A. increases cardiac output.
   B. controls cardiac irregularities.
   C. decreases the cardiac workload.
   D. sedates the patient.

75. Mr. Jaworski complains to the nurse, "Doesn't the hospital have any decent food? This meal is tasteless." The nurse explains that the soft, bulky diet
   A. helps to prevent an increased workload on the heart.
   B. is routine hospital food served to all patients.
   C. prevents constipation.
   D. eliminates the exertion needed to chew and digest fibrous foods.

76. On the first day after Mr. Jaworski's admission, he may do all of the following EXCEPT
   A. use a bedside commode.
   B. feed himself.
   C. give himself a complete bedbath.
   D. listen to the radio.

Roger Terry, a 40-year-old chronic alcoholic, enters a detoxification hospital for treatment. Two hours before entering, he consumes two double Scotches in order to steady his nerves.

77. A person who resorts to excessive use of alcohol as a method of adjustment can be accurately described as
A. lacking willpower.
B. emotionally immature.
C. extremely selfish.
D. having a chronic disease.

78. Which of the following would be BEST to include in the nursing plan in order to eliminate alcohol from Mr. Terry's body more quickly?
A. Give him large amounts of strong black coffee.
B. Have him take alternately hot and cold showers.
C. Allow him to sleep off the effects of the alcohol in a quiet, restful room.
D. Give him a noxious mixture that will cause him to vomit.

79. It is a rule of this hospital that upon admission every patient's luggage is searched for any item that may contain alcohol. Which of the following possessions of Mr. Terry will be confiscated by the nurse?
A. Aftershave lotion.
B. Dry-skin hand lotion.
C. Shaving cream.
D. Hair conditioner.

80. In obtaining a nursing history, the practical nurse questions Mr. Terry as to why he drinks the amount of alcohol that he does. It is expected that the answer will be
A. intentionally untruthful.
B. precisely correct.
C. boastful.
D. vague.

81. The nurse who can develop a good therapeutic relationship with Mr. Terry is one who
A. is strictly objective and uncommunicative.

B. is understanding and forgiving in nature.
C. is optimistic about all patients' good intentions.
D. is strictly moral and thinks that drinking alcohol is a sin.

82. Mr. Terry's physician will most likely order which of the following medications to aid in the withdrawal?
A. Morphine sulfate.
B. Haldol.
C. Chlordiazepoxide HCL (Librium).
D. Phenobarbital sodium (Luminal).

83. The second day after admission, Mr. Terry develops tremulousness, agitation, and restlessness. He is unable to hold a cup of coffee without spilling it. He asks the nurse how long it will be before his hands become steady. Which of the following responses should the nurse make?
A. "I will report your symptoms to the doctor, and she will probably order more medication for you."
B. "The tremulousness will go away in about 2 more days."
C. "You may have these tremors intermittently for 2 months. This reaction is common after a person has abstained from alcohol."
D. "You have sustained irreparable damage to the central nervous system, which will make these symptoms permanent."

84. Although Mr. Terry wants to withdraw from alcohol ingestion, he soon craves a drink and tries to devise ways to get one. What nursing intervention(s) will assist this patient?
A. Provide time for one-to-one interaction with staff.
B. Assess the patient's vital signs.
C. Offer the patient a prn Librium.
D. Do all of the above.

85. On one occasion, before coming to the hospital, Mr. Terry drank so much alcohol that he experienced delirium tremens. Symptoms of delirium tremens include all of the following EXCEPT
A. hypertension.
B. hallucination.

C. delusion.
D. extreme agitation.

86. When Mr. Terry is ready for discharge, Mrs. Terry asks the nurse what she should do to help her husband. Which of the following answers would be of the MOST value?
A. "Notify all his friends that Mr. Terry has undergone a detoxification program."
B. "Do not keep alcoholic beverages in the house."
C. "Be supportive when Mr. Terry needs help, and seek support for yourself from Al-Anon."
D. "Constantly monitor Mr. Terry's where-abouts."

87. In discussing Mr. Terry's nutrition, the nurse advises Mrs. Terry to administer multivita-mins as prescribed by the physician and to give her husband
A. a low-fat diet.
B. a low-protein diet.
C. a high-protein diet.
D. a high-carbohydrate diet.

Mrs. Mary O'Leary, 40 years old and obese, is admitted to the hospital complaining of upper right quadrant pain that radiates to the midback. A gallbladder series done on an outpatient basis had revealed cholecystitis with cholelithiasis. Upon Mrs. O'Leary's ad-mission to the hospital, the physician orders nitroglycerine, and morphine sulfate for the control of pain.

---

88. The practical nurse who gives the injections knows that nitroglycerine was ordered for Mrs. O'Leary because
A. it reduces nausea and vomiting.
B. it speeds up the action of the morphine sulfate.
C. it relaxes the gallbladder and its ducts.
D. it increases the secretion of gastric juice.

89. The physician has ordered a low-fat diet for Mrs. O'Leary. Which of the following dinners will the nurse pick for the patient?
A. Roast chicken, baked potato, steamed carrots, applesauce, tea.

B. Baked ham, baked macaroni and cheese, spinach, chocolate pudding, tea.
C. Roast beef, mashed potatoes with gra-vy, steamed carrots, apple pie, tea.
D. Barbecued spare ribs, French fries, tossed salad, fruit cup, tea.

90. Mrs. O'Leary is being prepared for surgery. The nurse explains that she must eat lightly and that no food or fluid is permitted after midnight before the surgery. The surgeon wrote that order because Mrs. O'Leary will have general anesthesia and withholding oral intake will prevent
A. gas and distension after surgery.
B. vomiting and possible aspiration of vomitus during surgery.
C. postoperative diarrhea.
D. postoperative constipation.

91. When Mrs. O'Leary returns from surgery, a T-tube has been sutured into her common bile duct. To maintain accurate intake and output records, the nurse must measure the T-tube drainage and
A. add it to the urinary output.
B. add it to the total intake for the day.
C. subtract it from the gastric drainage.
D. chart it separately on the output record.

92. Postoperatively a nasogastric tube is in-serted, which causes Mrs. O'Leary great throat discomfort. What nursing interven-tion will reduce the discomfort?
A. Having the patient take small sips of ice water.
B. Having the patient suck ice chips.
C. Having the patient suck anesthetic lozenges.
D. Gently moving the tube every 2 hours.

93. Mrs. O'Leary is soon to be discharged. In instructing her in regard to her future di-etary regimen, the nurse tells her to restrict her intake of
A. carbohydrates.
B. fats.
C. proteins.
D. vitamins.

Ten-year-old Mike breaks his right wrist while skiing and is taken to the emergency clinic at the bottom of the hill. After inspecting the X-ray, the doctor on duty casts the right arm. The doctor then gives Mike's father the X-rays and tells him to take Mike to the family doctor the next day.

94. As Mike and his father are leaving, the practical nurse on duty advises the father to take Mike to the emergency room of the local hospital immediately if
   A. the fingers on the casted arm feel cold and appear blue.
   B. the cast feels wet after 8 hours.
   C. the arm under the cast itches.
   D. the cast over the hand cracks a little.

95. The next day Mike's doctor reads the X-rays and inspects the cast. He tells Mike's father to return with Mike in 8 weeks. Before they leave, the nurse tells Mike all of the following EXCEPT
   A. he must do finger exercises regularly.
   B. he must keep his right arm in a sling.
   C. he must watch his fingers for swelling.
   D. he can use his skateboard.

Mrs. Singh, 45 years old, has been suffering pain and stiffness in her joints. She can now hardly walk. A tentative diagnosis of rheumatoid arthritis is made, and Mrs. Singh is admitted to the hospital for a complete work-up.

96. The actual cause of rheumatoid arthritis is unknown. Which of the following is considered to be a possible cause?
   A. The autoimmune process.
   B. Continuous poisoning from painkillers.
   C. Decreased blood supply to the brain.
   D. Avitaminosis.

97. Your understanding of the pathophysiology of rheumatoid arthritis is that it
   A. is a self-limiting disease.
   B. causes ankylosis of a joint.
   C. is a disease that is confined to the older age group.
   D. is chronic inflammation of a joint.

98. As part of your teaching about the disease, you advise Mrs. Singh that she should avoid
   A. regular exercise.
   B. fatigue.
   C. a great deal of rest.
   D. activity of any type.

99. You advise Mrs. Singh that in resting she should keep her affected joints
   A. well flexed.
   B. as straight as possible.
   C. elevated on a pillow.
   D. supported by sandbags.

James Izzo, a 49-year-old construction worker, is admitted to the hospital with a diagnosis of acute glomerulonephritis. When the nurse is obtaining his history, he states that for the past 2 weeks he has had a severe sore throat but didn't go to the doctor because he didn't want to lose time from work. His symptoms consist of extreme fatigue, swelling of his ankles, loss of appetite, and "bags" under his eyes. He also states that his urinations have decreased.

100. The production of scanty amounts of urine is called
   A. glycosuria.
   B. dysuria.
   C. anuria.
   D. oliguria.

101. The nurse knows that acute glomerulonephritis most frequently develops as a complication of an infection caused by
   A. streptococci.
   B. diplococci.
   C. spirochetes.
   D. Nesseria bacteria.

102. All of the following are primary nursing interventions for Mr. Izzo EXCEPT
   A. bedrest to promote kidney healing.
   B. control of previous infection by the administration of ordered antibiotics.
   C. a high-protein diet to restore good nutrition.
   D. scrupulous daily hygiene.

103. Mr. Izzo complains to the nurse, "I am very thirsty. The aide has not filled my water pitcher." The nurse knows that the physician has ordered Mr. Izzo's fluid intake to be restricted to 1000 ml per 24-hour period. The nurse offers him
   A. hot tea.
   B. lemonade.
   C. ice chips.
   D. Coca-Cola.

104. The nurse knows that all of the following foods are CONTRAINDICATED on Mr. Izzo's special diet EXCEPT
   A. fried pork chops.
   B. pancakes with syrup and butter.
   C. a double cheeseburger.
   D. barbecued spareribs.

105. In addition to the special diet, a nursing intervention for Mr. Izzo will be a
   A. daily CBC.
   B. daily urinalysis.
   C. daily weighing.
   D. daily BUN.

106. The physician orders Lasix for Mr. Izzo. The nurse will note the positive effect of the Lasix when the patient's
   A. blood pressure goes down.
   B. urine production increases.
   C. WBC decreases.
   D. Hb increases.

107. Upon taking Mr. Izzo's blood pressure, the nurse notices that it has suddenly elevated. Why does she report this to the supervisor immediately?
   A. It could be a sign that the Lasix is not working.
   B. It could be a sign of beginning renal failure.
   C. It could signify that the patient is going into cardiac failure.
   D. It could indicate that there is too much sodium in the patient's meals.

108. The purpose of keeping an intake and output record for a patient with acute glomerulonephritis is to determine
   A. infection.
   B. anuria.
   C. urinary retention.
   D. the degree of kidney damage.

Mrs. Regina Gold, a 75-year-old widow, is brought to the emergency room by ambulance from her co-op apartment, accompanied by a neighbor. Management had become concerned about Mrs. Gold's very peculiar behavior for the past 6 months; her speech and actions had become markedly inappropriate. After examination by the psychiatric resident, a tentative diagnosis of Alzheimer's disease is made. Mrs. Gold's brother, Mr. Ben Cohen, is notified and wants his sister to be placed in a nursing home.

109. Mrs. Gold repeatedly says, "Today is my anniversary, and I must prepare for the celebration." The practical nurse recognizes that this remark may
   A. indicate that Mrs. Gold's memory is unimpaired.
   B. be a symptom of Mrs. Gold's disease.
   C. be a plea for assistance.
   D. show an awareness of time and place.

110. To minimize Mrs. Gold's confusion, the MOST appropriate action for the nurse to take is to
   A. encourage dependent functioning.
   B. establish routine.
   C. reduce sensory input.
   D. increase participation in reality-orientation classes.

111. A reality-orientation program emphasizes
   A. orientation to reality for community living.
   B. conflict resolution and sharing of memories.
   C. participation and interest in the environment.
   D. orientation to time, place, and person.

112. Mrs. Gold's nutritional status requires regular monitoring. It is important for the nurse to know that this patient's
   A. protein requirements are less than when she was younger.
   B. fat requirements are greater than when she was younger.

C. caloric requirements are less than when she was younger.

D. nutritional requirements are less now that she is advancing in age.

113. To ensure that Mrs. Gold is eating a balanced diet, the nurse will
A. allow her to feed herself.
B. sit with her and feed her each meal.
C. assist her to eat the ordered diet.
D. permit her to snack whenever she asks for food.

114. Mrs. Gold's poor coordination interferes with her performing her own daily care. The practical nurse can best approach this problem by
A. encouraging participation and giving assistance when necessary.
B. reminding Mrs. Gold that she must bathe more thoroughly.
C. scheduling Mrs. Gold's bath to be done on a regular basis by staff.
D. giving Mrs. Gold extra time to perform daily care.

115. Which of the following explains Mr. Cohen's anger when he observes Mrs. Gold's urinary incontinence?
A. He has extreme guilt feelings.
B. He considers the staff neglectful and feels helpless to control the situation.
C. He doesn't fully understand the disease process.
D. All of the above.

116. Mr. Cohen refuses to discuss his sister's condition with anyone. The psychological defense mechanism he is displaying is
A. projection.
B. rationalization.
C. displacement.
D. repression.

The rest of the test consists of unrelated questions.

117. A 15-month-old toddler has been brought to the well-baby clinic. He is found to be normal, and the necessary immunizations are given. In counseling his mother, the practical nurse points out that
A. the child should be taken outdoors only on very warm, sunny days.
B. hazardous objects should be kept out of the child's reach.

C. the child should not be hugged or kissed too often.
D. the child may bite in showing affection.

118. A 10-month-old is brought into the clinic with a croupy cough. The diagnosis is upper respiratory infection. The nurse's advice to the mother includes all of the following EXCEPT to
A. prop the baby up in an infant seat or with pillows behind him.
B. put the baby in a humidified atmosphere, either by using a steam vaporizer or by keeping him in a steam-filled bathroom.
C. keep the baby in a dark room.
D. apply petroleum jelly around the baby's lips and nose to soothe irritation from mouth breathing.

119. Syphilis is a venereal disease that can affect
A. only the reproductive organs.
B. males only.
C. the entire body.
D. females only.

120. The outstanding symptom of monilial vaginitis is a vaginal discharge that is
A. purulent and foul-smelling.
B. white or watery and accompanied by itching and inflammation of the vulva.
C. bloody and occurs at the time of ovulation.
D. blood-tinged and occurs at regular monthly intervals.

121. Benign tumors of the uterus are commonly referred to as
A. sarcomas.
B. fibroids.
C. carcinomas.
D. lymphomas.

122. Potassium intoxication produces which of the following emergency situations?
A. Pulmonary edema.
B. Cardiac arrest.
C. Nausea and vomiting.
D. Severe jaundice.

123. Which of the following is NOT a sexually transmitted disease?
A. Hepatitis B infection.

    B.   Herpes zoster.
    C.   Genital warts.
    D.   Pediculosis pubis.

124. An oil retention enema has the effect of
    A.   cleansing the bowel.
    B.   softening fecal material.
    C.   soothing the lining of the intestine.
    D.   relieving abdominal distention.

125. A 65-year-old woman has lived alone since the death of her husband some years earlier. When she develops pneumonia, her physician decides to hospitalize her. During the course of her hospitalization it is discovered that she is diabetic, but the condition can be controlled by a change in diet. However, after the acute phase of her illness she remains in a severely weakened condition. Her physician suggests temporary placement in a nursing facility for observation and convalescence. The patient refuses, stating that she wants to be in her own home. The type of service of most value to this patient would be
    A.   homemaker-housekeeper service.
    B.   visiting nurse service.
    C.   hospital-based home care.
    D.   none of the above.

MASTERY TEST

ANSWER KEY—PART I

1.	B	26.	D	51.	A	76.	C	101.	A
2.	C	27.	D	52.	C	77.	D	102.	C
3.	B	28.	C	53.	B	78.	C	103.	C
4.	D	29.	C	54.	B	79.	A	104.	B
5.	C	30.	D	55.	B	80.	D	105.	C
6.	B	31.	C	56.	A	81.	B	106.	B
7.	C	32.	D	57.	A	82.	C	107.	B
8.	D	33.	D	58.	C	83.	C	108.	D
9.	A	34.	D	59.	D	84.	D	109.	B
10.	D	35.	D	60.	B	85.	A	110.	B
11.	D	36.	C	61.	A	86.	C	111.	D
12.	C	37.	C	62.	C	87.	D	112.	C
13.	A	38.	D	63.	A	88.	C	113.	C
14.	A	39.	A	64.	B	89.	A	114.	C
15.	B	40.	B	65.	B	90.	B	115.	D
16.	C	41.	D	66.	B	91.	D	116.	D
17.	A	42.	C	67.	B	92.	C	117.	B
18.	C	43.	B	68.	D	93.	B	118.	C
19.	B	44.	B	69.	B	94.	A	119.	C
20.	C	45.	B	70.	A	95.	D	120.	B
21.	D	46.	C	71.	C	96.	A	121.	B
22.	D	47.	A	72.	C	97.	D	122.	B
23.	B	48.	A	73.	C	98.	B	123.	B
24.	B	49.	C	74.	A	99.	B	124.	B
25.	D	50.	B	75.	A	100.	D	125.	C

EXPLANATIONS FOR ANSWERS—PART I

1. **B** Hemoglobin is found in mature red blood cells (erythrocytes). It is the hemoglobin that enables the red blood cells to carry oxygen all through the body.
2. **C** See the answer to question 1.
3. **B** The normal lower level for males is 13–18 gm. Mr. White's range is lower.
4. **D** Hipbone is the ilium; collarbone is the clavicle; shoulder blade is the scapula.
5. **C** The sternum is thin, and the blood cells in the marrow are more plentiful there than in other places.
6. **B** Anoxia is lack of oxygen. Cachexia is a weak and emaciated condition. Dyspnea is difficulty in breathing.
7. **C** A decrease in red blood cells results in a decrease in hemoglobin and therefore a decrease in oxygen.
8. **D** Because of a decrease in oxygen to the brain, changes in the heat-regulating mechanism of the body cause the anemia patient to feel cold.
9. **A** It is not safe to use hot-water bags. Also, external heat could be contraindicated because of disease processes.
10. **D** In anemia there are hemorrhagic tendencies of the mucous membranes of the mouth because of a reduction in the platelets of the blood. Platelets are essential for blood clotting.
11. **D** Stimulation of the gums will improve the circulation to them.
12. **C** The patient's comfort and self-respect are reasons enough to give the morning care before the transfusion.
13. **A** In leukemia, there is an excessive increase in white blood cells, many of which have become malignant. These malignant cells fill the bone marrow and bloodstream.
14. **A** See the answer to question 13.

15. **B** Tarry stools are suggestive of bleeding in the G.I. tract; smoky urine indicates bleeding somewhere in the urinary system; coffee-grounds-colored vomitus indicates peptic bleeding.

16. **C** Fatigue, generalized malaise, and bone pain may make the patient irritable; she feels miserable.

17. **A** Varicose veins are due to damaged valves that fail to prevent the backflow of blood. As a result the blood accumulates in the veins.

18. **C** See the answer to question 17. Varicose veins, more common in women than in men, are often associated with congenitally weak valves.

19. **B** Although hereditary weakness of the valves is a factor, long-standing distension of the veins brought about by pregnancy, obesity, or prolonged sitting or standing can cause these varicosities.

20. **C** A venogram is an X-ray film of veins. Venectomy and phlebectomy are surgical removal of a vein or part of a vein.

21. **A** A venotomy is a surgical incision into a vein. A varicosity is a swollen, tortuous vein.

22. **D** Recording the mother's vital signs and monitoring the fetus are part of the admissions procedure.

23. **B** In order to reduce anxiety it is good nursing practice to explain all procedures in advance.

24. **B** Hourly checks of the blood pressure help the nurse to assess the mother's condition.

25. **D** Sudden release of fluid may cause prolapse of the umbilical cord. Assessing the fetal heart sounds on admission will provide a baseline for subsequent assessments as labor progresses. Persistent bradycardia may be indicative of a serious fetal compromise.

26. **D** The area around the vulva has many bacterial colonies. Urine that is caught immediately after the vulva is cleansed and that is not allowed to touch the skin is relatively free of bacterial contamination.

27. **D** The strength, the character, and the frequency of the contractions are all indicative of the satisfactory progressions of labor, or the lack of such progress.

28. **C** The position, rate, and regularity of the fetal heart are important in determining the condition of the fetus.

29. **C** An important part of the nurse's duties is to allay the patient's preoperative anxiety. Allowing the patient to verbalize at the time she raises a question will decrease her anxiety and promote an environment conducive to patient education.

30. **D** Atropine sulfate is given to block the secretions of the mouth and respiratory tract. These secretions, if not controlled, could cause pulmonary complications.

31. **C** The most important nursing assessment when a patient first enters the recovery room is airway patency.

32. **D** This position favors drainage for the left arm, a necessity since the axillary lymph nodes have been removed.

33. **D** Because radiation causes cell damage, pneumonitis, radiodermatitis, and gastroenteritis may occur.

34. **D** Circulation in the affected area has been impaired. Therefore, Mrs. Dunn must avoid any activity such as gardening that may result in scratches, cuts, or bruises.

35. **D** To treat the reaction, the radiation will be discontinued, and steroid cream and antibiotic lotion ordered for the patient.

36. **C** Greasy foods, nuts, cheese, and raw vegetables are hard to digest and can be irritating to the gastrointestinal tract.

37. **C** Spaghetti with cheese sauce is the choice with the lowest residue.

38. **D** For today's office procedures, Dulcolax (Bisacodyl USP), a Fleet enema, and a light diet at breakfast will result in adequate preparation. The office nurse dispenses the medication with an explanation. Bisacodyl USP stimulates sensory nerve endings, thereby causing increased peristaltic contractions of the colon. The sigmoid colon and rectum must be evacuated to allow adequate viewing.

39. **A** If the barium remains in the intestine, it may cause severe constipation or fecal impaction.

MASTERY TEST

40. **B** Meat residue in the stool can lead to a false positive result when the stool is examined for blood. None of the other choices has this effect.

41. **D** In a permanent colostomy because of colon cancer, an opening (anus) is created in the abdominal wall. The tumor and the entire lower bowel are removed.

42. **C** Emotional support consists of reinforcing the patient's hope for a manageable future.

43. **B** Before any procedures are done, the nurse must be sure that the patient is breathing properly.

44. **B** The symptoms described may be indicative of a beginning allergic reaction to the blood. The infusion must be discontinued immediately.

45. **B** The passage of gas indicates that peristalsis has returned. The colostomy will therefore be functional.

46. **C** Ice cream is not a clear liquid.

47. **A** Once the patient has seen pictures of a colostomy, he will be able to relate to his condition and will be prepared for the site of the artificial opening that has been made in his abdomen.

48. **A** There is no sphincter in the colostomy. In order to control elimination naturally from the colostomy, it is necessary to stimulate peristalsis on a regular basis so that the lower intestinal tract is cleansed, the colon is emptied of its contents, and normal life activities can be pursued.

49. **C** Zinc oxide covers well and is adherent. Bacitracin ointment is not adherent and will be absorbed. Petrolatum is not adherent. Talcum powder could be irritating to the mucosa and cause the development of granulation tissue.

50. **B** Sitz baths can accomplish two things: bring heat and moisture to the perineal area, and cleanse the operative area.

51. **A** A diet high in fiber may be irritating to the bowel. Keeping a daily diary is the easiest way to make the diet individual and suited to the patient. Eliminating gas-forming foods will add to the patient's comfort.

52. **C** Although this answer is not specific, the aging process is the only cause that can be pinpointed.

53. **B** O.S. *(oculus sinister)* refers to the left eye.

54. **B** The sudden onset of double vision means that the implanted lens has slipped, and the supervising nurse must be notified immediately. The ophthalmologist must reposition the intraocular lens.

55. **B** The lens of the eye, a transparent, crystalline structure behind the pupil, focuses light rays on the retina.

56. **A** One week will give the eye time to heal under normal conditions.

57. **A** Mr. Steinfeld must do nothing to prevent the normal recovery of his eye muscles. Covering the eye will reduce the use of the eye muscles, resulting in a potential "lazy eye."

58. **C** Despite the increased appetite, children with diabetes mellitus tend to lose weight or otherwise fail to thrive.

59. **D** PZI has an onset of 4–8 hours, peaks in 14–20 hours, and has a duration of 24–36 hours. This time frame is excellent for the time constraints governing this family.

60. **B** For a child this age, the diet is kept as normal as possible except for the elimination of concentrated sweets such as ice cream.

61. **A** Early, independent assessment of a child's diabetes is essential to increasing patient's compliance. With the assistance of the school nurse, Marty can be helped to monitor his own blood glucose. In following the prescribed dietary regime, the patient would learn to avoid concentrated carbohydrates. His diet would be calculated utilizing the American Diabetic Association's food exchange lists, which would indicate a prescribed calorie intake dependent upon his growth needs. Daily, regular, planned exercise is important for good health in the diabetic.

62. **C** Eating a lump of sugar routinely is not indicated; this should be done only for a specific reason.

63. **A** Spadelike hands with simian (monkeylike) creases are diagnostic for mental retardation in the infant. The other choices are typical of normal infants.

64. **B** Because the child is so young, it is better for the parents first to come to terms with their own feelings about the child and then take the time to plan. It is too soon to think in terms of institutions. The family assessment will include a description of the family's feelings concerning Timmie.

65. **B** The high Fowler's position is the most comfortable for patients suffering from severe dyspnea.

66. **B** It is always best to explain truthfully to the patient exactly what the situation is. The other choices do not address the fact that Mr. Barrows should no longer smoke.

67. **B** Water acts to soften thick lung secretions and thus will lessen the patient's hacking cough.

68. **D** A leaning-forward, sitting position will help to lessen the patient's cough, drain the secretions, and reduce the chest pain, but will do nothing to reduce the infection.

69. **B** Reduced blood flow through one of the coronary arteries causes myocardial ischemia (decreased blood supply) and necrosis (death of an area of heart muscle).

70. **A** Arrhythmias such as premature ventricular contractions are the predominant problem during the first 48 hours after infarction and must be treated immediately with lidocaine. The other choices are not immediately effective in stopping PVCs.

71. **C** In this way, myocardial necrosis is minimized.

72. **C** Oxygen is not explosive or combustible, but it has the characteristic of supporting fire and causing it to spread rapidly.

73. **C** Promotion of the patient's comfort, rest, and emotional wellbeing is an important part of the treatment. Morphine sulfate does not serve the purposes mentioned in the other choices.

74. **A** This drug redistributes blood to the ischemic area of the myocardium, thus increasing cardiac output.

75. **A** A soft, bulky diet increases bulk, thus making defecation easier and preventing straining.

76. **C** It is less strenuous for the patient if the nurse gives him a complete bedbath on the first day after admission.

77. **D** Alcoholism is a chronic disease that affects 9–10 million people in the United States. It is considered to be the number 1 health problem facing our country today!

78. **C** Once the alcohol is absorbed into the blood stream, it is destroyed at a slow, steady rate. Therefore, the methods described in choices A, B, and D will not help.

79. **A** Aftershave lotion contains alcohol and therefore will be confiscated. The cetyl alcohol in hand lotion and hair conditioner does not pose a problem.

80. **D** The patient probably does not know why he drinks or how much he drinks daily. At this stage, he does not intend to be untruthful or boastful, and is unable to be precisely correct about the amount of alcohol consumed. This is part of the disease process and is termed denial.

81. **B** Understanding and forgiveness are necessary to deal with an alcoholic.

82. **C** Tranquilizers such as Librium are the drugs of choice today for use in withdrawal. Morphine sulfate is a cerebral depressant; Haldol is a sedative; Luminal is an anticonvulsant and sedative.

83. **C** Restlessness and tremors may persist for several days after the intake of alcohol has stopped. Choice A is too general, choice B is too specific, and choice D is not only callous but also untrue.

84. **D** Providing for one-to-one interaction of patient with staff will help to allay the patient's anxiety, which is often associated with alcohol withdrawal, and also to introduce a more positive coping mechanism. Assessing the patient's vital signs will identify clinical aspects of alcohol withdrawal: increased pulse rate, higher blood pressure, higher temperature. Finally, Librium, as needed, will decrease symptoms associated with alcohol withdrawal.

85. **A** A patient suffering from delirium tremens may be hypertensive, but hypertension is not a symptom of this syndrome.

86. **C** Alcoholism is a family disease. Mrs. Terry will need to support her husband in a constructive

manner. She will learn to cope more effectively if she involves herself in a twelve-step program.

87. **D** Many alcoholic patients are vitamin deficient and suffer from malnutrition. Carbohydrates help to stabilize the blood sugar and to promote glycogenesis. After the patient has been on the high-carbohydrate diet for some weeks, the nurse may tell Mrs. Terry that the doctor has ordered a regular well-balanced diet for her husband.

88. **C** The nitrites, including nitroglycerine, act on almost all smooth-muscle structures. The muscles of the biliary tract, including those of the gallbladder and biliary ducts, are effectively relaxed by nitroglycerine.

89. **A** All the other menus are high in fat.

90. **B** Oral intake is withheld preoperatively because under general anesthesia a patient who has eaten recently may become nauseous and vomit. The vomitus could then be aspirated and cause pulmonary problems.

91. **D** Separate charting is the only way to secure an accurate record.

92. **C** The nasogastric tube causes local irritation in the throat. Anesthetic lozenges will help reduce the resulting discomfort.

93. **B** Foods high in fats often cause nausea in patients with disorders of the biliary tract. A diet high in carbohydrates and proteins is recommended. Normal vitamin and mineral intake should be maintained.

94. **A** Coldness and blueness of the fingers indicate that there is some impairment to the circulation because the cast is too tight.

95. **D** There is a possibility of further injury if the patient falls, and skateboarding can be dangerous.

96. **A** The other choices are not considered to be causes of rheumatoid arthritis.

97. **D** Rheumatoid arthritis is not self-limited or confined to the aged. Ankylosis is rigidity of a joint and may be the result of rheumatoid arthritis.

98. **B** The patient should avoid becoming too tired. A regular program of exercise and rest is indicated in this condition, as are customary activities.

99. **B** The aim is to prevent contractures of the joints. Keeping the legs as straight as possible will help.

100. **D** Glycosuria refers to urinary sugar. Dysuria is painful urination. Anuria is the total suppression of urine.

101. **A** Acute glomerulonephritis is most often a complication of streptococcal infection. In giving his history, the patient said that he had had a sore throat for 2 weeks but neglected to seek medical attention. Sore throats are often caused by streptococci.

102. **C** Protein is restricted in cases of oliguria.

103. **C** Ice chips will help alleviate the patient's thirst while keeping the fluid intake low.

104. **B** Protein foods such as meat are limited in acute glomerulonephritis, but carbohydrates are encouraged.

105. **C** An increase in weight may indicate fluid retention due to inadequate kidney function.

106. **B** This type of diuretic (Lasix) increases the blood flow to the kidney, thereby increasing urine production.

107. **B** Early stages of renal failure are marked by rising blood pressure.

108. **D** The intake/output record is an excellent indicator of how the kidney functions. Any alteration in elimination indicates impairment.

109. **B** In Alzheimer's disease, the patient has no concept of present reality.

110. **B** The establishment of routine is necessary because memory loss is most prominent. In an established routine the patient's movements and actions become automatic, and this is the best way to achieve some control.

111. **D** Patients suffering from dementias are not oriented to time, place, and person. A reality-orientation program is of great help to them.

112. **C** Caloric requirements are less. Protein, fat, and nutritional requirements remain the same.

113. **C** It is not necessary to feed the patient. However, the best way for the nurse to ensure that Mrs.

Gold is eating a nutritionally balanced diet is to assist her to eat.

114. **C** Again, this question illustrates the need for a regular routine for patients with this diagnosis, as well as for assistance in accomplishing what is considered a positive patient outcome.

115. **D** Mr. Cohen's not understanding the disease process leads him to think that his sister is being neglected. He feels guilty and helpless.

116. **D** Mr. Cohen refuses to face (i.e., represses) the reality of his sister's condition. Repression is refusal to recognize the existence of urges and feelings that are painful or are in conflict with one's moral principles. Projection is the attribution of one's own unacceptable ideas or attitudes to another person. Rationalization is the justification of behavior by giving plausible but untrue reasons. Displacement is the transfer of feeling or action from the original object or person to another, more acceptable one.

117. **B** Children of this age are very curious and explore their environment constantly. They put everything into their mouths, and sharp objects can be a hazard.

118. **C** There is no reason to keep the baby in a dark room. However, he should be in a quiet, relaxed atmosphere.

119. **C** In syphilis, various parts of the body, including the heart, nervous system, and lungs may be affected. Either sex can contract the disease, which if untreated may result in death.

120. **B** In monilial vaginitis, the discharge is not bloody or malodorous.

121. **B** A fibroid is a fibromuscular benign tumor, usually in the uterus. A sarcoma is a malignant neoplasm in bone, muscle, or connective tissue. A carcinoma is a malignant growth in the skin, mucous membranes, or glands. A lymphoma is a neoplasm, usually malignant, of lymph tissue.

122. **B** Potassium is an electrolyte present in animal cells and is important for normal growth and muscle function. As the heart is a muscle, potassium intoxication can cause cardiac irritability, which may lead to cardiac arrest.

123. **B** Herpes zoster is an inflammatory condition in which a virus produces a painful vesicular eruption along the distribution of the nerves from one or more posterior ganglia.

124. **B** Oil has the effect of softening hard fecal matter. It is also less irritating to the bowel, so that it can be retained for a longer period of time before being expelled.

125. **C** Hospital-based home care would be ideal for this patient because her medical situation could be monitored while she was receiving home care services.

MASTERY TEST, PART II

Mrs. Anne Tanser is admitted to the hospital with a diagnosis of bleeding gastric ulcer. She has been taking a store-bought antacid for several months. Earlier on the day of admission, she attended a wedding where she drank two glasses of champagne. The physician's admission orders include the following:

Gastric analysis
Upper G.I. series
Aluminum hydroxide 8 ml q 2 h while awake
Cimetidine (Tagamet) 800 mg at bedtime

1. Shortly after admission, Mrs. Tanser vomits. The vomitus has a coffee-grounds appearance. The nurse knows from this that
   A. the ulcer is hemorrhaging.
   B. the hemorrhaging is not active.
   C. small-bowel obstruction is beginning.
   D. the ulcer is healing.

2. The nurse knows that in preparation for gastric analysis
   A. the evening meal the night before must be liquid.
   B. there is no special instruction regarding food and fluid intake before gastric analysis.
   C. fluids, food, and tobacco are withheld for at least 8 hours before gastric analysis.
   D. food and fluids, except water, are withheld for at least 8 hours before gastric analysis.

3. The practical nurse knows that, in order for an upper G.I. series to be done, it is necessary for Mrs. Tanser to take
   A. a cleansing enema.
   B. barium sulfate, given orally.
   C. a radiopaque dye, given intravenously.
   D. sodium phosphate.

4. Mrs. Tanser is on a bland diet. The practical nurse knows that the patient may have as a snack which of the following?

A. A piece of carrot cake.
B. A slice of pizza.
C. Baked custard.
D. Stewed fruit.

5. Since Mrs. Tanser is on a bland diet, which of the following should the nurse remove from the tray before serving the patient's dinner?
   A. Sugar.
   B. Pepper.
   C. Salt.
   D. Cream.

6. If Mrs. Tanser's gastric ulcer perforates, the MOST significant sign will be
   A. abdominal distension.
   B. extreme agitation.
   C. a rigid, boardlike abdomen.
   D. bloody projectile vomiting.

7. Mrs. Tanser is ready to be discharged from the hospital. In discussing dietary management with the patient, the nurse will advise her to eliminate all of the following EXCEPT
   A. artificially sweetened drinks.
   B. carbonated drinks.
   C. alcoholic drinks.
   D. tea.

Mr. Angelo Ferrari, aged 80 years, is admitted to a skilled nursing facility with a diagnosis of organic brain syndrome. He is ambulatory.

8. In planning for Mr. Ferrari's activities of daily living, the nurse must
   A. help him to become entirely responsible for his own care.
   B. assign him to help another patient.
   C. encourage him to carry out as much of his own care as possible.
   D. assume that he can't care for himself.

9. Mr. Ferrari suffers from orthostatic hypotension. In devising a care plan for him, the nursing staff must
   A. encourage him to get up very slowly.
   B. encourage him to exercise to get his muscles strong.
   C. not allow him in bed during the day.
   D. not allow him to go up the stairs.

10. Mr. Ferrari is often confused. This occurs
   A. when he leaves his room to go to the recreational area.
   B. when he awakens during the night to go to the bathroom.
   C. after he has eaten his dinner.
   D. after his visitors have left.

Mrs. Vivian Court, a 30-year-old primipara, is in active labor. Upon examining her, the nurse says, ''Call the doctor. The head is crowning.''

11. What does "crowning" mean?
   A. Elongation of the head.
   B. First appearance of the head at the vaginal opening.
   C. Full dilatation and effacement of the cervix.
   D. Lightening.

12. As Mrs. Court's infant descends during delivery, its face is directed toward the mother's sacrum and the physician's left hand. What is the designation for this position?
   A. Left occiput-posterior.
   B. Left occiput-anterior.
   C. Right occiput-posterior.
   D. Right occiput-anterior.

13. After the birth of Mrs. Court's baby, which of the following indicates that the placenta has separated?
   A. The mother has a sharp pain low down in her abdomen.
   B. The cord lengthens outside the vagina.
   C. The uterus becomes very firm.
   D. The cord stops pulsating.

Miss Ruby Clark is a 40-year-old nurse with chronic asthma. She is admitted to the hospital with a severe attack.

14. Asthma is thought to be caused by all of the following EXCEPT
   A. bacterial infection.
   B. fatigue.
   C. antigen-antibody reaction.
   D. respiratory alkalosis.

15. During the assessment of Miss Clark, the nurse understands that the characteristic sign of asthma is
   A. fever.
   B. nausea and vomiting.
   C. wheezing.
   D. severe cough.

16. When Miss Clark is put to bed, the nurse, noting her dyspnea, does all of the following EXCEPT
   A. placing the patient in Fowler's position.
   B. offering the patient her prn bronchodilator.
   C. starting the oxygen that has been ordered.
   D. turning on the air conditioning.

Jimmy Schmidt is born with bilateral cleft lip. His parents are upset when they see him for the first time and blame each other for the situation.

17. His mother asks the nurse, "What did I do to deserve this?" The practical nurse's BEST response would be
   A. "You can't cause cleft palate. It's a genetic fault."
   B. "Does cleft palate run in your family?"
   C. "Don't be upset. Surgery doesn't hurt babies."
   D. "I understand how you must be feeling."

18. In the nursing management of Jimmy, which of the following is MOST important in feeding him?
   A. Feeding him in the orthopneic position with frequent burpings.

B. Placing the feeding tube on the back of his tongue.

C. Holding him in a lying position with his head slightly elevated.

D. Feeding him small amounts at a time with frequent burpings.

19. After the lip is repaired, the nurse must prevent injury to the suture lines. All of the following procedures are recommended EXCEPT

A. preventing the infant from crying.

B. using elbow restraints.

C. tying the infant's hands down.

D. using an infant seat.

Mrs. Rose Winter, an 80-year-old widow, is admitted to a psychiatric hospital with a diagnosis of chronic brain syndrome. Her daughter states that Mrs. Winter has been confused and has been wandering away from home at every opportunity. Also, she has become increasingly careless about her appearance. However, there are days when she acts quite normal.

---

20. With a chronic brain syndrome such as Mrs. Winter's, the personality changes are most often manifested as

A. overt pleas for help.

B. suspicion and reticence.

C. an exaggeration of previous traits.

D. marked resistance and negativism.

21. Immediately after Mrs. Winter's admission, which of these nursing procedures would be BEST for her?

A. Providing a variety of new experiences.

B. Rotating staff assignments so that she will become acquainted with each member of the nursing staff.

C. Carrying out activities in the same order each day.

D. Insisting that she pay attention to present events.

22. When Mrs. Winter's daughter comes to see her the day after her admission, Mrs. Winter refuses to talk or to look at her. The daughter complains to the nurse, "My mother refuses to talk to me. She acts as though she doesn't know me. I couldn't keep her with us. Oh, I feel terrible!" Which of these responses by the nurse would be MOST appropriate initially?

A. "I'm sure you did the best you could under the circumstances."

B. "You feel guilty about having your mother here."

C. "This is a difficult situation for you and your mother."

D. "Your mother is having a little difficulty adjusting to the hospital."

23. Mrs. Winter's daughter asks the nurse whether she should come to see her mother again on the following day in view of the fact that the mother doesn't acknowledge her presence. Which of these responses would be BEST?

A. "It's not necessary for you to visit as long as someone else comes."

B. "The nursing staff will call you when your mother says she wants to see you."

C. "I'm sure your mother looks forward to your daily visit."

D. "It's okay not to come. Your mother doesn't miss you."

24. At about 3 P.M. one day, Mrs. Winter goes to the nurse and says, "I haven't had a thing to eat all day." The nurse knows that Mrs. Winter ate a large lunch. Which of the following should be a basis for the nurse's response?

A. Hunger is symbolic of a feeling of deprivation.

B. Confabulation is used by elderly clients as a means of relieving anxiety.

C. Loss of memory for recent events is characteristic of clients with chronic brain symdrome.

D. Retrospective falsification is a mechanism commonly used by elderly persons who are unhappy.

25. Mrs. Winter tells stories over and over about her children and past events. One day she keeps talking about holidays—how she used to cook for church suppers and family celebrations and baked huge quantities of cakes and cookies. Which of the following responses by the nurse would be BEST?

A. "Things are different now, Mrs. Winter. The church probably has a caterer to do the work."

B. "Those were the good old days, weren't they?"

C. "That must have been a lot of fun, Mrs. Winter. Will you help us to string popcorn for the unit party?"

D. "Those things were important to you, Mrs. Winter, but now we must talk about what is going on in the unit."

Six-year-old Jeannie Potter is admitted to the hospital for heart surgery for repair of tricuspid atresia. According to the history, she was deeply cyanotic at birth and suffered periods of anoxia. A palliative procedure was performed at the time because the infant was too young for the corrective surgery.

---

26. Tricuspid atresia
    A. is a form of congestive heart failure.
    B. is a congenital heart abnormality.
    C. is caused by anemia of the mother.
    D. can be cured by heavy antibiotic therapy.

27. Because of symptoms of congestive heart failure, Jeannie is placed on a low-sodium diet. Which of the following foods would be contraindicated for her?
    A. Milk.
    B. Candied sweet potatoes.
    C. Oranges and bananas.
    D. Frozen mixed vegetables.

28. Her father asks the nurse why Jeannie's fingers and toes are clublike. The nurse replies
    A. "There is edema in her extremities."
    B. "Not enough oxygen is going to the ends of the bones."
    C. "There is a decrease in the minerals of the bones."
    D. "Lack of oxygen has caused destruction of the red blood cells."

29. Her mother states that often, when Jeannie plays, she squats every few minutes, and asks, "Why does she do this?" The practical nurse answers
    A. "It is part of her play."
    B. "I don't know."
    C. "Jeannie probably finds that position restful."
    D. "She is bored."

30. The nurse notices that Jeannie is refusing to eat. When questioned, Jeannie states that she doesn't like the food and wants a hot dog. Which of the following responses by the nurse would be the BEST?
    A. Ask Jeannie if she would like her mother to bring food from home.
    B. Explain to Jeannie the reason for the diet.
    C. Tell Jeannie that her doctor will be very disappointed in her if she does not eat the food she is given.
    D. Promise her a large ice cream cone if she eats.

31. Before Jeannie's operation the nurse must do all of the following EXCEPT
    A. use nursing care procedures as teaching situations.
    B. use play to provide information.
    C. help Jeannie to take part in her own care.
    D. tell Jeannie that taking blood for laboratory examinations will not hurt.

32. When told that she will be out of school for an extended time, Jeannie, who likes school, says to the nurse, "Oh, dear, I'll forget how to read." The nurse's BEST answer would be
    A. "Once you learn, you never forget."
    B. "It will come back to you soon."
    C. "I'll ask your mother to bring you some puzzles and word games so that you can practice."
    D. "Don't worry about it. You have enough to think about the operation."

Paul Rosenthal, aged 36, suffers a fractured mandible after being thrown out of his car. The fracture is reduced and intermaxillary fixation applied.

---

33. What important procedure should the nurse implement as soon as Mr. Rosenthal is returned to his room?
    A. Ice bag placed on his head to reduce the headache.
    B. Eye on side of fracture patched because of edema.
    C. Scissors taped to side of bed.
    D. Chalk and chalkboard provided for communication.

34. What will be the nurse's BEST answer when Mrs. Rosenthal queries, "What shall I feed him? He is not able to chew or to even open his mouth with his jaws wired up that way"?
A. "He's overweight anyway. It won't hurt him to go without food for awhile."
B. "The nutritionist will provide a nutritious liquid diet that he can drink through a straw."
C. "Maybe you can cut his food up into tiny pieces that he can swallow without chewing."
D. "Buy a supply of baby foods."

35. Mr. Rosenthal's wife asks, "What should I do if he suddenly vomits?" The nurse's response is
A. "Call EMS immediately."
B. "Hold his head over the basin. He will just be taking fluids so the liquid will leak out."
C. "Cut the wires so that he can open his mouth."
D. "He won't vomit because there is no reason why he should."

> Jerry Kanofsky, a third-year college student, aged 21, is admitted to the hospital for staging of his non-Hodgkin's lymphoma. After completion of the staging, the oncologist orders intensive radiotherapy for the patient.

36. After radiation, it is important for the nurse to observe Jerry for
A. severe nosebleeds.
B. burning of affected areas of the skin.
C. increased blood pressure.
D. falling hair.

37. The physician orders that a unit of blood be given to Jerry. For which of these purposes is Jerry to receive a blood transfusion?
A. To increase his white blood count.
B. To fight impending infection.
C. To improve his liver function.
D. To reduce the possibility of jaundice.

38. After three treatments, Jerry tells the nurse that he doesn't feel like eating. All of the following nursing interventions will help combat this symptom EXCEPT
A. encouraging the patient to eat.
B. serving meals planned around foods that he likes.
C. serving him highly seasoned, spicy foods.
D. serving him small meals frequently.

39. As a complication of the massive radiation treatment, Jerry develops radiation pneumonitis. It is most important to take measures to
A. improve his respiratory function.
B. decrease discomfort.
C. distract his attention from his symptoms.
D. sedate him.

40. Oxygen is bubbled through water before being administered to Jerry. Why?
A. To purify the oxygen.
B. To adjust the pressure of the flow.
C. To assist the absorption of oxygen by the hemoglobin.
D. To prevent drying of the mucosa of the respiratory tract.

> John Smith, aged 70, has always lived alone and been self-sufficient. He suffers a sudden cerebrovascular accident, for which he is hospitalized. Physical examination reveals that he is suffering from a left hemiplegia, is aphasic, and has developed urinary and bowel incontinence. After 10 days his condition is considered stable. However, the residual conditions—hemiplegia, aphasia, and incontinence—continue. It is decided that he no longer needs acute hospital care and can be discharged to another institution or type of care for active rehabilitation and therapy.

41. The type of facility care prescribed is
A. an intermediate nursing facility.
B. a skilled nursing facility.
C. a chronic disease hospital.
D. domiciliary care.

42. After 3 months, Mr. Smith is evaluated by the utilization review committee. It is established that he can walk using a walker and can feed and dress himself, though he needs minor help in tying his shoelaces. Incontinence is no longer a problem after intensive therapy through a bladder and bowel training program. The type of facility care recommended by the attending physician and social service worker should be

A. an intermediate nursing facility.
B. a skilled nursing facility.
C. a chronic disease hospital.
D. domiciliary care.

> *Frank Sanchez, age 49, is helping a friend fix his car when it explodes. Mr. Sanchez is engulfed in flames, which his friend extinguishes by rolling him on the ground. When Mr. Sanchez is admitted to the hospital, about 30 percent of his skin is seen to be burned off. The rest of his body seems to be covered with large blisters.*

43. The FIRST thing that the nurse should do for Mr. Sanchez is to
    A. cover him with a damp sheet.
    B. apply Bacitracin ointment to his skin.
    C. assess his airway.
    D. sprinkle him with cool water.

44. The nurse records the burns, as described above, as being
    A. second-degree burns.
    B. third-degree burns.
    C. first- and second-degree burns.
    D. Second- and third-degree burns.

45. Important nursing interventions in the care of Mr. Sanchez are
    1. relief of pain.
    2. administration of intravenous fluids.
    3. encouraging a high-protein diet.
    4. recording urinary output.

    A. 1 and 3
    B. 1, 2, and 4
    C. 2 and 3
    D. 1 and 2

> *Ms. Nancy Winfield, aged 42, is admitted to the hospital for reevaluation of chronic multiple sclerosis, which was diagnosed 8 years previously. The practical nurse asks Ms. Winfield what her symptoms are at present. She states that at times she has double vision and that numbness in her hands is getting worse. The symptom that bothers her most, though, is increasing urinary incontinence. The nurse tells her that diagnostic tests will be done to assess the the present status of the disease.*

46. Which of the following diagnostic tests will be MOST helpful in confirming the diagnosis of chronic multiple sclerosis?
    A. Cerebrospinal fluid studies.
    B. Magnetic resonance imaging.
    C. Skull X-ray series.
    D. CAT scan.

47. Ms. Winfield says to the nurse, "I do hope that the tests will reveal something that can be improved." The nurse's reply, based on her understanding of the prognosis for multiple sclerosis, should be
    A. "I have not heard of any specific therapy."
    B. "There are many drugs now that can help to ease your symptoms."
    C. "You must try to prevent infections."
    D. "You must not allow yourself to become overfatigued."

48. In establishing a nursing care plan for Ms. Winfield, it is MOST important to
    A. improve her respiratory function.
    B. establish a routine pattern for urine elimination.
    C. increase her nutritional intake.
    D. establish an encouraging atmosphere.

49. While Ms. Winfield is in the hospital, all of the following are important nursing interventions for her EXCEPT
    A. improving functioning ability by muscle strengthening.
    B. establishing bladder control.
    C. preventing skin breakdown.
    D. encouraging the following of a special diet.

50. Ms. Winfield says to the nurse, "The doctor told me that so far there is no known cure for MS. That means that I am going to die from it." Which of the following responses would it be BEST for the nurse to make?
    A. "New drugs and treatments are being developed every day."
    B. "You must try to keep yourself self-sufficient by keeping your muscles strong and following all the orders of your physician."
    C. "You should avoid overwork and fatigue."
    D. "You must seek prompt treatment for infections."

> *Knowing that you are a practical nurse, a friend calls your house and asks you to come over. Her father, aged 65, is ill. When you arrive, you find Mr. Rosen unconscious and paralyzed on one side and you call for an ambulance. You think Mr. Rosen has had a stroke.*

51. Which of the following measures should be taken until the ambulance arrives?
1. Turn the patient's head to the affected side to keep the airway free of mucus.
2. Loosen tight clothing about the neck and waist.
3. Place the patient in Fowler's position to facilitate breathing.
4. Try to arouse the patient and give him sips of water.

A. 1, 2, 3, and 4
B. 1, 2, and 3.
C. 1 and 2 only.
D. 1, 2, and 4.

52. The medical term for stroke is
A. enuresis.
B. coronary occlusion.
C. subarachnoid hemorrhage.
D. cerebrovascular accident.

53. The most common effect of a stroke is
A. mental retardation.
B. paralysis of the lower extremities and deafness.
C. disturbance in speech and paralysis of one side of the body.
D. permanent paralysis of the upper extremities and blindness.

54. Careful attention must be paid to positioning Mr. Rosen, who has been hospitalized. The main objective in the nursing care of a stroke patient is to
A. prevent decubitus ulcers.
B. prevent complications that will make rehabilitation impossible.
C. provide adequate nutrition through tube feeding.
D. provide relief from pain and discomfort.

55. To prevent footdrop in Mr. Rosen, who has paralysis of a lower limb, it is most important to
A. provide adequate blankets.
B. use a footboard to keep the feet in a normal position.
C. massage the feet at least twice a day.
D. keep the feet clean and the toenails properly trimmed.

56. Use of a trochanter roll against the side of Mr. Rosen's paralyzed lower limb will prevent the limb from
A. developing ulcerations.
B. rotating outward from the hip.
C. rotating inward at the ankles.
D. developing footdrop.

57. Which of the following is a true statement in regard to the prognosis for stroke?
A. All stroke victims are permanently paralyzed.
B. Most stroke victims never speak understandably again.
C. Most stroke patients regain most of the use of their affected limbs if they receive proper care early.
D. Most stroke victims become physically and mentally handicapped by their illness.

> *Sarah Graham, aged 14 years, enters the hospital for surgical treatment of scoliosis. Her response to treatment by a brace has been unsatisfactory. For 1 week prior to the surgery, Sarah is placed in Cotrel traction and has to do prescribed muscle exercises for 10 minutes every hour.*

58. Sarah asks the nurse, "Why must I do these boring exercises?" The nurse's BEST answer is
A. "The doctor wants you to keep busy."
B. "You will be in a cast for awhile, so you must increase your muscle strength."
C. "The hospital policy is that you must do these exercises before back surgery. I don't know why."
D. "The exercises will help to control the pain after surgery."

59. After the surgery on her spine, Sarah is placed in a cast that covers her entire trunk. A cast that covers the trunk of the body is called
A. a spica.
B. a body cast.

C. a long-leg cast.

D. a walking cast.

60. A body cast is most often applied for the purpose of

A. preventing fractures.

B. immobilizing the spine.

C. protecting the skin.

D. preventing contamination of the operative site.

61. While the body cast is wet,

A. pillows should be placed to support the curves of the cast.

B. the patient should have a pillow under the buttocks.

C. the patient should have a pillow under the head and shoulders.

D. a heat cradle should be used to hasten drying of the cast.

62. The nurse must assess the casted patient for impaired circulation. Which of the following are signs of impaired circulation?

1. The skin has a bluish discoloration.

2. The skin looks inflamed.

3. The skin feels cold to the touch.

4. The skin looks swollen.

A. 1 and 4.

B. 1 and 3.

C. 2 and 3.

D. 2 and 4.

63. Sarah tells the practical nurse that she feels a tingling sensation under the cast. The nurse knows that

A. this feeling is a normal result of the casting.

B. this feeling will subside as soon as the cast is dry.

C. this feeling may be a sign of pressure and should be reported immediately to the supervising nurse.

D. this feeling will subside as soon as Sarah gets used to the cast.

64. When Sarah uses a bedpan, the nurse should

1. elevate the head of the bed slightly.

2. elevate the lumbosacral area with a small pillow.

3. protect the perineal area of the cast with waterproof material.

4. cleanse the perineum thoroughly after the bedpan use.

A. 1 and 3.

B. 1 and 2.

C. 1, 3, and 4.

D. 1, 2, 3, and 4.

65. The nurse turns Sarah four times a day, using the logrolling technique in order to

A. avoid twisting Sarah in the cast.

B. prevent strain on Sarah's back.

C. decrease the spaces between Sarah's vertebrae.

D. exercise Sarah's legs.

66. Sarah becomes very depressed when she realizes that she has to be in the cast for a few months. When she complains to the practical nurse about the extended time, the nurse's BEST reply is

A. "The cast is a better method than the brace."

B. "You wouldn't want to have the cast removed too soon."

C. "Think how nice you will look when your back is straight."

D. "The months will pass very quickly."

Five-year-old Eric Reilly is hospitalized with a diagnosis of nephrotic syndrome.

---

67. The most accurate description of this disease is

A. excessive loss of protein in the urine.

B. renal infection.

C. renal failure.

D. hematuria.

68. In planning the nursing care for Eric, the goal that should have priority is

A. maintaining complete bed rest.

B. promoting activity as tolerated.

C. preventing Eric from becoming bored.

D. providing Eric with playmates his own age.

69. Assessment of Eric should include

A. albuminuria, hypotension, pyuria.

B. albuminuria, hypertension, pyuria.

C. albuminuria, hypertension, edema.

D. albuminuria, hypotension, edema.

70. The nurse is ordered to obtain a 24-hour urine specimen from Eric. Which of the following methods is the proper one?

A. Have him void at 7 A.M. and collect all urine for the next 24 hours. Have him void again the following 7 A.M. and include this specimen. Send collected urine to the laboratory.

B. Have him void at 7 A.M. and collect this specimen. Discard all urine for the next 24 hours. Have him void at 7 A.M. the next day and collect his specimen. Send the two specimens to the laboratory.

C. Have him void at 7 A.M., discarding the specimen. Collect all urine for the next 24 hours. Have him void again at 7 A.M. the following day, adding this specimen to the container. Send collected urine to the laboratory.

D. Have him void at 7 A.M., discarding the specimen. Collect all urine for the next 24 hours. At 7 A.M. the next day have him void and discard this specimen. Send collected urine to the laboratory.

71. Eric has edema around his eyes. To help reduce the edema in Eric's eyelids it would be BEST for the nurse to
   A. apply cool compresses to Eric's face.
   B. elevate the head of Eric's bed.
   C. apply warm compresses to Eric's face.
   D. limit Eric's TV time.

72. In recording her assessment of Eric, which of the following signs will the nurse record if Eric begins to develop renal failure?
   A. Headache.
   B. Anorexia.
   C. Hypotension.
   D. Hyperactivity.

73. In planning the activities of daily living, it is MOST important for the nurse to give Eric
   A. a comb and brush.
   B. a mirror.
   C. a washcloth and towel.
   D. a toothbrush.

74. Of the following, the one that has been most effective in the treatment of children with nephrotic syndrome is
   A. vitamin D.
   B. erythromycin.
   C. prednisone.
   D. streptomycin.

75. In the treatment of Eric, all of the following nursing interventions are to be carried out EXCEPT
   A. relieving edema.
   B. observing for hematuria.
   C. protecting from infection.
   D. providing emotional support for the child and his family.

76. The nurse assigned to Eric is careful to observe for signs of complications resulting from the therapy. A possible complication is
   A. hematuria.
   B. loss of hair.
   C. loss of bladder control.
   D. dehydration.

Mr. Sebastian Canning, aged 65, comes to the clinic complaining of increasing inability to hear well. After examination a diagnosis of otosclerosis is made.

---

77. The nurse knows that otosclerosis produces loss of hearing because of
   A. accumulation of a waxy plug in the affected ear.
   B. disease in the auditory nerve.
   C. hardening of the small bones of the inner ear and loss of vibration.
   D. disease in the mastoid process.

78. The treatment of otosclerosis is
   A. to use a hearing aid.
   B. to remove the waxy plug from the ear.
   C. perform a fenestration operation.
   D. to accept the situation and make the best of it.

Matthew Raines, a 32-year-old licensed practical nurse, has accepted a position in a psychiatric unit of a large Veterans Administration hospital. Questions 70–85 relate to some of the relationships, situations, and responsibilities with which he must deal in the course of his work.

---

79. One of the MOST important requirements for the practical nurse who is assigned to a psychiatric unit is
   A. the ability to prevent accidents.

B. the ability to detect early signs of mental illness.

C. the recognition of mentally ill patients as persons who are sick and in need of help.

D. a knowledge of the classification of all mental illness.

80. If a patient refuses to talk with Matthew Raines and avoids him whenever possible, Matthew's BEST approach would be to
A. ignore the patient.
B. confront the patient and validate his thinking.
C. insist that the patient talk to him.
D. refuse to take care of the patient.

81. Mr. White is a very quiet patient who sits alone in a corner of the ward most of the day. To help Mr. White it would be best for Matthew Raines to
A. encourage Mr. White to associate with the patients near him.
B. take a few minutes each day to sit with Mr. White and listen to him when he wants to talk.
C. ignore Mr. White until he is ready to talk.
D. tell the other patients to stay away from Mr. White.

82. One day Matthew Raines becomes angry with a supervisor and takes his anger out on the nurse's aide with whom he works. On this occasion the practical nurse is exhibiting the defense mechanism called:
A. displacement.
B. identification.
C. rationalization.
D. compensation.

83. When approaching a patient who is showing great overactivity it is important for Matthew Raines to:
A. permit the patient to choose the activities in which he wishes to participate.
B. use a firm, friendly, consistent approach.
C. control the patient's hyperactivity.
D. encourage the patient to talk about his activities.

84. Which of the following would BEST help an overactive patient in Matthew Raines's unit?

A. A game of basketball or softball.
B. A game of checkers or cards.
C. A quiet room to himself.
D. Isolation.

85. For many nurses, including Matthew Raines, the most difficult part of the nurse-patient relationship is
A. being professional at all times.
B. being able to accept the patient's behavior at all times.
C. being able to understand the patient.
D. developing an awareness of self and the nurse's role in the relationship.

> Juan Hernandez, a 4-month-old infant, is admitted to the hospital pediatric unit, with a diagnosis of bronchiolitis. He is placed in a croup tent.

86. The practical nurse would expect Juan to display all of the following symptoms EXCEPT
A. dyspnea.
B. stridor.
C. rhonchi.
D. constipation.

87. The practical nurse knows that the purpose of placing Juan in the croup tent is to relieve his
A. dyspnea.
B. irritability.
C. anorexia.
D. tachypnea.

88. Juan's temperature is 101.8. The physician has written an order to administer Tylenol liquid 40 mg po q4h prn for temperature >101. The practical nurse will FIRST
A. administer Tylenol liquid 40 mg by mouth to Juan.
B. check Juan's medication record to see when he last received Tylenol.
C. check the original physician's order in Juan's chart.
D. call the physician to clarify the Tylenol order.

89. The nurse has available Tylenol liquid 10 mg/cc. She will administer how many cubic centimeters to Juan?
A. 4 cc.
B. 3 cc.

C. 2 cc.
D. ½ cc.

90. In managing the nursing care for Juan, the practical nurse would expect to carry out all of the following interventions EXCEPT to
A. elevate the head of the bed.
B. encourage po fluid intake.
C. assess repiratory status.
D. take axillary temperatures.

91. Mrs. Hernandez speaks and understands very little English. Which method of communication will the practical nurse use with Mrs. Hernandez?
1. maintaining eye contact.
2. speaking slowly.
3. speaking loudly.
4. using gestures.
A. 1 and 2.
B. 2, 3, and 4.
C. 3 and 4.
D. 1, 2, and 4.

92. Juan is improving and is becoming more interested in playing. Which of the following should the practical nurse provide for Juan?
A. A jigsaw puzzle.
B. A soft, plush rattle.
C. Wooden blocks.
D. A pull toy.

Ms. Donna Lewis, aged 28 and G2P2, delivered a full-term, 8-pound female infant less than 15 minutes ago. The baby girl has been admitted to the newborn nursery.

93. The practical nurse knows that on admission to the nursery Baby Girl Lewis's Apgar score was recorded as 9 at 1 minute and 10 at 5 minutes. These Apgar scores on Baby Girl Lewis
A. indicate a high incidence of neurologic defects in the infant.
B. are associated with a high infant-mortality rate.
C. indicate a good infant condition post-delivery.
D. have no significance to the practical nurse in the nursery.

94. Baby Girl Lewis's body temperature is an extremely important nursing consideration because

A. infants lose heat by convection and evaporation.
B. infants lose heat solely by evaporation.
C. infants lose heat solely by convection.
D. infants have no fat stores to assist in temperature regulation.

95. During the first 24 hours that Baby Girl Lewis spends in the nursery, the practical nurse will expect to see
A. a decrease in her serum glucose.
B. a rise in her red blood cells.
C. the passage of meconium.
D. a decrease in her body temperature.

96. Vitamin K 1 mg is given intramuscularly to Baby Girl Lewis. The practical nurse knows that she is administering this drug because it
A. allows for less infant irritability following delivery.
B. prevents hemorrhagic disease in the newborn.
C. prophylactically treats ophthalmia neonatorium.
D. increases the heart rate.

97. The practical nurse notes during the admission assessment into the newborn nursery that Baby Girl Lewis's heart rate is 132 and her respiratory rate is 32. Which of the following should the practical nurse do?
A. Report these findings to the charge nurse.
B. Report these findings to the pediatrician.
C. Start oxygen at 50%.
D. Take no action because these findings are normal.

Steven Brodsky, a 26-year-old carpenter, is diagnosed as having an acute appendicitis. An appendectomy is performed. After surgery, Mr. Brodsky is returned to the medical unit with a nasogastric tube connected to low Gomco, an intravenous infusion running, and a drain inserted into the incision site because the appendix has ruptured.

98. The practical nurse admitting Mr. Brodsky to the medical unit would immediately assess
   A. the dressing site.
   B. the patient's blood pressure.
   C. the patient's respirations.
   D. the patency of the nasogastric tube.

99. The nasogastric tube was inserted to
   1. relieve nausea and vomiting.
   2. remove fluids and gas.
   3. measure the stomach contents.
   4. promote peristalsis.
   A. 1 and 2.
   B. 1, 2, and 3.
   C. 3 and 4.
   D. 2, 3, and 4.

100. As the practical nurse is assessing Mr. Brodsky's intravenous equipment, she notices that the patient is receiving 8 drops per minute rather than the required 24 drops per minute. Before reporting this to the charge nurse, the practical nurse should
   A. insert 3 cc of saline into the I.V. site to clear the tubing.
   B. pinch the I.V. tubing to clear it.
   C. open the clamp on the I.V. tubing to clear the tubing.
   D. check the site of the I.V. infusion.

101. The physician has ordered Keflin, 500 mg, an antibiotic, to be added to Mr. Brodsky's intravenous fluids. The practical nurse will monitor the patient for which of the following untoward effects of this drug?
   A. Urinary retention.
   B. Urticaria.
   C. Hypertension.
   D. Constipation.

102. Mr. Brodsky's nasogastric tube is removed. Peristalsis has returned, and Steve is started on a clear-fluid diet. Which of the following diets would the practical nurse expect her patient to have for breakfast?
   A. Soft-boiled egg, orange juice, and tea.
   B. Farina, cranberry juice, and tea.
   C. Beef broth, Jello-O, and tea.
   D. Oatmeal, milk, and tea.

Mrs. Linda O'Neill brings her 2-month-old daughter, Ellen, into the pediatrician's office for her monthly visit. During this visit, Ellen is to begin receiving her first series of TOPV (trivalent oral polio vaccine) immunizations.

103. Mrs. O'Neill confides to the practical nurse that she is concerned Ellen will become ill after receiving the vaccine. Which of the following is the BEST response that the practical nurse can make?
   A. "Mrs. O'Neill, have more faith in us. We wouldn't give Ellen anything that would make her ill."
   B. "Have you discussed this concern with the pediatrician?"
   C. "Ellen may run a slight fever after receiving the vaccine. If she does, we can treat this with children's Tylenol."
   D. "You're right. Ellen may get polio."

104. Before administering the vaccine, the practical nurse will assess for which of the following?
   A. Whether the infant has an acute febrile illness.
   B. Whether the infant is breast fed.
   C. Whether the infant is gaining weight.
   D. Whether the infant is developmentally delayed.

105. Mrs. O'Neill asks the practical nurse when Ellen will be given measles vaccine. The practical nurse's reply is that Ellen will receive the measles vaccine at
   A. 4–6 months of age.
   B. 6–8 months of age.
   C. 8–10 months of age.
   D. 12–15 months of age.

Jen Svenson, a 19-year-old college sophomore, has been admitted to the hospital with a diagnosis of R/O (rule-out) paranoid schizophrenia. Although Jen achieved academic honors in high school, she had to leave college because of failure in all subjects. Jen speaks to the admitting nurse in a pressured, flat, toneless voice. She is unable to answer questions directly and has flight of ideas. She hears voices and thinks the FBI is after her.

106. The initial nursing care plan should include
- A. development of a discharge plan.
- B. assistance with stabilization of the patient.
- C. regulation of drug therapy.
- D. testing of intellectual capacity.

107. During the nursing assessment, Jen's speech is described as showing flight of ideas. Which of the following defines "flight of ideas"?
- A. Patient talks rapidly, is distracted by stimuli, and has rapid ideation. Ideas can be following by the listener.
- B. Patient talks rapidly, is distracted by stimuli, and has rapid ideation. Ideas cannot be followed by the listener.
- C. Patient fills in gaps in memory with fabrications of his/her own invention.
- D. Patient meaninglessly repeats another person's words or phrases.

108. Jen's diagnosis is confirmed. She is placed on a major tranquilizer, Thorazine (chlorpromazine HCP). The nurse observes Jen for all of the following side effects EXCEPT
- A. orthostatic hypotension.
- B. akathisia.
- C. urinary retention.
- D. diarrhea.

109. Jen approaches the practical nurse caring for her and says, "I have something important to tell you, but I want you to promise not to tell anyone." The nurse's BEST response would be
- A. "Okay, I promise not to tell anyone."
- B. "Nothing is so important that it can't be shared with the whole treatment team."
- C. "If it's important, maybe you should tell your doctor."
- D. "I understand that anything you tell me is confidential. However, all information is shared with the treatment team, who are here to help you, although not with anyone else."

110. In assisting Jen to deal with auditory hallucinations, the nursing care plan will include which of the following goals for the patient?
- A. To deal more effectively with reality versus unreality.

- B. To develop interpersonal skills.
- C. To improve verbal communication.
- D. To promote complex skills and activities.

Patricia Hollis, a 17-year-old black female, is admitted to the pediatric unit in sickle-cell crisis.

---

111. Pat's hemoglobin is returned from the lab at 5 grams/100 ml. On the basis of her knowledge of sickle-cell crisis, the practical nurse would expect the physician to issue an order to
- A. administer iron injections.
- B. administer platelets.
- C. administer whole blood.
- D. administer packed red blood cells.

112. Pat is complaining of pain in her joints and abdomen. The practical nurse understands that this pain is caused by
- A. intracellular bleeding.
- B. arthritis secondary to the sickle-cell process.
- C. extracellular bleeding.
- D. clumping of red blood cells.

113. Pat's mood is depressed, and she is noncommunicative to the nursing staff. Which nursing approach will be most beneficial?
- A. Assure Pat that she is improving.
- B. Provide a peer who also has sickle-cell anemia to talk to Pat.
- C. Spend additional time with Pat for the sole purpose of allowing her an opportunity to talk.
- D. Take no special action. Depression is a common symptom of sickle-cell anemia.

114. Pat says to her nurse, "I hope I will outgrow these crises." The BEST nursing response will be
- A. "Sickle-cell anemia is considered cured once the patient reaches young adulthood."
- B. "Sickle-cell anemia is a chronic illness with periods of remission and exacerbation."
- C. "Sickle-cell anemia can be controlled if the patient takes iron daily."
- D. "Sickle-cell anemia can be controlled with periodic blood transfusions."

115. As Pat gets ready to go home, she says to the practical nurse, "I guess I won't be able to go away to college next year because I have this disease." The BEST response for the nurse to make is
  A. "You're right. It would be better for you to stay home."
  B. "Have you discussed this with your doctor?"
  C. "Sickle-cell anemia will not prevent you from going away to school. However, you should explore the medical facilities available near the college you choose."
  D. "You should be able to go away to school if your disease is in remission."

The rest of the test consists of unrelated questions

116. The human personality grows and develops as a result of
  A. environmental influence.
  B. cultural influence.
  C. hereditary influence.
  D. all of the above.

117. Temper tantrums are usually a result of
  A. lack of love.
  B. frustration.
  C. jealousy.
  D. lack of willpower.

118. Which of the following terms means "painful menstruation"?
  A. Amenorrhea.
  B. Dysmenorrhea.
  C. Metrorrhagia.
  D. Hypermenorrhea.

119. Relief from minor menstrual discomforts can best be obtained by
  A. eliminating the daily bath and taking a daily laxative.
  B. taking a cold shower and applying an ice bag to the abdomen.
  C. avoiding exercise and remaining in bed as much as possible.
  D. taking moderate exercise, avoiding tight clothing, and eating a well-balanced nonconstipating diet.

120. Rationalization, one of the most common defense mechanisms, is dangerous when used to extreme primarily because

  A. the person who rationalizes is copying the behavior of another.
  B. it leads to immature and childish behavior.
  C. it leads to suppression of feelings that should be brought to the surface.
  D. it is a form of lying in which the individual justifies his/her behavior with falsehoods and does not face conflicts honestly.

121. A 20-year-old woman at a fertility clinic is confused about the administration of the estrogen-progesterone pills that she takes for birth control 20 days of each month. She asks the nurse, "Suppose I miss a couple of days. Should I take two or three pills the next day?" The nurse's answer should be
  A. "Yes, that way you will get back on schedule."
  B. "No, it doesn't matter. Just be sure to take one tomorrow."
  C. "No, You should abstain from intercourse, wait until your next period, and then start all over again."
  D. "No, just start the 20-day sequence again, immediately."

122. When a patient is admitted to the hospital, she tells the practical nurse that the rash on her face and hands is due to an allergy to certain medications. The nurse should
  A. record this, together with her observations of the rash, in the patient's chart.
  B. tell the patient not to worry, that everything will be taken care of.
  C. tell the patient that most people have allergies.
  D. report this immediately to the supervisor.

123. In collecting a specimen for sputum examination, the nurse must be sure that the specimen contains
  A. nasal secretions.
  B. material coughed up from the bronchi and lungs.
  C. saliva.
  D. material from the stomach.

124. When the nurse is preparing to catheterize a patient, she discovers that the wrapper around the tray is wet. She considers the equipment to be

A. unsterile and unsafe to use.
B. unsterile but usable.
C. sterile.
D. safe to use once the wrapper is removed.

125. When the nurse tries to take a rectal temperature in the newborn, she finds that she is unable to insert the thermometer. She reports this to the supervising nurse immediately. What may be wrong?

A. Pyloric stenosis.
B. Imperforate anus.
C. Intussception.
D. Patent foramen ovale.

ANSWER KEY—PART II

1.	B	26.	B	51.	B	76.	B	101.	B
2.	C	27.	D	52.	D	77.	C	102.	C
3.	B	28.	B	53.	C	78.	C	103.	C
4.	C	29.	C	54.	B	79.	C	104.	A
5.	B	30.	A	55.	B	80.	B	105.	D
6.	C	31.	D	56.	B	81.	B	106.	B
7.	A	32.	C	57.	C	82.	A	107.	A
8.	C	33.	C	58.	B	83.	B	108.	D
9.	A	34.	B	59.	B	84.	A	109.	D
10.	B	35.	C	60.	B	85.	D	110.	A
11.	B	36.	B	61.	A	86.	D	111.	D
12.	B	37.	A	62.	B	87.	A	112.	D
13.	B	38.	C	63.	C	88.	C	113.	C
14.	D	39.	A	64.	D	89.	A	114.	B
15.	C	40.	D	65.	A	90.	D	115.	C
16.	C	41.	B	66.	D	91.	D	116.	D
17.	D	42.	A	67.	A	92.	B	117.	B
18.	A	43.	C	68.	B	93.	C	118.	B
19.	C	44.	D	69.	D	94.	A	119.	D
20.	B	45.	B	70.	C	95.	C	120.	D
21.	C	46.	B	71.	B	96.	B	121.	C
22.	C	47.	D	72.	C	97.	D	122.	A
23.	C	48.	B	73.	B	98.	C	123.	B
24.	C	49.	D	74.	C	99.	B	124.	A
25.	C	50.	B	75.	B	100.	D	125.	B

EXPLANATIONS FOR ANSWERS—PART II

1. **B** If the ulcer were hemorrhaging, the vomitus would have shown bright red blood. The other choices are irrelevant.
2. **C** For an accurate analysis, it is necessary to obtain a specimen that is free of tobacco, food and all fluid, including water.
3. **B** Barium sulfate is given by mouth before X-ray of the upper G.I. tract. The compound is radiopaque and is not digested, so that it provides an outline of the G.I. tract on the X-ray film.
4. **C** Baked custard is very bland, easy to digest, and soothing to the gastric mucosa. The other choices are contraindicated for a patient with bleeding gastric ulcer.
5. **B** Pepper is irritating to the gastrointestinal mucosa.
6. **C** The abdomen reacts to the severe pain of the perforation by becoming rigid. The patient lies as still as possible and even declines to breathe deeply, so as not to move the tender abdomen.
7. **A** Carbonated drinks contain carbon dioxide, which causes gastric distension and discomfort. Alcohol is irritating to the gastric mucosa as is tea, which contains tannic acid and caffeine.
8. **C** This is the best procedure for helping Mr. Ferrari keep some independence. He is incapable of assuming entire responsibility for his care.
9. **A** Orthostatic hypotension is an excessive fall in blood pressure on assuming the upright position. It is not a specific disease but rather a manifestation of abnormal blood pressure regulation due to a variety of causes.
10. **B** At night things appear different. It is best to keep a dim night light on. Also, Mr. Ferrari can be guided.
11. **B** Crowning is the phase in the second stage of labor when a large segment of the fetal scalp is visible at the vaginal orifice, with the perineum distended and the anus opened.

12. **B** LOA is considered to be the most favorable position for delivery.

13. **B** The lengthening of the cord outside the vagina indicates that the placenta has separated.

14. **D** Each case of asthma differs as to the cause. Some cases are brought on by fatigue or stress. Others can be caused by infection, allergies, irritants, etc.

15. **C** Bronchial asthma is a reversible condition that manifests itself by alternating episodes of wheezing and dyspnea. Wheezing is due to constriction of the bronchioles.

16. **C** Fowler's position with the upper part of the body elevated is the most comfortable for dyspneic patients and makes breathing easier. The head of the bed is raised 18–20 inches above the level. The knees are also raised. The air conditioner is turned on to control the environment and thereby reduce the quantity of allergens and regulate temperature and humidity. Oxygen is not started to increase the oxygenation of lungs because of blockage from the increased mucus.

17. **D** Sympathizing with the parents at this time is important. Allowing them to grieve is initially what is essential. After the shock is absorbed, patient/parent teaching would be appropriate.

18. **A** Feeding the child in the upright (orthopneic) position will prevent aspiration. Frequent burpings are necessary to bring up the swallowed air.

19. **C** Tying the infant's hands down so that he/she cannot move them will increase frustration, causing the infant to cry.

20. **B** Chronic brain syndrome results in impaired capacity for abstract thinking. Suspicion and reticence are symptoms of this impairment.

21. **C** Routine is the best thing for these patients. Rotating staff assignments and providing a variety of new experiences will only increase their confusion.

22. **C** The nurse must realize that both the mother and the daughter have feelings about the situation, and choice C reflects this. Even though the mother is suffering from a dementia, there are periods of lucidity in which she can assess her situation.

23. **C** Again the daily routine is important. The mother may not remember her reaction of the previous day but may be upset if the daughter does not visit.

24. **C** Mrs. Winter remembers things that happened 50 years ago, but recent events are a blank to her. Short-term memory loss is characteristic of chronic brain syndrome.

25. **C** Stringing popcorn is a task at which Mrs. Winter can succeed. This will help her self-esteem. Validation of past events is important to the older patient.

26. **B** Tricuspid atresia is a congenital heart abnormality. It is characterized by a small right ventricle, large left ventricle, and diminished circulation.

27. **D** Frozen mixed vegetables are processed with a sodium compound.

28. **B** Because of insufficient oxygen, the bones develop abnormally.

29. **C** Children who suffer from oxygen deficiency often assume a squatting position when tired. It is not known why.

30. **A** This can be a learning situation for the mother, who can be instructed as to the kinds of food the child should have.

31. **D** To gain and keep the child's confidence, it is best to be truthful at all times.

32. **C** This is the best answer because puzzles and games are things that the child can visualize. The other answers are abstractions that will mean little to a 6-year-old. In addition, choice D is faintly ominous.

33. **C** If Paul Rosenthal has to open his mouth in an emergency, it is necessary to be able to release the fixating wires.

34. **B** Mr. Rosenthal will be able to suck through a straw. Solid food is not indicated because he is unable to chew with the fixation. Choice A is facetious and unhelpful; choice D, rather flip.

35. **C** In an emergency the wires must be cut so that Mr. Rosenthal can open his mouth. He must not be allowed to aspirate any food or fluid.

36. **B** Radiation treatment causes skin reactions that can be severe.

37. **A** Many times these patients develop an anemia with a corresponding decrease in the white cell count.

38. **C** Highly seasoned, spicy foods will further decrease the patient's appetite. The patient must be adequately nourished, and choices A, B, and D will help to achieve this goal.

39. **A** Radiation pneumonitis is a severe inflammation of the lung tissue, causing respiratory distress. This condition can cause respiratory arrest, and thus be fatal, if not treated.

40. **D** Oxygen can be drying to the mucosa. This in turn can lead to infection.

41. **B** Mr. Smith needs skilled nursing care and active rehabilitation and therapy.

42. **A** After successful treatment in the skilled facility, Mr. Smith can now be placed in a facility in which he can perform some of his own care and thus will need less nursing care.

43. **C** The nurse must be sure that Mr. Sanchez can breathe before any treatments can be undertaken.

44. **D** Second-degree burns are characterized by vesiculation (blisters). In third-degree burns, the skin is destroyed.

45. **B** Mr. Freeman will be given I.V. fluids at this stage and will be unable to eat. Choices 1, 2, and 4 are important interventions. Fluid/electrolyte replacement immediately is important because of the fluid loss caused by the burn. Urinary output is measured to assess fluid replacement and kidney function. Relief of pain is essential to patient comfort.

46. **B** Although all of the listed diagnostic tests will be helpful, magnetic resonance imaging will be most valuable because it is the most sensitive imaging technique and may show demyelination in the brain and spinal cord.

47. **D** The prognosis for multiple sclerosis is unfavorable. In order to maintain the patient's present level, she must not become overfatigued. Choice D is the best answer that the nurse can give. Choices A, B, and C serve no purpose.

48. **B** Ms. Winfield is distressed by her urinary incontinence. The nurse must work with her to try to establish bladder control.

49. **D** There is no need for a special diet.

50. **B** At present there is no specific treatment for multiple sclerosis. Therefore the patient must try to maintain her present condition and to prevent further deterioration for as long as possible. Choice B is the most positive, while truthful, response the nurse can make.

51. **B** Turning the patient's head to the affected side and loosening tight clothing around his neck wil help to keep his airway open. Fowler's position will make breathing easier.

52. **D** The term means "pertaining to the blood vessels of the brain."

53. **C** Stroke is a focal neurologic disorder that disturbs the nerve pathways involved in speech and in motion of the paralyzed side.

54. **B** Prevention of contractures is most important.

55. **B** Unless the foot is adequately supported by a footboard until the muscles regain their strength, footdrop will occur.

56. **B** The affected leg of a patient who suffers hemiplegia generally falls into external rotation unless preventive measures are taken.

57. **C** The sooner proper care is given and improvement begins, the better is the prognosis. The eventual extent of recovery depends also on the patient's state of health and age.

58. **B** It is necessary for the patient to increase her muscle strength because she will lose some strength while in the cast.

59. **B** A cast that covers the trunk of the body is a body cast. A spica includes one limb. A long-leg cast includes the leg from the foot to the groin. A walking cast is constructed with the concept that some weight bearing helps the formation of new bone.

60. **B** The spine is immobilized to promote healing.

61. **A** All curves should be supported in order to maintain the stability of the cast.

62. **B** If the skin looks bluish and feels cold, circulation is impaired.

63. **C** The practical nurse must be very aware of possibly abnormal signs, such as the tingling sensation Sarah is experiencing, and report them immediately to the supervising nurse.

64. **D** All these procedures constitute good nursing practice.

65. **A** All measures must be taken to prevent the twisting of Sarah's body. To prevent skin breakdown, she should be logrolled about four times daily.

66. **D** The nurse must always maintain a positive attitude. Choice C implies that Sarah's appearance was bad before the surgery.

67. **A** Nephrotic syndrome is not a disease in itself. The condition, marked by large amounts of

protein in the urine, results from a specific glomerular defect and indicates renal damage.

68. **B** There is no need for complete bedrest. It's important not to fatigue the child, but activity should be encouraged as tolerated.

69. **D** Blood pressure should be monitored in both the supine and standing situations. A drop in blood pressure that exceeds 20 mg Hg should be reported to the supervising nurse immediately. Edema and albuminuria are signs of the syndrome.

70. **C** This method will give a true 24-hour urinary specimen. By discarding the first 7 A.M. specimen, the nurse is discarding urine from the previous 24 hours. The next 7 A.M. specimen should be included.

71. **B** When the head of the bed is elevated, gravity will help to decrease the edema in the eyelids.

72. **C** Hypotension is one of the indicators of beginning renal failure.

73. **B** It is necessary for Eric to notice daily changes in his facial appearance. The degree of edema will change the way he looks.

74. **C** Corticosteroid therapy has been found to be helpful in the treatment of nephrotic syndrome.

75. **B** Hematuria is not a sign of nephrotic syndrome.

76. **B** Loss of hair can result from the steroid therapy. The other choices are not complications of the therapy.

77. **C** Hardening of the small bones is accompanied by the formation of spongy bone at the footplate of the stapes. This causes a conduction-type deafness.

78. **C** The operation consists of making a little window through the hardened bone so that sound can be transmitted.

79. **C** The psychiatric nurse must remember to include the patient, and not just the disease, in the plan of treatment.

80. **B** The best nursing approach would be to confront the patient and validate the assessment of the situation. On the basis of this experience, Nurse Raines would develop a plan of action to establish a better care plan for the patient.

81. **B** It is necessary for the nurse to secure the confidence of Mr. White. In sitting with the patient, the nurse expresses his belief in the patient's worth and in this way helps to control the patient's environment.

82. **A** By using this defense mechanism, the individual's equilibrium may be preserved for a long time. Frustrations are relieved. Hopefully, once the anger has subsided, the person will gain insight into his/her behavior and address the issue in a more appropriate manner.

83. **B** Activity has to do with motivation. Overactivity is best channeled into a firm, scheduled routine. If the channeling is not firm, the patient's activities will merely be divided and nothing will be accomplished.

84. **A** These physical games will help to channel constructively some of the patient's activity.

85. **D** It is difficult at times for the nurse to divorce him-/herself from the situation. It is necessary to be aware of the nurse's professional role in the relationship. It is not possible to understand all patients, and some patient behavior cannot and should not be accepted. Choice A is narrower than choice D and therefore not as good.

86. **D** Bronchiolitis is an inflammation of the bronchioles. Therefore the symptoms of this disease are focused on the respiratory system, not the gastrointestinal system, and constipation is not a symptom to be expected.

87. **A** Bronchiolitis causes the formation of copious amounts of mucus, resulting in obstruction of the bronchioles. In turn, this blockage causes dyspnea, or difficulty in breathing.

88. **C** The practical nurse should check the physician's original order first. This assures safe, competent practice validating that the physicians's written order is the same as the order on the medication sheet. Then the practical nurse would note on the patient's medication sheet when Tylenol 40 mg was last given to decide whether it can safely be given again at this time. Lastly, the medication would be administered. There is no need to call Juan's physician at this time, as the order is explicit.

89. **A** The formula the practical nurse would use to determine the amount of medication to be given is

$$\frac{\text{desired amount}}{\text{available amount}} = \text{amount to be administered}$$

$$\frac{40 \text{ mg}}{10 \text{ mg/cc}} = 4 \text{ cc}$$

90. **D** The nursing care plan focuses on maintaining the respiratory integrity of this patient: elevating the head of the bed, encouraging fluid intake by mouth, and assessing respiratory status. Rectal temperatures are the most accurate indicators of body temperature; and since there is no contraindication for rectal temperatures in this case, axillary temperatures are not indicated.

91. **D** Direct eye contact, slow speech, and the use of nonverbal communication, such as gestures, are good ways of communicating with Mrs. Hernandez. Speaking loudly will serve no useful purpose and may excite, frighten, or anger the listener.

92. **B** A soft, plush rattle is appropriate for this age group. A 4-month-old is able to grasp and reach for objects. However, motor coordination is still unrefined. Sharp, hard toys such as blocks would be unsafe. Juan is not ready for jigsaw puzzles or pull toys.

93. **C** The Apgar score is the beginning infant assessment of the newborn. It is a numerical expression of the newborn's condition, being the sum of points given for heart rate, crying power, muscle tone, plantar reflex, and skin color. The assessments are made 1 minute and 5 minutes after birth and, for the nursery nurse, prove to be important indicators of the newborn's condition and status.

94. **A** All infants can potentially have reduced body temperature because of heat loss by convection and evaporation. Therefore, it is important to keep the newborn's skin dry and regulate the environment to maintain warmth.

95. **C** Meconium is the dark green-to-black stool that is normally passed in the first 24 hours of life. The practical nurse observes for passage of meconium to rule out abnormalities of the gastrointestinal tract. Serum hypoglycemia (decrease in serum glucose), serum polycythemia (a rise in red blood cells), and a low body temperature are expected when dealing with a preterm, low-body-weight infant, rather than a full-term, average-weight newborn.

96. **B** Vitamin K prevents hemorrhagic tendencies, since the liver's ability to produce clotting factors is dependent on this vitamin.

97. **D** The normal apical pulse in the newborn is 120–140 per minute, and the respirations are 30–40 per minute. Therefore Baby Girl Lewis's pulse and respirations fall within normal limits, and no action is needed.

98. **C** Respiratory integrity is the first concern. Therefore the immediate nursing response when a patient is returned postoperatively is to assess respirations, and thereby determine whether the patient has a patent airway.

99. **B** A nasogastric tube is used after bowel surgery to deflate the bowel and promote intestinal healing. By relieving stomach contents, the nasogastric tube helps to eliminate nausea and vomiting and decreases the buildup of fluids and gas. By relieving bowel distension, the nasogastric tube actually prevents the return of peristaltic activity.

100. **D** Before taking further action, the practical nurse should assess the I.V. site to determine whether infiltration has occurred. If the I.V. has infiltrated, the practical nurse will expect to see a swollen and painful I.V. site.

101. **B** A hivelike rash, or urticaria, is the most common side effect to antibiotic therapy. Other untoward effects may include hypotension, diarrhea, vomiting, and respiratory distress leading to anaphylaxis.

102. **C** A clear-liquid diet consists of only clear fluids that do not contain a milk base. Eggs, farina, and oatmeal would be added for a soft diet.

103. **C** Live trivalent oral polio vaccine is preferred to the inactivated form because administration is

easier and the immunologic effects are broader and longer. This TOPV vaccine may cause a slight elevation of temperature and irritability in the infant, effects that are easily controlled with an antipyretic, such as Tylenol.

104. **A** Immunizations should be delayed if the child has an acute febrile infection or illness. The common cold, without fever, does not contraindicate immunizations.

105. **D** The measles vaccine is most effective when given at about 12–15 months. At this age, all maternal transplacental antibiotics have been catabolized.

106. **B** Inpatient psychiatric hospitalizations are short term in nature. The nursing care focuses on assisting with stabilization of the patient's problems so that the patient is not a danger to him-/herself or others. In-depth psychotherapy is done on an outpatient basis.

107. **A** *Flight of ideas:* Patient talks rapidly, is distracted by stimuli, and has rapid ideation. Ideas can be followed by the listener. *Associative looseness:* Patient talks rapidly, is distracted by stimuli, and has rapid ideation. Ideas cannot be followed by the listener. *Confabulation:* Patient fills in gaps in memory with fabrications of his/her own invention. *Echolalia:* Patient meaninglessly repeats another person's words or phrases.

108. **D** Diarrhea is not a side effect of Thorazine. Urinary retention is an untoward effect of this drug. Akathisia (inability to sit still) and orthostatic hypotension (a drop in blood pressure when standing) may also be caused by Thorazine.

109. **D** The practical nurse wants to communicate the fact that she recognizes Jen's need for confidentiality. However, the nurse also must let the patient know that all information is shared with the treatment team; that is, all caregivers who render direct patient care and contribute toward generating a focused care plan for that patient.

110. **A** When a patient is hallucinating, the nursing goal is to reassure him/her that the hallucinations are not part of reality.

111. **D** A normal female hemoglobin value is 14 ± 2 grams/100 ml. The nurse would expect the physician to order packed red blood cells to increase the hemoglobin level. Hemoglobin is the oxygen-carrying matter in red blood cells.

112. **D** The joint and abdominal pain results from clumping of red blood cells. This causes blockage of the affected capillaries and thereby a decrease in oxygen to the surrounding cells.

113. **C** Dealing with a chronic illness is difficult for an adolescent. Spending extra time with the patient will allow her an opportunity to discuss her concerns and feelings.

114. **B** The best nursing response is direct and truthful. Sickle-cell anemia is a chronic disease marked by periods of remission and exacerbation.

115. **C** Sickle-cell anemia needn't prevent travel or other new experiences. However, it would be prudent for a patient to ascertain whether medical facilities will be available to him/her.

116. **D** The human personality develops from infancy to old age. Choices A, B, and C all have effects on its development.

117. **B** Temper tantrums usually indicate that the individual, regardless of age, has not learned to cope with frustration.

118. **B** Amenorrhea is the absence of menstruation. Metrorrhagia is uterine bleeding, usually of normal amount, occurring at completely irregular intervals. Hypermenorrhea (menorrhagia) is abnormally heavy or prolonged menstrual bleeding.

119. **D** This is an excellent regimen to relieve minor menstrual discomfort.

120. **D** Without facing his/her conflicts, the patient will never be able to resolve them.

121. **C** The estrogen-progesterone pills must be taken with regularity. This combination is given continuously for 3 weeks. Nothing is given the 4th week. The starting point is the menstrual bleeding.

122. **A** It is necessary to record both the nurse's observation and the patient's statement.

123. **B** It is the lung and bronchus secretions that make up the sputum specimen.

124. **A** The tray should be discarded and another obtained.

125. **B** Imperforate anus is a complication that must be taken care of immediately in the newborn. There are different degrees of imperforate anus.

APPENDIX: IMMUNIZATION SCHEDULES AND REQUIREMENTS

Table 1. Recommendations for Hepatitis B Immunization

A. Persons for Whom Hepatitis B Vaccine Is Recomended or Should Be Considered

---

Pre-exposure

Persons for whom vaccine is recommended:
- health-care workers likely to have blood or needle-stick exposures
- clients and staff of institutions for the developmentally disabled
- hemodialysis patients
- homosexually active men
- users of illicit injectable drugs
- recipients of certain blood products
- household members and sexual contacts of HBV* carriers
- special high-risk populations

Persons for whom vaccine should be considered:
- inmates of long-term correctional facilities
- heterosexually active persons with multiple sexual partners
- international travelers to HBV endemic areas

Postexposure

Persons for whom immunization is recommended:
- infants born to HBV-positive mothers
- health-care workers having needle-stick exposures to human blood

*Hepatitis B virus.

B. Hepatitis B Virus Postexposure Recommendations

Exposure	HBIG*		and	Hepatitis B Vaccine†	
	Dose	Recommended timing		Dose	Recommended timing
Perinatal	0.5 ml IM	Within 12 hours	and	0.5 ml (5μg) IM at birth	Within 7 days of birth‡; repeat at 1 and 6 months
Sexual§	0.06 ml/kg IM	Single dose within 14 days of sexual contact	and	1.0 ml (10μg) IM	Within 14 days of exposure; repeat at 1 and 6 months

*Hepatitis B immune globulin.
†Recombinant vaccines.
‡It is preferable to give the first dose with HBIG within 12 hours of birth, administered at different sites.
§Vaccine is recommended for homosexual men and for regular sexual contacts of HBV carriers and is optional in initial treatment of heterosexual contacts of persons with acute HBV.

C. Recommendations for Hepatitis B Prophylaxis Following Percutaneous Exposure

Source	Exposed Person	
	Unvaccinated	Vaccinated
HBsAg-positive	1. HBIG x 1 immediately* 2. Initiate HB vaccine† series.	1. Test exposed person for anti-HBs. 2. If inadequate antibody,‡ HBIG (x1) immediately plus HB vaccine booster dose.

Known source
  High-risk
    HBsAg-positive
	1. Initiate HB vaccine series
	2. Test source for HBsAg. If positive, HBIG x 1.
		1. Test source for HBsAg only if exposed is vaccine non-responder; if source is HBsAg-positive, give HBIG x 1 immediately plus HB vaccine booster dose.

Low-risk HBsAg-positive	Initiate HB vaccine series.	Nothing required.
Unknown source	Initiate HB vaccine series.	Nothing required.

*HBIG dose 0.06 ml/kg IM.
†HB vaccine dose 20 μg IM for adults; 10 μg IM for infants or children under 10 years of age.
First dose within 1 week; second and third doses, 1 and 6 months later.
‡Less than 10 SRU by RIA, negative by BIA

Table 2. Recommended Schedules for Active Immunization, Beginning in Infancy, of Normal Infants and Children

Recommended Age	Vaccine(s)	Comments
2 months	DTP-1, OPV*-1	Can be given earlier in areas of high endemnicity.
4 months	DTP-2, OPV-2	6–week to 2–month interval desired between OPV doses to avoid interference.
6 months	DTP-3	An additional dose of OPV at this time is optional in areas with a high risk of polio exposure.
15 months††	DTP-4, MMR-1, OPV-3	Completion of primary series of DTP and OPV.
18 months	HbCV†	Conjugate preferred over polysaccharide vaccine.
4-6 years	DTP-5, OPV-4 MMR-2	Preferably at or before school entry.
14-16 years	Td	Repeat every 10 years throughout life.

*OPV: oral polio vaccine.
†HbCV: Haemophilius influenzae vaccine, type b.

Table 3. Immunization Schedule for Children Not Immunized as Infants,* as Recommended by the New York State Department of Health

Timing	Vaccine(s)	Comments
First visit	DTP-1, OPV-1 (If child is ≥ 15 months of age, MMR; if child is 18 months to 5 years of age, HbCV)	DTP, OPV and MMR can be administered simultaneously to children ≥ 15 months of age. HbCV can be administered simultaneously with DTP, OPV, and MMR to children 18 months to 5 years of age.
2 months after first DTP, OPV	DTP-2, OPV-2	
3 months after first MMR	MMR-2 (if child is ≥ 4 years of age)	MMR can be administered as soon as 30 days after the first dose.
2 months after second DTP	DTP-3	An additional dose of OPV at this time is optional in areas with a high risk of polio exposure.
6–12 months after third DTP	DTP-4, OPV-3	
Preschool (4–6 years) (not necessary if the fourth DPT and the third OPV are administered after the fourth birthday)	DTP-5, OPV-4	Preferably at or before school entry.
14–16 years	Td	Repeat every 10 years throughout life.

*If initiated in the first year of life, give DTP-1, 2 and 3, OPV-1, 2 and 3 according to this schedule, MMR when the child becomes 15 months old and HbCV at 18 months of age.

Contraindications

1. Current illness with something more serious than a cold.

2. Immunosuppressive therapy (radiation, corticosteroids, antimetabolites, alkylating agents, and cytotoxic agents).

3. Recent (within 3 months) immune globulin (IG), plasma, or blood transfusion.

4. Immunodeficiency disorders; see routine immunization of HIV-infected children (Table 4).

5. Leukemia, lymphoma, or generalized malignancy.

6. Prior allergic reaction to the same vaccine.

Precautions

1. Specific severe allergic conditions must be considered for each antigen; consult manufacturer's package insert.

2. Infants and young children who may have underlying neurologic disorders should be further evaluated before administering pertussis-containing preparations.

Table 4. Recommendations for Routine Immunization of HIV-Infected Children

	Type of HIV Infection	
Vaccine	Asymptomatic	Symptomatic
DTP	Yes	Yes
OPV	No	No
IPV	Yes	Yes
MMR	Yes	Yes
HbCV	Yes	Yes
Pneumococcal	Yes	Yes

Table 5. New York State Immunization Requirements for School Attendance

A. School and Preschool Program Requirements

Beginning January 1, 1990, all children attending a school, a day care center, or other preschool program must be immunized against the following diseases:

diphtheria   measles   rubella
polio   mumps   Haemophilus influenzae b

The minimum requirements are as follows:
1. 3 doses of diphtheria toxoid
2. 3 doses of oral polio vaccine
3. 1 dose of live measles vaccine administered after 12 months of age
4. 1 dose of live mumps vaccine administered after 12 months of age
5. 1 dose of live rubella vaccine administered after 12 months of age
6. 1 dose of HbCV administered between the ages of 18 months and 5 years

B. Postsecondary Requirements

Beginning August 1, 1990, students attending colleges and universities (postsecondary) must demonstrate immunity against measles, mumps, and rubella. These requirements will eventually apply to full- and part-time graduate and undergraduate students born on or after January 1, 1957.

Table 6. Tetanus Prophylaxis in Wound Management

History of Tetanus Immunizations	Clean, Minor Wounds		All Other Wounds	
	TIG*		Adult TIG	
Uncertain or <3	Yes	No	Yes	Yes
3 or more	No†	No	No†	No

*TIG: tetanus immune globulin.
†Unless more than 10 years since last dose.
‡Unless more than 5 years since last dose.

NOTE: Tetanus immune globulin and Td may be given simultaneously but in different sites. Substitute DTP vaccine for children under 7 years of age.